"Everyone wins in
the game of infertility—

it just might not be the way
you always planned.

Keep an open mind and
the family you so desire

will be yours."

—Julie Vargo and Maureen Regan

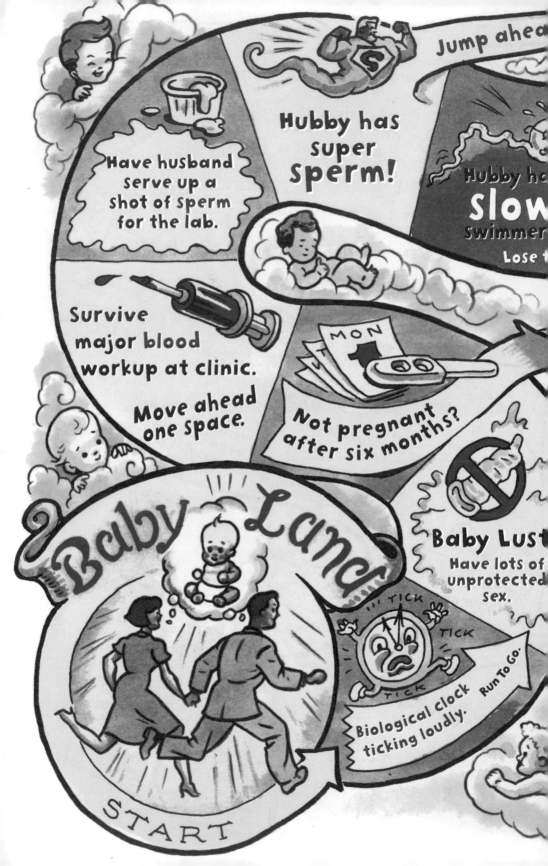

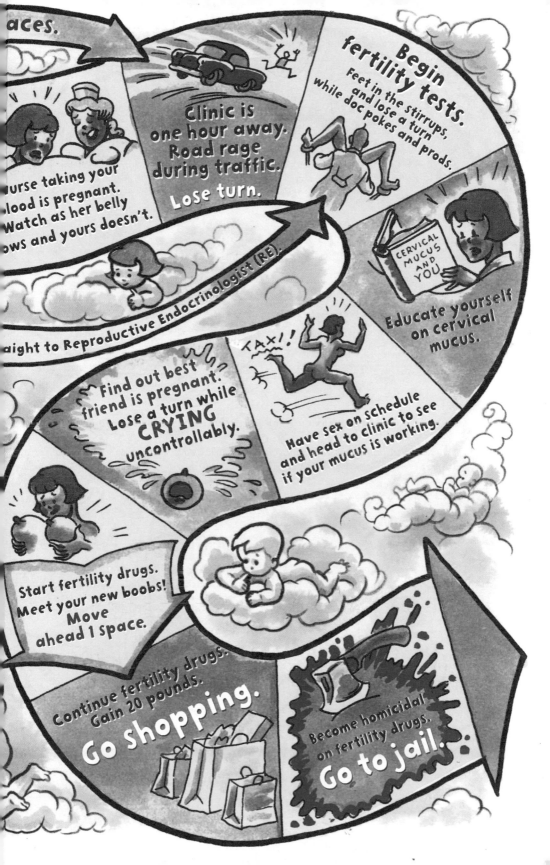

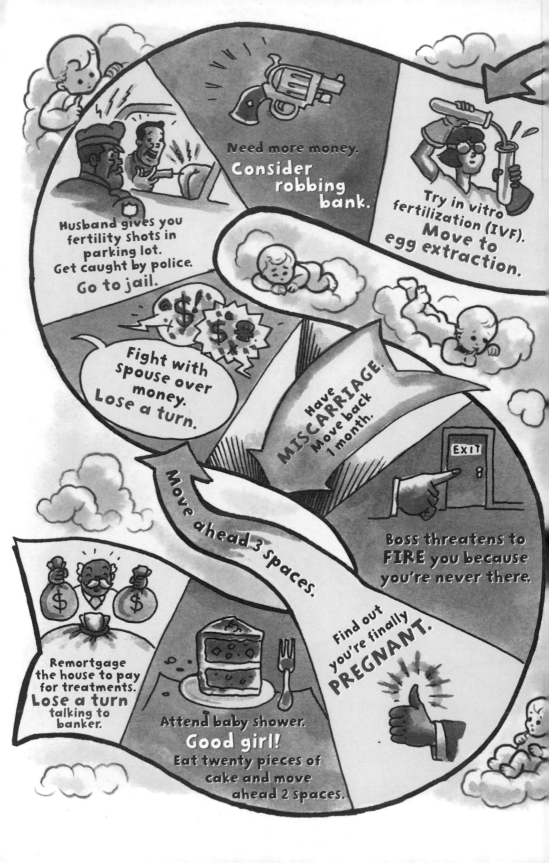

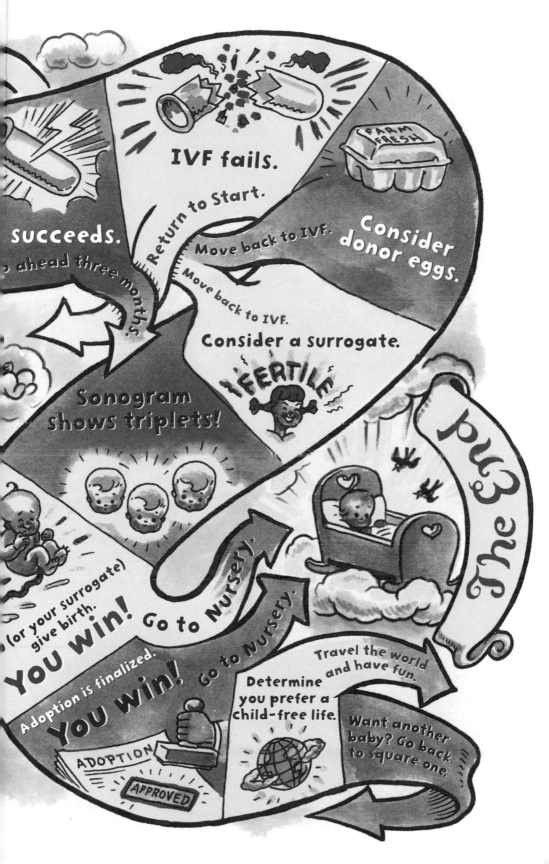

A Few
Good Eggs

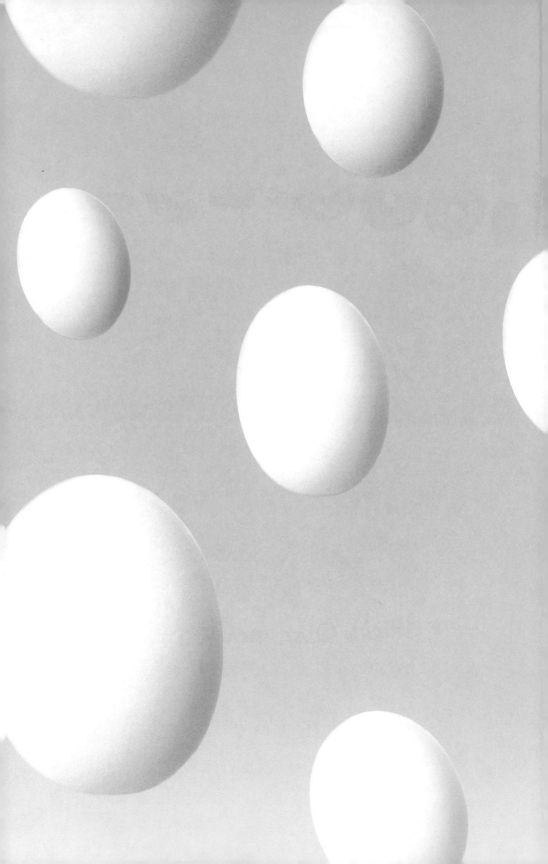

A Few Good Eggs

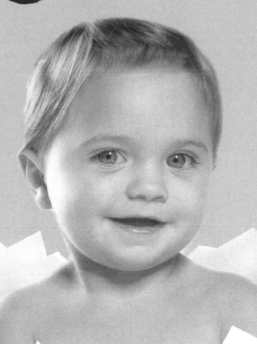

Two Chicks Dish on Overcoming the INSANITY of

INFERTILITY

Julie Vargo and Maureen Regan

COLLINS LIVING
An Imprint of HarperCollins Publishers

This book contains advice and information relating to health care. It is not intended to replace medical advice and should be used to supplement rather than replace regular care by your doctor. It is recommended that you seek your physician's advice before embarking on any medical program or treatment. All efforts have been made to assure the accuracy of the information contained in this book as of the date of publication. The publisher and the author disclaim liability for any medical outcomes that may occur as a result of applying the methods suggested in this book.

A hardcover edition of this book was published in 2005 by HarperCollins Publishers.

HarperCollins books may be purchased for educational, business, or sales promotional use. For information please write: Special Markets Department, HarperCollins Publishers Inc., 10 East 53rd Street, New York, NY 10022.

FIRST PAPERBACK EDITION PUBLISHED 2006

Art direction by Michelle Ishay
Endpaper illustration by Ross MacDonald
Designed by Laura Klynstra Blost

The Library of Congress has catalogued the hardcover edition as follows:

Vargo, Julie, 1959–
    A few good eggs : two chicks dish on overcoming the insanity of infertility / Julie Vargo and Maureen Regan—1st ed.
    p. cm.
    Includes Index.
    ISBN 0-06-077681-1
    1. Infertility, Female. 2. Infertility, Female—Psychological aspects. I. Regan, Maureen, 1961– II. Title.

RG201.V37 2005
618.1'78—dc22

2005042664

ISBN 13 978-0-06-083440-1 (pbk.)
ISBN 10 0-06-083440-4 (pbk.)

08   09   10   RRD   10   9   8   7   6   5   4   3   2

DEDICATION

To Family.

CONTENTS

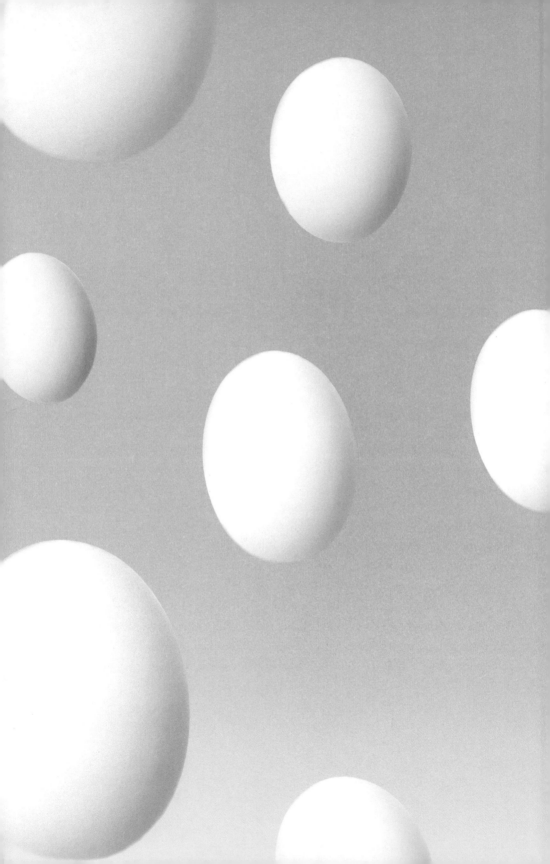

FOREWORD
by Dr. BRIAN M. COHEN

I originally read the manuscript for this book out of curiosity because one of its authors had been my patient a few years earlier, and I was curious to see what she was up to. I started reading it while flying home from a conference, and when I looked up again, we had landed. That rarely happens to me with any kind of writing.

In my thirty-five years of practicing medicine, I have worked with countless couples. I have witnessed the development of reproductive endocrinology from the isolation and development of antibodies for the radio immuno assay of many reproductive hormones through the era of tubal microsurgery and sophisticated ovulation induction techniques. In recent years we've had the advent of assisted reproductive technology and the many aspects of in vitro fertilization, which have truly changed the options available to all couples.

But no matter which infertility treatments are available, it is most important that health care providers be totally honest and ethical with patients who have infertility because the intense desire for a child renders many people far more vulnerable to infertility entrepreneurs. The advent of managed care and the growth of large infertility centers has unfortunately brought with it the loss of the direct, detailed, personalized patient care given by an individual physician. I remain convinced that every couple must be assessed individually, rather than following a generic protocol that conforms to the masses. A doctor cannot achieve pregnancy in every couple. But once we know that we are up against an incurable problem, it is incumbent upon us to level with them as soon as possible to resolve their needs in a timely and in the least painful manner.

This book is refreshing by virtue of its honesty, integrity, and the straightforward presentation of the facts of infertility. Julie Vargo and Maureen Regan talk about taboo topics—with personal admissions regarding everything from career versus commitment to motherhood, personal choices and consequences, the male partner and his feelings, and the realities of marital stress. Julie and Maureen even remind us that most first-time mothers who conceive after age forty-two have accomplished the dream with donor eggs—and that's cool, if that's what you want. However, if you want your own biological baby, early and prompt assessment by a specialist is strongly advised.

This is good stuff. These are things women need to hear.

Both Julie and Maureen went through assessment and treatment for infertility. So did many of their friends. They don't talk like doctors. They tell it like it is—woman to woman. Reading this book, I felt as if I were sitting at the table, too, listening to the "girl talk" that professionals rarely, if ever, hear. Their perspective was not new to me, for I pride myself in spending adequate time listening to each patient's individual concerns and needs with much compassion and sensitivity. But the frankness and transparency with which Julie and Maureen talk about their experiences gave me a lot of insights, and I believe this book will be a truly positive inspiration to other women and men facing infertility.

A Few Good Eggs is written with much wisdom. It is a direct, serious—and yet humorous—review of the many factors that truly affect couples who are pursuing their dreams of having children. The book contains a very timely message about the pandemic of infertility, which affects one in six couples. It emphasizes the challenges to women who are facing their ticking biological clocks, and it stresses that earlier motherhood is easiest and probably best. Julie and Maureen strongly advise the need for a balanced and healthy lifestyle, both mentally and physically. They emphasize the need to be well-informed and to ask the right questions of their physicians. An excellent chapter reviews the monetary issues, focusing on the immense burden of financial stress upon a couple, and how to create realistic financial expectations.

These two women say things in their book that medical professionals don't, can't, or won't say. They make it clear that OB/GYNs are not necessarily trained in infertility. They describe why women should seek the expertise of reproductive endocrinologists sooner rather than later. This is particularly important if you are over thirty-five—yet no one has really said it so straightforwardly before. Women should have reasonable, but justifiable, expectations from the physicians who are caring for them. Many patients don't know that legitimate fertility doctors are truly available 365 days a year—including weekends and holidays. Julie and Maureen not only realize it—they want the rest of the world to know as well.

The authors intimately report their own personal responses, anxieties, and mood swings as they went through the barrage of fertility tests and drug therapies one must endure. They also offer some ingenious ways of coping with the hormonal changes and expectations throughout the menstrual cycle. The need for couple and partner communication throughout infertility treatment is expressed in great detail, as well as the importance of counselors, ministers, and professional therapists. With much humor, they earnestly remind us all that "your sister, cousin, or best friend may not be your best adviser" during this difficult period. There are even positive ideas for couples as they go through sperm collection and insemination!

To me, the most important part of this book is its message that you should do for yourself what must be done. Couples should have sufficient knowledge to ask the questions and expect reasonable explanations for delays in success. As Julie and Maureen point out, no couple should accept a persistent response of "Just keep trying," "It's bad luck," or "We'll get it right some time."

With its great wisdom, good humor, and sensitive and detailed presentation, *A Few Good Eggs* is a must-read for all couples struggling with infertility—and highly recommended reading for all young women who need to make informed decisions about their long-term life aspirations to balance career with motherhood.

Brian M. Cohen, M.B.Ch.B., M.D. (postdoctoral)
Diplomat A.B. O. G.—Subspecialty Reproductive Endocrinology
F.A.C.O.G., F.R.C.O.G. (London), F.C.O.G. (S.A.), F.A.C.E., F.I.C.S.
Clinical Professor, Department of Obstetrics and Gynecology at University of Texas,
Southwestern Medical School
Director, National Fertility Center of Texas, P.A., Dallas

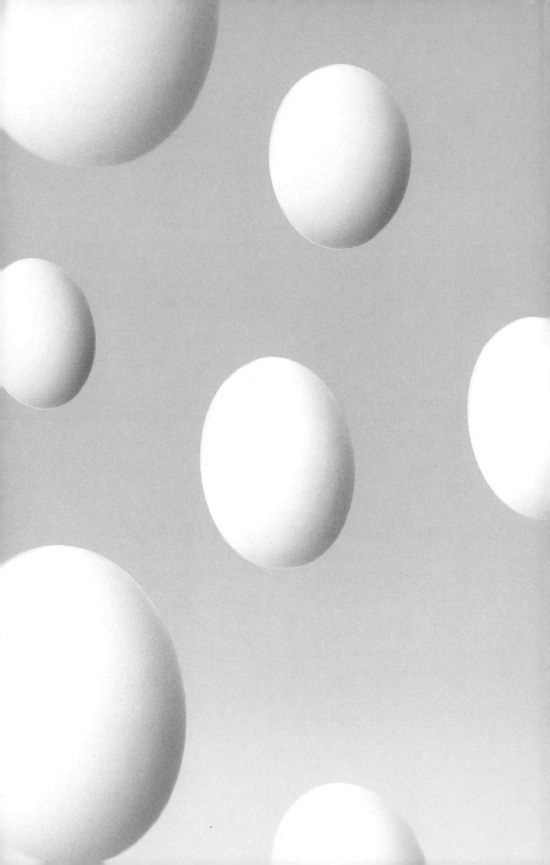

FOREWORD
by Dr. W. MICHAEL YARBROUGH

I practiced obstetrics and gynecology for twenty-two years in Dallas, Texas. From about 1987 on, an amazing trend developed: A large majority of my patients elected to delay childbearing until they had finished their education and established their professional careers. Many waited until they were in their late thirties before attempting to conceive.

This shift became even more dramatic during my last seven years in practice, when almost all of my pregnant patients were over thirty-five—and many were forty. Also, the number of patients with twins or triplets dramatically increased, directly due to advances in reproductive technology, coupled with the increase in infertility associated with increased maternal age. Very few of my younger gynecological patients worried about problems having children when they were ready—they just put childbearing off into the future when they would be prepared financially. Whenever I would mention that they should consider having their children sooner than later, I would get a laundry list of reasons for waiting. None believed infertility would be a problem for them.

Just try to imagine the advances made in medicine over the past twenty years, especially in reproductive medicine. It's pretty mind-boggling if you think about it. When I started private practice in 1980, the options available for women with infertility were few. Now, the news media is full of examples of women in their late forties having children. I think this is giving women a false sense of security and making it seem as if modern technology such as IVF, GIFT, or ZIFT will solve any problems they may have.

If only it were that easy. It's not.

Often their own doctors don't move them along fast enough. I know it's probably not politically correct to say, but unfortunately, many obstetricians/gynecologists have minimal training in reproductive medicine. They frequently do not appreciate all the intricacies and complexities of infertility and often refer their patients to infertility specialists later rather than sooner, resulting in only further frustration and loss of valuable time for the infertile couple. Most resident physicians in obstetrics/gynecology finish their training with only minimal exposure to reproductive medicine, yet often present themselves to the public as doctors who practice obstetrics, gynecology, and infertility. The majority of their training is spent learning basic gynecologic surgery, obstetrics, and women's health. Even the majority of residents finishing their training have not mastered advanced laparoscopic surgery.

Whether we like it or not, this is the age of medical specialization. It may be inconvenient to see more than one doctor, but it is something all of us have to live with. One physician cannot remain current in all fields of medicine with all the rapid changes taking place. We cannot be experts in everything, and we owe it to our patients to accept our limits and refer them to those who are the most qualified to give them their best chances of having children. While many obstetricians/gynecologists are qualified to perform a basic infertility workup, it is impossible for them to keep up with all the advances being made in reproductive medicine. By the way, fertility experts such as reproductive endocrinologists also do not deliver babies. They leave that to the experts: obstetricians.

I was a solo practitioner; I was fortunate enough to not participate in any form of managed care. I had an incredible office staff that had been with me for many years. A real live person answered the telephone, and we knew the majority of our patients very well and considered them not only patients, but also friends. I made myself available to my patients even when I was not on call. Unfortunately, we now live in the world of managed care, with HMOs and PPOs that limit access to physicians and hospitals, since all are not on every plan. Very few physicians have the luxury I had. With decreasing reimbursement for physicians and hospitals, an unbelievable amount of stress is being placed on physicians, their offices, and hospitals.

This is huge when we talk about infertility—as Julie and Maureen point out. Physicians are forced to see more patients in less time, and the patient is the ultimate loser. Have you noticed that your costs of health insurance keep increasing, even with decreasing reimbursement to physicians and hospitals? Only the insurance companies and their stockholders are benefiting. Managed care not only dictates which physicians you may see and which hospitals you may use, but also often dictates treatment plans and medications available to you. In other words, managed care limits access and treatment options, or even more often, offers no reimbursement for infertility treatments.

My advice is to seek out a physician who is not only an expert, but who also will be your advocate. Pursuing the dream of having children is very stressful, and *A Few Good Eggs* lets you know just how stressful it can be—and that others in your situation have the same frustrations as you do. You need a physician who appreciates and understands just how stressful infertility can be. Your physician should be supportive and receptive to your questions and concerns. If your physician does not thoroughly explain to you what is happening and why, does not give you enough time, appears irritated or threatened by your questions or blows you off, change physicians. You are not a number, not just one of a thundering herd of patients. Physicians and their offices owe it to you to be responsive, to know who you are and why you are seeing them. Remember, you also have to be an advocate for yourself, and you want people on your team who have your same goals.

I wish I had had *A Few Good Eggs* fifteen years ago. I would have made it required reading for those who never thought it could happen to them. Never before have I read a book from a layperson's point of view that explores the world of infertility as Julie and Maureen do. While introducing the world to the vocabulary of assisted reproduction and offering an excellent source of basic information, they demonstrate in depth the emotions many women are experiencing as they fight infertility. Indeed, infertility discussion among friends has been almost taboo, and many infertility patients feel they have a stigma attached to them. Infertility is an unbelievably stressful situation. On more than one occasion, couples I referred for fertility treatment soon divorced.

So here's what I say now—if you or a friend is experiencing infertility, there is much you can do. Find a support group or someone who has experienced infertility to help you through your journey. Most people who have never experienced infertility have no concept of what you are experiencing and are not familiar with all the available options. Find a good doctor.

If you want children, do not wait until your situation is perfect to start trying. You can always find a reason to wait, and then it might be too late. Educate yourself, know your options, find out who has the best results. And most important, read this book.

—W. MICHAEL YARBROUGH, M.D.
Diplomat A.B.D.G., F.A.C.O.G.
Emeritus Status at Presbyterian Hospital of Dallas

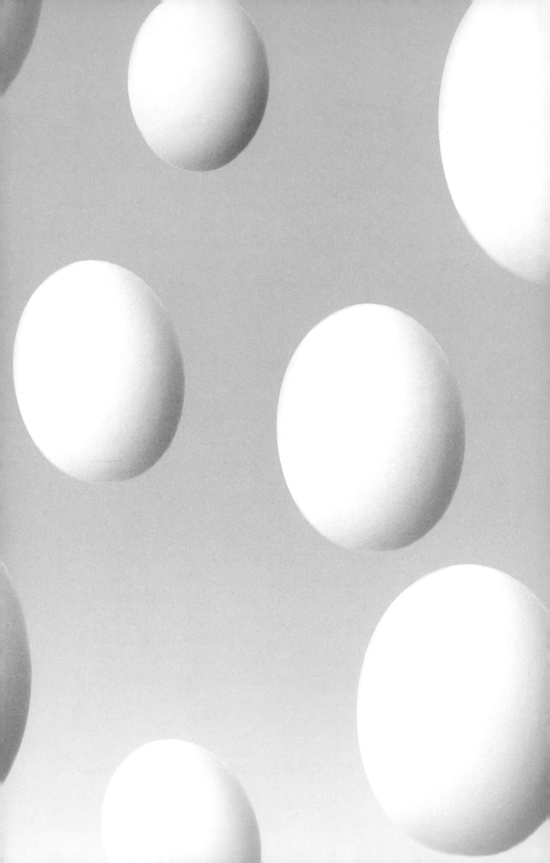

INTRODUCTION: Why We WROTE This BOOK

From the moment a woman decides she wants a baby, trying to conceive takes on new meaning. For most women, becoming a mother is easy. For others, it's not.

One in six American couples experiences infertility. For a woman lost in baby lust, the very word stings like a slap in the face. The unfair part? (As if there could be anything more unfair than not being able to have the family you've always wanted.) Infertility blasts the baby dreams of everyone, regardless of age, class, or economic standing—from teachers, nurses, and sales clerks to CEOs and celebs like Jane Seymour, Celine Dion, Brooke Shields, and Joan Lunden. Even couples already potty training a child may experience secondary infertility when they try to give Junior a sibling.

We know the pain and panic of infertility. We also know the blessed joy of pregnancy and motherhood. Somehow we and our marriages survived the incredible journey from there to here. Along the way, we learned more about our bodies and how they function, how babies really come into the world (more complex than high school sex-ed classes lead you to believe), and what to expect when you're *trying* to expect than we ever imagined.

As infertility patients, we have lived and researched almost every aspect of this topic. Both of us spent several years trying to get pregnant, with and without fertility specialists. We've endured fertility treatments and the anguish of multiple miscarriages and secondary infertility, as well as the joy of pregnancy, birth, and motherhood. Between the two of us, there's little we haven't seen or experienced firsthand.

In retrospect, surviving the insanity of infertility allowed us to compile plenty of research for this book. While in the midst of it all, however, we simply felt alone and left out—as if Mother Nature were playing a sick joke on us while God was busy working miracles elsewhere.

Faced with infertility's unknowns, Julie, a journalist, searched for books to help her cope with her situation. She did find some useful scientific and medically based books written by doctors and resource groups, but she didn't find what she needed most—the wisdom and insights of women who had been through infertility and would share the nitty-gritty, the secrets, the must-knows that only good friends share with one another. Face it—while doctors experience infertility through their patients' involvement, unless they are also infertility patients *themselves* or have truly committed to many hours of counseling their patients for many years, they cannot truly know how this whole process affects your life.

Halfway across the country, Maureen was searching for similar material—to no avail.

When we met thanks to our mutual friend Jill Novack Lynch, we rejoiced at finding a kindred spirit—another woman who had suffered in silence and wanted to speak out, to help other women going through the same things we have experienced. Our personalities clicked. Our talents meshed.

Maureen's experience in the publishing world corroborated what we felt: No book existed that shared the things our mothers didn't know and our doctors wouldn't or couldn't tell us. We wanted someone to speak to us just as we were speaking to each other—candidly, honestly, and passionately. So we decided to write the book we couldn't find and so desperately wanted. This book is based on personal experiences—our experiences, the experiences of friends, and the experiences of medical professionals. It is an amalgam of ideas, opinions, concerns, criticisms, advice, and anecdotes. In addition to experiencing infertility ourselves, we have interviewed infertile women and men as well as infertility specialists. The thoughts and information included in this book are the things we—and our friends—had to find out on our own, including the emotional challenges, activities, and solutions even our doctors didn't think to mention.

We want to break the silence surrounding infertility by providing information for everything from the logistics of actually getting pregnant—about which many women are surprisingly ignorant—to facing infertility. More important, we look at what goes on in the mind as well as the body. While pregnant women worry about decorating nurseries and timing contractions, women who are trying to conceive fret over ovulation kits, body temperatures, and calendars. Infertile women stress over hormone shots, sperm counts, and internal allergies to parts of their bodies that they didn't know even existed. It's overwhelming to say the least.

We will be the first to tell you this is not a medical guide or reference book. This book should also not be considered in any way a substitute for your doctor's advice. Doctors are an essential component of the infertility team. They spearhead the treatments, answer our questions, calm our medical fears, write the prescriptions, and perform the tests and surgeries. We cannot "do" infertility without them. No book can replace them—although we hope this one will provide some opportunities for increased dialogue or inspire questions like "Why do you think it's better for my husband to give me those shots than for me to come in here every day where a professional can do it?"

We're not doctors—nor are we looking to replace yours. We are women like you, and we tell it like it is. Think of this book as a surrogate support group tucked between two covers, a circle of pals who have already had their ride on the infertility roller coaster and who will help you realize you aren't the only infertile woman who is confused, anxious, vulnerable, or manic. We've all been there. Let us help. For the strictly medical details of infertility, talk to a doctor. For the down and dirty scoop, read this book.

To be sure we aren't leading you astray, however, we did have two extremely knowledgeable, well-respected, and highly credentialed doctors review our text. Dr. Brian Cohen is a renowned reproductive endocrinologist with the Dallas-based National Fertility Center of Texas. Dr. W. Michael Yarbrough recently retired from his private OB/GYN practice in Dallas where he spent twenty-two years specializing in high-risk pregnancies. Both men are experts in their respective fields, and we are fortunate to have them on our team.

We hope this book helps you on your journey. Fasten your seatbelts. It's a bumpy road ahead.

Julie Vargo and Maureen Regan

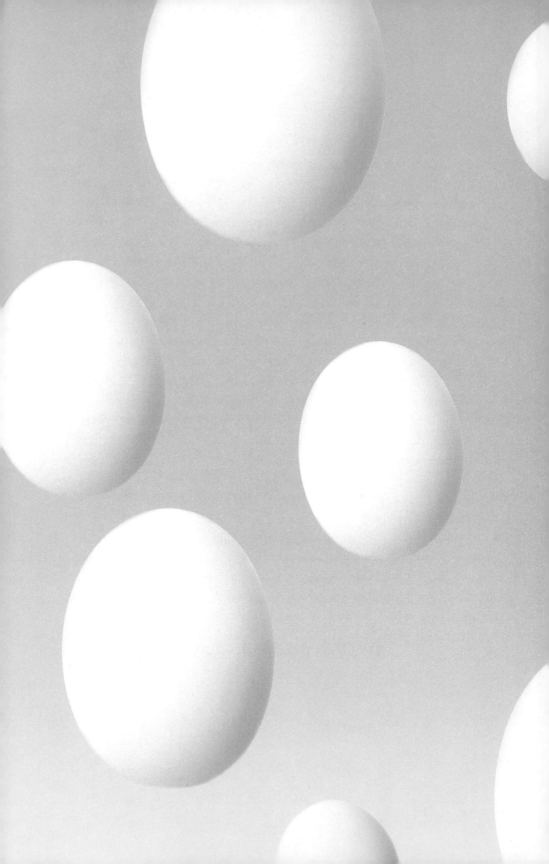

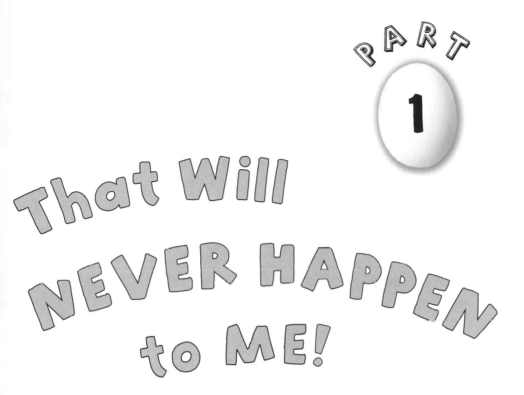

PART 1

That Will NEVER HAPPEN to ME!

I won't be the one who doesn't find Mr. Right. I won't be the one who can't get pregnant. I won't be the one who always attends baby showers but never gets one thrown for me. I won't be the infertile one.

That will never happen to me.

Yep, that's what we thought, too. We were so wrong.

We share our infertility stories throughout this book so you will believe us when we say we know where you're coming from. We've lived the insanity of infertility and survived.

But our stories—and those of our friends—illustrate a larger point: Infertility knows no boundaries. It happened to us. It can happen to you.

We went through hell to build our family units, but most importantly, we did it.

So can you.

Julie's Story

I put off marriage and a family to pursue my career. For the first fifteen years following college, I had a slew of glamour jobs—fashion editor for a major metropolitan newspaper, creative director for a video production company, and freelance journalist and speechwriter. Along the way, I met and married my husband, Robert. We spent the go-go eighties and still-pretty-busy nineties overachieving in our careers, traveling, and having fun. Having kids was the last thing on my mind.

When we reached our early thirties, Robert and I slowed down enough to notice we were still child-free. It was time to start a family. So, I stopped taking the Pill and assumed Mother Nature would take over. She didn't. That's how I found my thirty-six-year-old self sitting in the pale pink lobby of a fertility clinic, unaware I was about to bare my soul and open my body to strangers who would quickly become as intimate as family.

Suddenly, I became a walking science experiment. I spent more time at the fertility clinic than I did at work. I took my temperature constantly and ingested prescription drugs with price tags that gave me sticker shock. I endured uterine scrapings, learned to read fuzzy sonograms, and braved shots administered by my husband. I quit exercising, gained weight, and made love according to the calendar. To add insult to fertility-injury, I even added up the amount of money I obviously could have saved on contraception over the past sixteen years. It's about $3,840, and I still think of what I could have done with that extra $20 a month during the lean years.

How could this have happened to me?!

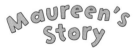

Maureen's Story

I married my husband, Will, when I was thirty years old, and I promised myself I would have a baby before I was thirty-two.

Thirty-two was important to me because I am the youngest of five kids, born when my mother was thirty-two. As a result, I always complained to her that she was an old mother. Back then, my friends' mothers were ten years younger than mine. My, how times have changed, right? Anyway, five months after I got married—on New Year's Eve without even "trying"—we conceived our son, Quinn. The pregnancy was delightful, the birth horrible, and the child amazing. I gave birth to Quinn four months shy of my thirty-second birthday. I had beaten my deadline and was convinced I would never be labeled as an "Old Mom."

Fast-forward five years. At thirty-seven, I got pregnant again—only to suffer what would be the first of several miscarriages. What was happening? I didn't know where to turn, so I stood still. I was confused, disappointed, and angry as I kept trying to get pregnant, only to lose babies.

In July 2001, our family of three moved from San Francisco back to New York. At that point, I received a proposal from Julie for a book about infertility. In the proposal, Julie urged the reader to find a good reproductive endocrinologist. A what? I'd never even heard of that kind of doctor. I called Julie right away and asked her for more information. She urged me to see someone locally. The new doctor explained I was suffering secondary infertility—the inability to conceive or carry a child to term when you already have one child.

Infertility? How could this have happened to me?!

CHAPTER 1
JOIN the CLUB

Julie

We started trying to conceive when I was thirty-four, and I think I knew right away we were in trouble. I guess it was instinct or maybe just a gut reaction to each period's arrival when I knew we were having more than enough sex to satisfy the conception quotient.

My husband didn't believe we were having a problem—at first. When I lamented the fact we weren't pregnant yet, Robert would toss out comments like "Well, we haven't really given it enough time yet," or "I'll bet it will work next month," or "I'm not worried yet, why are you?" I think this is called denial.

Finally, after more than a year, I went to my OB/GYN who wondered why I hadn't gotten in there sooner.

Maureen

Although he was a delight, my son, Quinn, was active and didn't sleep through the night for four years. This made me delay having another child. It never occurred to me I would have any difficulty because Quinn's conception was effortless. So I waited . . . and waited . . . and put it off longer and longer.

Nobody, not even my hip, cool, Harvard-educated Marin County gynecologist, bothered to inform me of the effect my age may have on my reproductive biology. So I didn't think twice about putting off another pregnancy. I thought

I had all the time in the world—at least until I was forty. Why not? All these celebrities were having their babies late, right?

My gynecologist never told me I was infertile. It was a conclusion I came to on my own after my second miscarriage. I begged her to test my fertility, but she brushed me off. To her, I was just a case of advanced maternal age—not a fertility issue. I shudder to think what would have happened if I hadn't met Julie and gone to a fertility specialist. Well, I wouldn't have had my daughter, Ava. Quinn would have been an only child.

The moral of my story is that "all the time in the world" is really not much time at all. I almost missed the boat. What a humbling experience.

10 Mis(sed)-Conceptions About Infertility

1. Infertility won't happen to *me*.
2. I can't be infertile. I already have a baby!
3. I can *get* pregnant, so I don't have fertility issues. I just have miscarriages.
4. I'm too young to have fertility issues!
5. My doctor told me I didn't need to see a fertility specialist until I had three miscarriages.
6. I'm in great shape. I exercise all the time. I can't be infertile.
7. I'm not infertile. I'm just not having enough sex.
8. You *can* wait a long time to have a baby.
9. Men can't be infertile. They make sperm all the time.
10. Normal is a miracle.

Welcome to the wild, wacky world of infertility, where insanity reigns supreme, where the path to parenthood doesn't follow the prescribed "normal" route.

Oh, well. What's normal anyhow?

In reproductive terms, some women get pregnant so easily. They decide it's time to start a family, stop taking the Pill or toss out the diaphragm and—WHAM—a few weeks later, they're on the nine-month path to motherhood. Those women drive us crazy. Call it envy.

The biggest mistake we make as women is to assume that we can get pregnant. We take it for granted really, the miracle that it is. We don't know about you, but we spent most of our precious fertile years—the twentysomethings—trying NOT to get pregnant. Wish we knew then what we know now!

The easily impregnated don't understand what the rest of us go through to have our children. They just smile their motherly smiles, shrug their shoulders, and pat the tousled heads of the wriggling tots dangling from their perfect pre-pregnancy Gap outfits. At least that's how we see it.

Meanwhile, the rest of us labor like construction workers to build our families. Mother Nature sure isn't fair. We guess she never faced any fertility challenges, so she can't relate. But really, she's a mother, so we personally think she should be a bit more understanding.

The Silent Sisterhood

When women get pregnant, they tell everyone. They have parties. People bring them gifts. They are pampered. Cute, witty books are written about their condition. They even get a new name—Mommy. Pregnant women are so expansive—not only in their girth, but also in their personalities and their outlooks.

When women find out they are infertile, they tell no one. If they have a party, it's a pity party they host for themselves. The one gift they want, a baby, they've been told they can't have easily. The books and research about their condition are scientific, focused, and sometimes depressing. The medical procedures can be daunting—surgeries, inseminations, blood tests, needles, needles, and more needles. And what about the bills?

It's no wonder infertile women are withdrawn. Infertility is a crisis! It affects our identity. We feel like big losers. It's like this big secret sorority—a silent sisterhood—because no one talks.

Here's what we think: Women don't talk about being infertile because we feel guilty. We feel "less than." We are pissed off about it, too. We're obsessed about something we feel bad about. Who wants to share that with the world? Well, it's time to get over that.

We know a woman who has suffered from unexplained infertility for many years and just doesn't want to talk about it anymore. Everyone around Frieda has babies, and she has passed through disappointment, self-pity, and even anger. She has gotten to the point where she is beginning not to feel anything at all about it—thus her disinterest in even discussing it. Her infertility has become such a deep and personal thing. Unfortunately, she is suffering even more by keeping her feelings so suppressed and never talking about it.

Then there's our forty-year-old friend Clara, who doesn't want to talk about infertility because she doesn't think that word has anything to do with her. Clara had her first child at thirty-eight and a miscarriage a few months ago. Because she is forty, we suggested she consider taking a more aggressive approach toward getting pregnant. But she refused to believe that *she* could have any fertility issues. She just did not want to go *there* . . . and *there* was a place, given her age, she needed to get to sooner rather than later. The time she spends in denial may cost her the second baby that she wants. Unfortunately this happens more often than not.

We have discovered that the topic of infertility is like miscarriage. If one woman has the guts to break the ice in confessing to a miscarriage, they will come to find many other women have suffered the same fate. Infertility is no different. Share your thoughts and experiences, and perhaps someone else will open up. We both learned a great deal by being open and honest about our infertility issues.

Infertility is a medical condition—actually a compendium of various physical malfunctions and/or diseases. It is nothing to be ashamed of. If you want to take it even further, infertility doesn't even mean you won't become parents someday. We have come to think of infertility as a game—The Infertility Game. It is a game in which, believe it or not, everyone is a winner. We know you don't feel like a winner right now (who would?), but the truth is if you want a baby in your family, you will have one. Go ahead, read that line again. If you want a baby, you will have one. Now you may not actually *have* a baby the biological way—or maybe you will, thanks to drugs, in vitro fertilization, intrauterine insemination, or some other technical assistance. Maybe you will use a surrogate, donor eggs, or donor sperm or maybe you will adopt or foster parent.

The bottom line is this—if you want a family, you can have a family. You may not have the experience of being pregnant, or the children may come into your life in a way you never dreamed of as a little girl, but you and your partner can be parents. Everyone can have a baby . . . no matter what age you are. You just might not have it biologically.

If you need a doctor's approval to speak up, listen to what Julie's reproductive endocrinologist had to say. "Fifteen or twenty years ago, I knew without asking patients that if I saw them in public or at a civic function, I was not to recognize or greet them because of the perceived public stigma attached to infertility," says Dr. Brian Cohen, Director of the National Fertility Center in Dallas, board-certified reproductive endocrinologist, and a clinical professor at University of Texas Southwest Medical Center. "Today, people are less sensitive about that, perhaps because patients today are more mature women who have postponed childbearing."

You Aren't Alone (Although You May Feel Like It!)

Okay. So, you've established that you can't have a baby the old-fashioned way (with very little planning, a bottle of wine, and a lot of sex). Just because infertility is the reality doesn't make you a bad person or even mean you're alone. Facing infertility is a lot like being a member of one of the biggest clubs in this country—except no one wears a uniform, there's no secret handshake, and you probably wouldn't recognize another member if you sat next to her on the bus. In addition to being isolating and emotionally and physically exhausting, it is heartrending to belong to this secret club. And boy, oh boy, do you pay your dues!

To let you know just how NOT alone you are, here are some startling statistics from The National Survey on Family Growth, published in 1995: About 6.1 million women faced fertility challenges in 1995, compared with 4.9 million in 1988. The exact percentages were 8.4 percent of the reproductive-age population in 1988 compared with an increase to 10.2 percent in 1995.

Want some more proof? Look here.

- About 2 percent of American women (1.2 million) visited a doctor about infertility in the past year, and another 13 percent (7.6 million) reported an infertility visit at some point earlier in their lives.
- One in six American couples experiences infertility and spends billions of dollars annually on treatment.
- In 2002, 20 percent of women ages thirty-five through thirty-nine were childless, up from 10 percent in 1976, according to the U.S. Census Report on Fertility in American Women.
- Approximately 90 to 95 percent of childless couples turn to fertility doctors for help.
- According to a 1995 government survey, 3.3 million Americans reported suffering from secondary infertility after already having one child.

That's a lot of people. It is our unscientific bet that the numbers are up even more from the time these statistics came out. We can't go anywhere that we don't stumble across someone pushing an in vitro baby in a stroller, someone in the throes of infertility, or someone tiptoeing around the issue because they are still in denial.

JULIE

Every summer, Robert and I haul the kids up to Vermont to stay at this wonderful family resort—The Tyler Place. For one idyllic week, sixty-eight families converge near the Canadian border to relax, eat fabulous food, participate in activities, and watch their kids enjoy a camp experience. We started going during a week informally reserved for couples with babies and really small children when our two children were still tots.

One afternoon when I looked up from the hammock, here's what I noticed— lots of older parents like us, several sets of twins, and Chinese and Korean babies with Anglo parents. I was surrounded by infertile women who'd not built their families the old-fashioned way. This family resort is not inexpensive, so I was also surrounded by a certain demographic strata. That strata was chock-full of late-thirty to early forty-something women like me who had waited to have their children—all the more interesting.

I started to ask questions and discovered tales of hormone injections, in vitro fertilizations (IVFs), miscarriages, and adoptions. Surprisingly, fertile women were in the minority during our week's stay. It was refreshing and reassuring to me to see these women and hear their stories. Many of them are included in this book.

Most importantly, it showed me that I was not an anomaly, and I was certainly not alone. My Tyler Place friends joined the chorus of women lamenting about waiting so long to find Prince Charming, to get their careers in gear, and to have kids—only to find it was not as easy as expected. These were well-educated, well-informed, traveled women—some doctors, some lawyers, and even some home full-time with the babies they worked so hard to have. And they almost missed the boat, too.

It was an eye-opener. Although I knew I was part of a growing trend—those who were having so much fun in life that they almost forgot to have their kids—here in this bucolic bit of Vermont countryside, it was physically, and therefore visually, apparent en masse. I enjoyed my advanced maternal age, my midlife motherhood, and my better-late-than-never babies, even more that week.

Nothing assuages guilt more than being part of a crowd.

Even the guy who fixed Maureen's dishwasher got into a conversation with her about his and his wife's infertility issues. Let us tell you, when an appliance repairman feels like talking about how he and his wife can't conceive, well, you almost feel as if infertility is the norm.

There are many theories about why we are seeing an increase in infertility. First—and some would say foremost—there is the whole age thing. Most infertility experts will tell you that the trend to postpone parenthood until the thirties and forties accounts for a large portion of the problem. The term is "advanced maternal age"—old mommies and mommy wannabes.

"I'm seeing more people with infertility at a later age than ever before," says Dr. Michael Yarbrough, Julie's OB/GYN who spent more than two decades in private practice specializing in high-risk patients. "They get out of school, they're career-oriented, [and] they delay marriage and childbirth into their thirties. Then, they don't have many childbearing years left; they have greater instances of endometriosis and other problems."

What else? There has been an increase in sexually transmitted disease since the advent of the sexual revolution in the seventies. Women are exercising more, which can deplete fat and mess up reproductive hormones. And let's not forget the laundry list of "typical" causes for infertility—uterine irregularities, hormonal disorders, abnormal ovulation, polycystic ovary syndrome, recurrent miscarriage, blocked Fallopian tubes, thyroid problems, and abnormal sperm.

Then there are all the infertility "what-ifs?"—those things totally unproven, but suspected or wondered about. Some doctors ponder how intense childhood athletic teams and increased muscle mass on preadolescent girls who have not yet had a period might affect their future ability to conceive. It doesn't look good for women with extremely low body fat or anorexia.

There are whispered concerns about what effect the menstruation-suppressing birth control pills, such as Depo-Provera or Seasonale, may have on future conception rates among women who take them for too long. Others comment about the amount of hormones and antibiotics and preservatives in our food, the pollution in our air and water, and the mercury in our fish, and what all that is doing to our internal systems.

There is also the dreaded unexplained infertility, in which there just doesn't seem to be a reason why you aren't able to conceive yet. When our girlfriend Lynne, now forty-two and finally pregnant with twins after six artificial inseminations and three IVFs, first married her husband, Leonard, in 1996, she thought they were healthy, normal people.

"I was thirty-five at the time and had never been pregnant before. We did know, however, that Leo was fertile—he had gotten a woman pregnant years ago, but she had had an abortion. I wanted a year to settle into marriage before we started trying."

When she was thirty-six, Lynne and Leo tossed out the condoms and got down to business. "After two years of not conceiving, I knew something was wrong," she says. "I was thirty-eight. I know I should have been more concerned, but really I never had that maternal clock thing going on. I always just assumed I would have kids and everything would be great, so when it wasn't happening for us, I didn't feel pressed to push it. I also had a spiritual belief that God would grant us our kids when we got them.

"Anyhow, after two years, I did tell Leo we should look into our infertility coverage with our insurance company and figure out what we were going to do. So we found a doctor and had some tests. When the tests came back, both our fertilities were fine, except Leo's sperm was a little slow—he had low motility. He was stressed at the time, so I figured that was causing it; no big deal. But after more testing, the doctors still couldn't figure out why we were not getting pregnant. They told us we were in that small fraction of people who have unexplained infertility. Suddenly, it dawned on us—others had correctable infertility, but not us. Unexplained infertility. That was hard to take."

Don't Take a Guilt Trip

Women who face infertility feel unnecessarily guilty—everything from "I made God mad at me" to "I've saddled my spouse with this unattractive, barren woman." We feel guilty and awful when someone in the office gets pregnant (and we can't), then feel guilty because we don't want to go to the shower or toss money into the kitty for her shower gift. We feel guilty for lusting over her baby when she brings it to the office. Guilt is like this never-ending merry-go-round ride.

"My wife frequently has feelings of being 'defective' and 'inadequate,'" says Terry, a forty-four-year-old dentist who is married to thirty-six-year-old Marlie. "She gets pretty depressed at times. She feels that I won't love her because she can't make me a father. But infertility is no one's fault—it's a medical condition. I think the problem lies in the stigma associated with infertility. It is still not widely considered a medical condition, and insurance doesn't really cover it. Most people don't understand what infertility is.

"I think my wife feels guilty because she feels like it's normal to be able to conceive easily," he adds. "She has this timeline in her head of how she wants things to go. Get married, buy a house, [and]have babies. It's not working out as planned. It seems like all of our friends are getting pregnant so easily. We're happy for them when it happens, but deep down we're jealous of them having it so normal. Then we feel guilty for being jealous. It's insane."

JULIE

Guilt heaping is not reserved simply for spouses. Like most women who face infertility for the first time, I did a pretty good job of blaming myself for not being able to achieve the holy grail of womanhood. Was it because I screwed my body up by taking birth control pills for sixteen years? (The doctor said it wasn't, but if I had to do it all over again, I wouldn't have stayed on the Pill all that time.)

Or was it because I began running track in seventh grade, before my periods were fully established? (The jury is still out on that one—although many are questioning the wisdom of exercise-obsessed adolescents.)

Could it have been my focus on athletics through college, and after, joining a gym before even finding my first job? (The lower the body fat, the harder it can be to get pregnant. Facts show skinny women obsessed with lowering their body fat via excessive exercise are losing not only their periods, but also diminishing their ovarian reserve.)

Was it because I spent all my really fertile years styling photo shoots, writing copy, traveling all over the place, and NOT thinking about starting a family? (Getting older is never great for egg production.)

Robert's tests were dandy: power sperm and lots of speedy swimmers. So I felt guilty about that. I even told my husband that he was free to leave me if he wanted to go find someone "normal." It's funny, because in talking with my hard-to-conceive friends, it seems most of us thought we would give our husbands carte blanches to divorce us once their fertility tests came back fine—even if we never told them so.

So how do you get rid of guilt? You admit there are some problems—but NOT problems with either of you—and you work to fix them. Acknowledge the feeling, accept it for what it is, and show it the door. We admit right here that this may be easier said than done. But guilt makes you second-guess yourself. It makes you feel like a failure, and while you may have a few body parts that aren't quite with the program, you *as a person* are not a failure. Wallowing in guilt is a big time waster. Finally, when you are trying to get pregnant, it's important to rid yourself of all toxicity. Guilt is toxic. Guilt has got to go!

Start by stopping the "blame game." Find a support group. Visit a therapist. Determine to give up the guilt. Then, get as aggressive as you are willing to be to get pregnant. Do everything necessary—from the scientific to the stress-reducing and from doctor-ordered to alternative options. You can't feel guilty for trying. Then, prepare yourself to accept the outcome. Remember that no matter what, there is a child somewhere waiting for you—whether biological, donor egg or sperm, adoptive, or foster. Infertility is a tough game, but it is a game that you will win. Hey, then you can feel guilty for being so happy!

Guilt is as exhausting as all the medical procedures you are doing (or are going to do, depending where in the infertility cycle you are). Your first goal is to get back to some semblance of normalcy. You can't be the great mom (or dad) you will be some day if you can't take care of yourself.

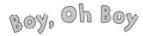

Ditching guilt is also important for the man in your life. In about 40 percent of infertile couples, the male is either the sole or a contributing cause of infertility. For men, the diagnosis of infertility with *them as the cause* is horrifying, guilt-inducing, esteem-eroding, and just plain awful. Talk about feeling like an absolute loser—in the eyes of the woman you love, not to mention the peers with whom you watch football.

Guy problems can range from having too few sperm (oligospermia), no sperm (azoospermia), or malformed sperm (with two tails or two heads, for example), to sperm that couldn't swim to save their lives, much less impregnate women. He might have a hormonal or antibody problem, blocked sperm ducts, or a varicose vein in his testicle called a varicocele. Maybe he sits in a hot tub every day at the gym or wears his undies too tight—both of which can raise the temperature of his testicles and overheat the sperm, killing or damaging them. Perhaps he is one of the few who has retrograde ejaculation—where the semen actually slips back into the bladder during orgasm instead of skyrocketing out the correct end of the penis. He could even have a urinary tract infection.

More crushing is a diagnosis that appears to have been avoidable. We have another friend, Dr. A. (for Anonymous, of course), who didn't want to be identified for certain ego-related reasons but who did want his tale told. Dr. A. is a surgeon. He is married. He and his wife had no problem conceiving their first child when he was fresh out of medical school and smack in the middle of residency (let's say the conception part was easy, but according to his wife, finding time to actually have sex was the trick). Fast-forward seven years. When they began trying to conceive a sibling for their daughter, they began having problems. After tests, the good doctor discovered he had a low sperm count due to the cumulative buildup of all the radiation he's been exposed to in the operating room.

"It's not like I would have changed my job if someone told me being a doctor could affect me like this," says Dr. A. "But I would have taken some precautions to protect myself. My wife says I should have worn lead underwear. I just didn't know."

We have no reason to doubt him—he is a doctor, after all. But to bolster his point with a researched factoid, we read about a study in the April 2004 edition of *Parents* magazine on this topic. According to the *Journal of Industrial Health* quoted in the article, exposure to not only radiation but also pesticides and other harmful chemicals in the workplace can significantly reduce a man's sperm count. While a doctor can't control radiation in the workplace, it does make us regular people want to go organic in the yard if our guy mows the lawn.

And remember stress? This study also determined that men who had job burnout and emotional, mental, and physical exhaustion were also more likely to have trouble impregnating their wives. Other doctors have told us that when guys are stressed out, their hormone levels test flat. Fortunately, low hormone levels can be treated.

Once you determine what your partner's particular problem may be, you can consider options for treating it. For some, it's surgery or simply cooling off the testicles. For others, it's jumping right to the big technological guns such as in vitro fertilization.

Sylvia, a thirty-three-year-old actress married to a Los Angeles developer, was very fertile. But after several tests, her handsome hubby was diagnosed with low sperm count. He had been married once before and had experienced trouble getting his wife pregnant then. The couple had just assumed it was her fault; they never did any fertility workups and adopted a child. When he married Sylvia, she was determined to have biological children. Sylvia was told that IVF was their only hope of conceiving, so after more than $100,000 in IVF, they finally had success. Most of it was all of her effort—which she admits was hard to swallow sometimes, as her fertility was intact, but she loved her husband and she wanted biological children with him, so she was a trooper about it. And she never made him feel like a guilty loser.

MAUREEN

I was angry because with each day that passed I was losing time. I felt as if I had let my husband down, but never beat myself up too much for that. Unlike Julie, I never thought to tell my husband he could leave me, probably because we already had one child. Regardless, I believe in loyalty and love. I knew that although my body was failing me, *I was not the failure*. I just had to figure out WHY? If I could just get that WHY answered, I would feel so much better.

Finally, my fertility doctor found the answer: low progesterone. Lower levels of progesterone, the hormone necessary for sustaining a pregnancy, can be brought on by stress. I needed to de-stress, while running my business, caring for my family, and everything else in between. Now that's funny.

Double Whammy

In the grand scheme of things, a blocked Fallopian tube, low progesterone, or poor sperm motility doesn't sound so bad. Why? It's one thing to fix. But 25 percent of infertile couples have more than one factor contributing to their infertility.

What could be happening? Oh, myriad things. Just pick and choose from the above reasons, and assign one problem to yourself and one to your partner. For example, he could have a blocked sperm duct, and you could have scarred Fallopian tubes caused by a past pelvic infection. Or you could be allergic to his I-can't-swim-for-nothing sperm. The list becomes endless when you consider the combination of problems that could exist.

We Have No Idea What's Wrong

Unexplained infertility means just that: Doctors cannot determine the source of your particular problem. Unexplained infertility accounts for 5 to 20 percent of all fertility cases. Why the wide range? It's dependent on your doctor's degree of knowledge, as well as how much testing and history-taking/making on you and your partner he or she is willing to do that really determines the diagnosis. If you or your doctor (or your insurance company, for that matter) won't invest the time it takes to figure out your fertility issues, you will be placed in the "unexplained infertility" category—even if yours is not really unexplained, just un-figured out.

While there are many cases in which doctors really cannot figure out why you are not getting pregnant, for others slapping an "unexplained infertility" diagnosis is much easier than really digging in and doing the work to find out what is really going on. There is really no reason that unexplained infertility should be a diagnosis in more than 5 percent of all cases.

Being told you have unexplained infertility is a real sock-in-the-belly. This is the diagnosis that makes you want to pull out your hair and run screaming into the streets, "What do you mean you can't figure it out—with all the old-fashioned poking and prodding, all the newfangled high-tech equipment, how can this be?" Or it makes you sulk under the covers for a few days in stunned disbelief.

JULIE

After a year of testing and treatment, Dr. Cohen sat us down and explained our options. Robert was fine: great sperm, lots of them. I obviously had some hormonal and uterine issues, but nothing that should have been insurmountable. I had quit working out intensely, I had gained some weight, and we were having sex like rabbits. I was taking a cocktail of fertility drugs and giving enough blood to win a blue ribbon from the Red Cross. We were doing something.

At this point, he said he would have to classify me as "unexplained" infertility. We could do IVF, but he wasn't sure it would work given my slightly scarred uterus and inability to build a cushy lining in which to snuggle a few fertilized eggs. Maybe we should consider a surrogate.

To be fair, Robert and I had given him a one-year time frame in which to work any high-tech fertility wizardry. There was more he could do, but after 365 days, this was his diagnosis. That diagnosis really sucked. There is no other polite way to say it. I hate uncertainty. How do you fight that? I would have rather been told something—because something else, anything else, is definitive. It can or can't be fixed. What the heck can you do with "unexplained?"

Nothing.

That aside, nothing is more of a bummer than unexplained infertility. We can fight something if we can see it or know what it is, but how do you address the unknown? Something is wrong, but no one can figure out just what and you have to live with it—how unfair.

Getting Started

You've determined you're infertile . . . or you just think you might be. Before you do anything else—before you even call the doctor—sit your partner down for a family discussion. Discuss your goals, dreams, and desires when it comes to kids—your kids.

Not many people do this. Neither of us had these conversations until we were up to our ovaries in fertility treatments. Kinda late to be discussing an overall game plan when the team is already on the field and the ball is in the air. To avoid pain and suffering later, sit down and talk now.

Here are some other questions to ask.

1. What are your familial goals?
2. Do you have to have a biological child? Is it more important to be pregnant or to be a parent?
3. If you can't have biological kids, will you regret it in the future?
4. How many kids did you think you might have someday?
5. How do you feel about the experimental aspect of fertility drugs?
6. How committed are you to this marriage relationship?
7. Do you understand the time and financial commitment infertility involves?
8. How far are you willing to go—emotionally, physically, and financially—to have "your" baby?
9. How do you feel about this whole infertility thing?
10. To achieve your individual goals of family, do you need to be with other people?
11. When is enough enough?
12. What do you think/know about assisted reproductive technologies?
13. Have you ever heard of donor eggs? donor sperm? surrogacy? gestational carriers?

14. Are you willing to consider donor eggs? donor sperm? surrogacy? gestational carriers?
15. Do you understand the time commitment of infertility treatment?

Our pal Rachel, a dynamic Southwest headhunter, did it right. After trying to get pregnant for six months with no luck, she sat her husband down and broached the whole possibility of infertility with him. Thirty-eight at the time, she had thought about the whole process. Rachel was fine with being child-free, was willing to go through infertility treatments, and wasn't interested in using donor eggs, but she had no clue how her husband, Ed, felt.

"I told him—I need to know if my infertility is a deal breaker," says the now forty-three-year-old, who just gave birth to IVF twins. "Far be it from me to keep him from getting his own child. I told him that, and I said I was serious. I said, 'If you need to have your own child with a woman you love, it might not be me.' I spent an hour communicating my fears to him and digging to find out his feelings. Astonishingly, none of it had ever occurred to him. He had no idea of the ramifications of infertility."

When you ask questions like these, you have to know yourself well enough to be able to handle the answers, too. What if your husband does only want a biological child with a woman he loves? What if he HAS to have his sperm involved, but doesn't care about who's egg is used? What if the roles are reversed, and your husband has the problem? How would *you* answer these questions? Do you feel the need to be pregnant, or are you more interested in being a parent as soon as possible?

Discussions must occur, and now is the time. Go out to a café and start communicating.

CHAPTER 2
The FACTS About INFERTILITY

Maureen

Infertile women waste a lot of time, not to mention energy, when we engage in self-pity, blame, resentment, and the "oh, woe is me" syndrome. Fortunately, I am not good at denial (I leave that to my husband!), and I don't spend too much time weeping over what ifs. Instead, I jump right in and face things immediately. I try to challenge each problem with fortitude and courage.

So when I found out I was suffering secondary infertility, I just got down to business and worked to solve the problem. Okay, I'll admit it—my way hurts more. But for me, the sooner I challenge a problem, the sooner I come to a resolution. As it was, it took several years before I gave birth to my daughter.

Julie

Once we accepted that our doctor was right and began infertility treatments, we moved into the emotionally guilt-ridden "whose fault is this anyway" stage.

In the search for someone to blame, the easiest target is usually your partner. Robert, usually a pretty understanding fellow, wanted to know what *I* did to get us in this situation. What?! I countered with maybe if *he* hadn't wanted to wait so long to start a family, we'd already have one. We beat ourselves—and each other—up for all the years we focused on career-building rather than conceiving kids. If we hadn't been so intently scaling the corporate ladder and building companies, would we now be busy climbing jungle gyms and organizing play groups?

Ah, the blame game—ever so fun and *sooooo* productive.

Ten Tips for Facing Infertility

1. Keep reminding yourself that you are not alone.
2. Realize that dealing with infertility is an all-consuming process.
3. Stay calm.
4. Remind yourself you are not a failure if a procedure doesn't work.
5. Have a sense of humor about this—even if it doesn't seem at all funny right now.
6. Do your research. Then do some more.
7. Listen to your body and your inner self. If you really listen, you'll learn those two are rarely wrong.
8. Don't rule anything out—from antibiotics to acupuncture and from yoga headstands to standing on your head during sex.
9. Find the right doctor.
10. Don't get angry at your partner for not nurturing you—he is hurting and confused, too.

Infertility Happens

No woman believes she could possibly be infertile until the doctor tells her so. Even then, we still don't *really* believe it. Even when faced with what appears to be a classic case of infertility, many couples struggle to admit they might have a problem. It's not uncommon. It's called denial.

Technically, infertility is considered a medical problem of the reproductive system that may or may not be able to be treated. About 50 percent of couples who seek infertility treatment will have a successful pregnancy, depending on the problem with which they are diagnosed. If you are younger when you seek treatment, your odds of getting pregnant are higher. If you are older when you first visit a fertility specialist, your chance of getting pregnant is lower. About 5 percent of infertile couples who don't seek medical help spontaneously conceive after a year of trying. We don't even have to ask a Las Vegas bookmaker to see where the odds are in our favor. Get thee to a doctor.

By the way, infertility is not just a woman's problem, either. Various studies show that about 40 percent of infertility can be traced to a female problem and 40 percent to a male problem. In the rest of couples, infertility results from problems in both partners or the cause cannot be explained. So drag your partner along to that first infertility consultation because sooner, rather than later, he's going to have to be tested, too.

How Did This Happen?

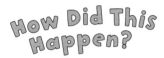

Infertility has the ability to encompass your whole life and swallow you up if you allow it. It is totally normal to feel shocked at discovering yourself on the journey. It's also normal to experience this first sensation of failure that infertility has chosen to roost in your reproductive system for some reason that surely revolves solely around you. (It doesn't.)

Infertility and its treatment is all about hope and failure. We can assure you there will be plenty of other things to punch holes in your self-esteem and knock the wind out of your self-confidence as you progress through treatment, so don't allow yourself to get too derailed in the beginning. If you realize right now that some days will be better than others, you won't be surprised. If you realize that this kind of insanity is normal for the fertility-challenged, you won't go insane.

We promise you will survive this initial shock. While all infertility cases may be slightly different physically, the emotional process is pretty much the same. Learning that you are infertile means relinquishing the traditional dreams of how you will create a family—dreams you may have held since you were a child. But it doesn't mean you won't have a family. This is a growth process that demands you consider and do things you could not have dreamed possible to build the family you deserve.

Once confronted with their own infertility, the first reaction most couples have is disbelief. When your doctor suggests something might be wrong, you're stunned. For a few weeks, you will be sure the doctor is wrong, that he mixed you up with that other couple in the waiting room. He simply read the wrong charts. He couldn't possibly mean you.

Denial and disbelief are okay places in which to start this trip emotionally. But don't delay the journey by hanging around there too long. Pretending you aren't infertile doesn't make you so, and therefore it sure doesn't get you pregnant.

Couples can waste precious baby-making time in denial or debate on this topic. Look, it happened, and it's crappy that it happened to you. But the faster you move on, the faster you can be parents.

What Do You Mean "Infertility?"

So, just what is infertility? We think it is a silent epidemic. We think it is a medical condition. We think it is unfair and more pervasive than most women realize. But here's the "textbook" definition.

Infertility, in the most basic terms, is defined as the inability to conceive after one year of regular, unprotected intercourse.

What this textbook definition doesn't tell you is that infertility is like an onion. From the outside, it looks pretty simple—it's an onion. From the outside, infertility looks pretty simple, too—you can't get pregnant. But when you start to peel it, you discover how the onion is actually made up of multiple layers. The same is true with infertility. Once you start looking beyond the "can't get pregnant" part, you find that there are many causes of infertility, many layers to each cause, many drugs, and many options. The textbook definition of infertility doesn't even begin to cover miscarriage and the women who cannot carry babies to term. These women are suffering infertility, too. Unlike the onion, which ends at its core, infertility's layers can continue to peel back until you either reach success or decide to try something else, like adoption, surrogacy, or child-free living.

Like most women we know, we both stumbled into our infertility. None of us woke up one morning and said, "Hey, I think I'm infertile"—not even those of us with medical backgrounds. Our friend Angela tried unsuccessfully to get pregnant for seven months. Angie is thirty-seven years old and a doctor, for God's sake—a podiatrist to

JULIE

My rector had a good thought, a thought that is worth passing on. When I went to him in search of solace and someone to blame for my infertility, my miscarriages, and my feeling bad, he told me to blame God. Father Chuck said it wasn't His fault, but His shoulders were big enough for the burden. He was right. That helped us. I also respected what Father Chuck had to say because he is the adoptive father of three. He and his wife had been where Robert and I were. He had perspective—as well as a solution for me.

You can modify this thought to include Mother Nature, Father Time, Allah, Buddha, or whoever you want. This suggestion gives couples a third party they can trash together.

be exact. You would think a doctor would be the first to make the connection between not getting pregnant and having infertility. No!

Instead, Angie made an appointment with her gynecologist, but only got to see the nurse practitioner who told her not to worry and to just keep trying. Angie didn't think this was good advice and asked to be tested for any problems. The nurse practitioner refused, pooh-poohing her concerns. Angie then made an appointment with a fertility specialist. After first trying to simply give her fertility drugs, this doctor finally ordered some tests. When the tests came back, Angie was told that one of her Fallopian tubes was tied up like a pretzel, and the other was obstructed by a cyst. Uh-oh. Not good. Even though Angie is a doctor, she had no idea what this meant to her fertility. When we told her it meant the egg could not get to the sperm, she was flabbergasted. She started asking us more and more and more questions. What are the side effects of fertility drugs? Should she go straight to in vitro fertilization? How could she tell when she was ovulating? Could she ovulate with mangled Fallopian tubes?

Newly infertile women are a lot like newly pregnant women in that they are both hungry for information and clueless as to how much their lives are about to change. Most of us stumble onto the idea that we might be facing fertility challenges the same way Angie did. We begin to sense something might be wrong when, after a few months of well-coordinated, unprotected sex, we're still not in the family way. For some reason, we women seem to tune into this sooner than our men. Maybe it's our famous women's intuition. Maybe it's because it's our bodies, and we know what should be happening. Maybe it's because our biological clocks are ticking so loudly.

Here are a few general rules for figuring out if it's time to get some help.

- If you are over thirty and not pregnant within six months of trying to conceive, see a fertility expert.
- If you are in your twenties, run, don't walk, to the doctor's office if you aren't pregnant within a year.
- If you can get pregnant, but keep having miscarriages, you need to see a fertility specialist—even if you already have a child.
- If you've been pregnant once, but can't seem to get pregnant again, you are experiencing secondary infertility and need to see a specialist.

Just to make it more complicated, here are some other considerations that might hinder fertility: If you have a history of pelvic inflammatory disease (PID), painful periods, irregular cycles, or anything else health-wise you think might possibly hinder your chances to conceive, we suggest you ask your OB/GYN to refer you to a fertility specialist as soon as possible for a medical opinion.

Our friend Kay had menstrual problems as a teen that actually heralded her diagnosis of polycystic ovary syndrome (PCOS) eleven years later. PCOS is caused by a hormonal disorder in which too much luteinizing hormone (LH) is produced, causing the ovaries to begin to release too much testosterone, the male hormone. Luteinizing hormone is normally released as a surge right before ovulation. In turn, LH overdrive lowers the amount of follicle-stimulating hormone (FSH) released, which is produced by the pituitary gland and causes the egg follicle to develop. This creates an abnormal rhythm of ovulation. (We know this is technical stuff. For more information on ovulation, the pituitary gland, and hormones, see chapter 6.)

PCOS is a very common cause of infertility. Here's what happens: If you have produced some, but not enough, FSH, you might have several partially formed cysts cropping up on the ovary—as opposed to one cystic follicle that grows normally and ruptures to let an egg burst forth—each month. Instead, the small developing follicles remain trapped inside the ovary each month. The resulting cysts over time remain in the ovary just below the surface. Left untreated or undiscovered, these cysts might thicken the outer ovary and hinder successful ovulation. If you can't ovulate, you sure as heck can't get pregnant, as Kay eventually found out.

In addition to screwed-up periods, Kay also had more body and facial hair than other girls—probably due to the excess testosterone she was producting. She was a little heavier, as well, although she exercised and ate well, both as a child and as an adult. Both of these are possible red flags for PCOS, but it wasn't until she was almost thirty and trying to get pregnant that doctors figured out what was causing the problem. (Her mom kept saying being hairy was just hereditary, part of being French-Canadian, so Kay never thought anything about it and just waxed her upper lip for years until laser treatment made waxing obsolete. Who knew?)

Daria, another pal, got a clue about future fertility problems when she suffered severe endometriosis throughout her teens and twenties. Endometriosis happens when the endometrial tissue that is supposed to line the uterus each month in preparation for a possible pregnancy actually begins to grow outside the uterus somewhere else in the body—such as the abdominal cavity or around the outside of the uterus and/or ovaries and/or Fallopian tubes. If this endometrial tissue enters the ovaries through an opening, it can even create an endometrial growth of tissue, like a cyst (or endometrioma), inside the ovary. Endometriosis can be in a small spot or pervasive, wrapping around and across organs like a cobweb. While getting pregnant actually helps limit endometriosis, endometriosis ironically makes getting pregnant difficult.

While doctors warned her about the potential problems for getting pregnant, Daria put off childbearing until her thirties. That's when the trouble—as predicted—started, and Daria found herself in a fertility clinic trying to straighten it all out. Hormonal treatment, surgery, and two IVFs later, Daria achieved the moniker "Mom."

While these various conditions foreshadowed problems for Kay and Daria, this may not be the case for you. All the symptoms that Kay and Daria experienced—alone or teamed with something else—may not mean infertility for you. Every *body* (and thus *everybody*) is different, which makes infertility such a tricky medical condition. But, menstrual cycles are supposed to follow a certain pattern. If you have experienced anything that seems a little different from your friends' cycles, and you can't seem to conceive, go to the doctor and get it checked out.

JULIE

What else could send you scuttling to the doctor sooner rather than later? Well, sometimes Mother Nature provides a few clues along the way that, had we known what to look for, we might have noticed.

Here are a few flashing red lights that might have made me consider I had a problem earlier.

1. Light, irregular periods that continued long after I stopped taking the Pill;
2. A blocked Fallopian tube caused by a ruptured ovarian cyst in my mid-twenties (a doctor had mentioned the clogged tube after fixing the damage done by that messy, exploding cyst, but it slipped my mind for the next decade. Oops.);
3. Lower-than-average body fat and higher-than-average muscle mass from decades of working out.

If you have any of the above, tell your doctor. They could be nothing. They could be everything.

If you have been on the Pill for years and have had your periods "controlled" by these hormones, it may take a month or so for them to get reregulated. It may take no time. It may take forever. No one *really* knows. So play it safe and see a specialist if your periods don't seem textbook and you don't get pregnant within a few months of unprotected sex.

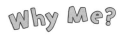

Why Me?

This is what's known as a rhetorical question. No one can answer it. Why you and why not that chick in the office no one can stand? Because sometimes crummy things happen to good people. As much as you will want to find an answer, it is not because you are a bad person or undeserving of a child. It is not because you were mean to your own mother, skipped confession all through high school, or smoked that joint in college. So don't wallow in needless guilt. There's enough time for that later.

While we can't answer the "Why me?" question, we can tell you nearly every infertile couple asks it. We should also warn you that most also get into at least one fight discussing this question.

Julie and her husband got into it when Robert wanted to know just how many times she was going to ask him that stupid "Why me?" question. Well, you can figure out where the conversation went from there. When it came to "Why me?" Maureen's husband wouldn't even go there with her. No pity allowed. Will's response: "You can't look back, and you can't give up. You have to look forward."

Our research, however, assures us this is pretty typical of other couples' conversations on this topic—and its corollary "Why us?" question as well.

Listen to this: After weeks of answering "I don't know" (the husband's always safe answer), our friend Anne's husband made the mistake of answering the "Why me?" question with some ideas of his own. He began ticking off things from Anne's past—she smoked pot in high school, had multiple sex partners, and had an abortion in college. Maybe, he reasoned helpfully, these were possible reasons for the dilemma?

It makes us question why Anne bothered sharing those silly, little stories of her past with her husband in the first place. She should have realized she'd hear about them again! No need to share the gory details of how Anne's tête-à-tête with her husband ended. Suffice it to say everyone learned his or her lesson and moved on to bigger and better things.

Sometimes infertility seems especially cruel. Our pal Kay lives in a small Texas town and has two sisters. One sister has eight (yes, you read that right) kids. The other sister has two children, both conceived while she was taking the Pill.

Kay, however, has PCOS, racked up a decade of infertility treatments, and is currently suffering secondary infertility after the birth of her daughter a few years ago. "I come from a very fertile family," says Kay. "I can't tell you how many times I cried on my mom's shoulder, wondering what's wrong with me."

The crying might have allowed Kay to bond more firmly with her mother, but it isn't what eventually got her pregnant. "I had to get over that 'why me?' attitude if I was going to be able to get through this whole thing," she says. "Once I got that behind me, I was able to get down to business and focus on what was important—finding a way to have a child."

To add insult to injury, Kay had miscarried as a teen. "I had to deal with a lot of guilt," she says. "I took my infertility at first as punishment for something I had done as a kid when I was coming out of a rebellious stage. Support groups helped me to deal with the guilt. But I still struggle with the fact that it's my fault we can't get pregnant. It's hard when your body doesn't do what it's supposed to do."

For some, determining just what part of your reproductive system is out of sync helps refocus the energy. Julie had a faulty uterus. Maureen had messed-up hormones. Daria had endometriosis. Kay had polycystic ovary syndrome.

"Just giving it a name made a big difference," says Kay. "At least I knew the reason I was having problems, could research PCOS, and find others with the same problem. Suddenly, I wasn't so weird."

Why you? We don't know. Why us? We still wonder about that, even after the fact. The point here is to learn from these stories and not waste your time with the unanswerable "why me?" question. But you probably *will* ask yourself the question, so go ahead and get it out of your system. Just promise us you won't spend *too* much time worrying about it.

Normal Is a Miracle

When you consider the precision ballet of ovaries, Fallopian tubes, and uterus necessary to create a favorable environment for conception, it's a wonder any of us were conceived to begin with! Add to that the act of getting the sperm to the egg, multiplied by stress, post-poned parenthood, environmental factors, and the whole process of keeping the baby safely inside you and flourishing for nine months. Well, it's certainly easy to see why normal conception, pregnancy, and birth are actually miracles.

When you aren't expecting to have problems (and who really thinks they'll have problems?), you take nor-mal for granted. We did. We thought it would be a snap—our birthright, something that would come naturally and normally, and without much effort at all. And it would all happen when *we* were ready.

What we never thought about

MAUREEN

With my son, it never occurred to me that anything could go wrong, and it didn't. It was a normal pregnancy. Everyone has those, right?

By the time I was ready to give birth to my daughter ten years later, there hadn't been a day that passed during the pregnancy that I didn't pray for a healthy child. My naïveté had disappeared after my battle with infertility. I am wiser. I will never again take for granted the blessing of a normal, healthy pregnancy and child.

was the whole complicated process of creating a life and all the things that could go wrong. We discovered infertility, a medical condition that demands you be a bit of a detective—as well as an investigative journalist and a crackerjack researcher. Suddenly, normal is not so normal. But we think you are entitled to put those skills on your résumé once you've survived this whole process.

Reality Check

Get out your calculator. We're going to do a little fertility math to show you why you need to get a parenthood plan in place sooner rather than later.

12 months = 12 chances per year to get pregnant.

1 day per month your egg is available and ready for the sperm = 1 day per month you can get pregnant

12 months x 1 day = 12 days per year you can get pregnant.

5 days = life span of sperm inside your body

Of course, this is not totally scientific, but here's what we are basing this on. Once you have ovulated, an egg remains viable for impregnation for twelve to thirty-six hours, depending on who you listen to. Let's average that out to one day.

Regular menstrual cycles can average in length from twenty-eight days (which is considered "average") to as many as thirty-four to thirty-six days. Some months, ovulation may not occur for reasons like illness or stress. Some months, it may actually occur twice! But we feel safe saying it is roughly one ovulation per one cycle per month. Under the right conditions, sperm can live inside a woman's body for up to five days. So working around the egg's time frame, you have seven days surrounding ovulation in which to get the sperm to the finish line—five before ovulation and two during and after.

Everyone is different, so there might be a give or take of a few days over the course of a year. But the whole point of this example is that out of 365 days, twelve is not very many at all—twelve chances a year.

Now let's say you hit it right on. Sperm and egg are in the right place at the right time. How often does that happen? Not every time you have sex on the right days. Statistics vary, but a *normal* couple with *normal* fertility actually conceives only 25 percent of the time during one month of trying. That's a one in four chance. Whoa.

So now, let's divide 12 months by 4 (25 percent of 12) to see the average ability to get pregnant in a year . . . if you are "normal."

$12 \div 4 = 3$

Three great shots per year to conceive. That's all. And that's for someone who doesn't have fertility issues. But for those of us with fertility challenges, even those odds sound great. You'd take them, wouldn't you?

This shows that the monthly window of opportunity in which to get pregnant is small—whether you are facing infertility or not.

We think the biological clock must be a Timex because it keeps ticking no matter what. So don't waste another precious second of your childbearing years wondering what to do.

It's time to get to work.

CHAPTER 3

You Look GREAT, but Your EGGS Don't

Julie

I don't care what the media leads you to believe—women don't have an unlimited amount of time to make a family. Yeah, I know. I bought into that balogna, too.

Even though I met Robert in my mid-twenties and married him when I was thirty-two, we didn't even think about kids until I was thirty-six years old, didn't bother discussing or considering it. We figured we'd get around to it. Sound like anyone you know?

Like many women today, I put off having a family to pursue my career. Robert built his business, and we bought a house. We snickered smugly when friends had babies before they had their own houses, furniture, or job security. We were the smart ones, waiting until everything was just "right." I started freelancing, so I could be home and still work if we ever had kids. We had it all figured out. It was going to be "perfect" when we had kids.

I thought we had plenty of time. I was so delusional even at age thirty-six. Ha, ha, ha! That was Mother Nature nudging Father Time in the side with her elbow and laughing at me. Too bad I didn't hear her back then. I might have asked what the joke was and found out it was on me!

Maureen

I learned the hard way that a woman's body acts its age. At thirty-seven, I thought I was still young, but then suffered a miscarriage. When I quizzed my

OB/GYN, she got exasperated and finally just dismissed me by saying, "Look, it's old eggs, Maureen, old eggs."

Wow. Here I am, an educated woman, and no one had ever told me my eggs would get old. I was floored. Then I got mad. Why didn't this doctor, who I had been with for eight years, tell me about this possibility earlier? Is that why I wasn't getting pregnant? Old eggs?

This doctor never tested me to find out if my eggs were really old. Okay, I know now she was no fertility specialist, but if you are going to give someone a diagnosis like old eggs, you should give them some solution or at least a test. Given my age, old eggs was a good guess. But it wasn't my problem, as I later found out.

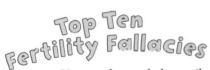

Top Ten Fertility Fallacies

1. You can have a baby easily until you're at least forty-five.
2. Menopause happens to women in their fifties.
3. If you are young at heart, so is your body.
4. If _____ (fill in the blank with your favorite post-forty pregnant celeb) can do it, so can I.
5. Once I stop using birth control and have unprotected sex, I'll get pregnant right away.
6. If I eat right, exercise regularly, and don't smoke, my body will be able to carry a baby whenever I am ready.
7. It's no big deal if I can't get pregnant. My doctor can always get me there.
8. You can never be too thin.
9. Nobody *I* know would ever use donor eggs!
10. When I want to get pregnant, it will just happen.

You've come a long way, baby. We can't remember who first said "Forty is the new twenty-five." Or maybe it was "Fifty is the new thirty." No matter. The point is women no longer have to look or act their age. Thank God!

Thanks to new attitudes and cool clothes—not to mention hair color and extensions, skin care, Botox, push-up bras, plastic surgery, and twenty-four-hour fitness clubs strategically located just about everywhere—you might look and feel better at thirty-five or forty than you did at twenty-two. In fact, it's difficult sometimes to tell a woman's age anymore just by looking at her.

But just because we've stopped the clock on our surface doesn't mean we've beaten Mother Nature at the game she invented or that Father Time has stopped the clock inside our bodies. You may look great on the outside, but you are still old on the inside, which means everything when it comes to reproduction.

While guys produce fresh sperm constantly, scientists seem to think that each woman is apparently born with all the eggs we'll ever have—about one million egg cells in each ovary. And just like the ones in your refrigerator at home, those eggs eventually run out or get so old you have to toss them away.

Science is always working to remedy this. There are studies that tout the possibilities of specialized ovarian stem cells in mice that generate new eggs daily. Or women rendered infertile by chemotherapy giving birth after having an ovarian tissue transplant. For now we're going with conventional wisdom, which says you are born with all the eggs you get and there is no way to turn the clock back. This means age really does matter if you want to get pregnant no matter what our youth-oriented, you-can-have-it-all society tells us. So if you look twenty-five but are really thirty-eight, you're operating with thirty-eight-year-old eggs—not to mention a thirty-eight-year-old uterus and Fallopian tubes that may have more scars on them than antique furniture. Unfortunately, nobody seems to believe it.

Case in point: We went to lunch the other day with a woman we will call Editor at Big Magazine (EBM). EBM is twenty-eight years old. We were chatting about the whole age and baby topic, a personal fave of ours. EBM wanted us to tell her why she should quit living the "good life," as she called it, to start worrying about kids.

"Sell me," she said, between bites of arugula. "I'm only twenty-eight. I want to have my career and travel and have all the fun now. I want to be like Carrie Bradshaw in *Sex and The City*. Why shouldn't I wait to have kids?"

We love opening lines like this. We told her about egg quality and other age-related fertility issues. We told her about finding a guy who was Mr. Ready, not just Mr. Ready-to-Party. We told her if she wanted grandchildren when she was in her golden years, she needed to be sure she didn't miss her golden opportunity to have kids soon. We told her the biological clock waits for no one, not even fresh, young EBMs having all the fun—like her.

As Julie remembers it, Maureen specifically told the diminutive editor that her egg quality "was slipping away faster than that salad you're eating—right now, while you're sitting here talking to us, your eggs are getting old, old, old."

EBM turned white. "You guys are freaking me out," she said. "I don't want to be seen as a woman looking for a man to settle down. I don't have time to figure out a plan. I don't want to have to think about this now."

Then she paused and sighed. "I don't want to think about it," she said. "But I have to, don't I?"

Yes, honey, you sure do.

Age Matters

While reading the morning paper one sunny September day, Julie came across a headline in the *Dallas Morning News* that captured our attention: "Material Girl Wants Another Bundle of Joy."

Apparently, Madonna, the then forty-six-year-old singer and pop icon, wanted another child. Madonna, who at the time had two children ages four and seven, and a decade-younger, film-director husband, told the *Times of London* that she was consulting with doctors about having another baby.

The gym-trim and yoga-toned Madonna was quoted as saying, "Because of my exercising and this, that, and the other, I've kind of screwed up my cycle a bit, and I'm going to the doctors to make sure I'm okay to have a baby, so wish me luck."

Several months later, after finishing a world singing tour in fall 2004, the pop icon told *People* magazine she wouldn't mind getting pregnant again. She's not making any definite plans, mind you, just planning to "have fun with my husband and see what happens."

Good luck. Not to rain on anyone's parental parade, but getting pregnant after age forty is difficult. After age forty-five, very difficult. The statistics don't change, not even for multimillionaire pop stars.

Here are the stats.

> When women are thirty to thirty-four years old, one in seven couples faces
> infertility.
> If women are thirty-five to thirty-nine, one in five couples has a problem.
> For couples in which the woman is forty to forty-four, one in four couples
> has a problem.

Want some more cold, hard numbers? Almost 95 percent of women ages forty-five and older are unable to conceive on their own. Let's make that crystal clear— only 5 percent are going to get pregnant using their own eggs, and only a fraction of those are going to be viable pregnancies. Why? Their own eggs are just too old to create healthy pregnancies. Hence the term "old eggs." Pretty straightforward.

Our friend Cindi, who lives in Texas, heard the same "old eggs" comment from her fertility specialist. Although she had a teenage daughter from a first marriage, she wanted to have a baby with her new husband. She started seeing a fertility doctor when she was thirty-five, after trying to conceive for a year. She then suffered through several miscarriages, three fertility specialists, and one IVF when a doctor told her perhaps her eggs were "old and stressed out." At that point, she was thirty-nine years old. The comment devastated her. She was so emotional that, without talking to anyone, she had her tubes tied the next week. Tied her tubes! That was her solution to old eggs. It also ended the possibility of ever having another baby. Does she regret that rash decision? She won't say.

Wouldn't it be great if every doctor made it their mission to tell women at least once that their eggs were aging? Like maybe during your annual exam the year you turn thirty?

"Hey Mary, look it's none of my business, but you are getting older. Those eggs are not going to last forever. You need to start thinking if you want to have a family. Just didn't want you to be surprised about old eggs later on."

If this was medical protocol, women wouldn't necessarily rush out and try to get pregnant the next day, but we'll bet many of them wouldn't wait as long as we did. We'd all know about old eggs. We'd be prepared. We'd make more informed choices.

Sometime during the infertility process, you may be told that you have old eggs. Do not take it personally, do not crumble, and do not think the baby book just slammed shut. Do what women with old eggs do. Consider your options.

Option One: Find a Doc
If you want to get pregnant, find a good reproductive endocrinologist or an RE (a fertility specialist, NOT a gynecologist) and get tested. (More on why you want an RE rather than a gyn doc later on in the book. Just trust us for now.)

Option Two: Find Some Other Eggs
If you really do have old eggs that cannot create a viable pregnancy, consider finding a younger woman to act as an egg donor. At forty, your chances of getting pregnant with a healthy baby via IVF are ten times higher if you use the eggs of a younger woman and your partner's sperm. This is a great option for women who actually want to be pregnant, control the prenatal environment,

and don't care that the baby is not their biological child—although there is a genetic connection to the father.

Option Three: Find a Surrogate

If you can't carry a pregnancy to term for whatever reason, you can find a surrogate. Soap opera star Deidre Hall, who was forty-five when her first son, David, was born, used a surrogate inseminated with her husband's sperm to carry the baby. The couple used the same surrogate to carry their second son, Tully, two years later. We don't know about the eggs.

Option Four: Adopt

Finally, older women who don't want to fiddle around adopt. Sandra was forty-one when she and her husband, Victor, finally got around to baby talk.

Victor, a physician savvy on the science of conception and older women, asked her point blank, "What's more important to you—being a mom or having a baby?"

When Sandra answered, "Being a mom," he suggested they bypass trying to conceive and start the adoption process immediately, which they did. Today, the two are parents of a beautiful, gregarious kindergartener they adopted shortly after she was born in China. To round out their family, the couple returned from China in 2004 with their child and their new one-year-old daughter. Sandra is forty-seven. Victor just turned forty-five. They couldn't be more ecstatic.

JULIE

There are always exceptions to the rules. When I was growing up, my neighbor got pregnant by surprise (!) at the ripe old age of forty-four. I was in high school at the time with her youngest son, and Mrs. T. was the talk of the town for nine months. No one could believe this old lady was having a baby—just when she had almost gotten the last one out the door.

Back then, a pregnant forty-something was an oddity—not like today, where you see women in their forties birthing babies all around you. But in the mid-seventies, a midlife pregnancy was referred to as a "change-of-life baby." I suspect Mrs. T. assumed she was so close to menopause there was no way she could get pregnant, so she didn't bother with birth control. Your cycles can get irregular in your forties, or if you are stressed out or sick.

Maybe Mrs. T. figured she was safe . . . that she had old eggs. But she didn't, and Maureen didn't, and maybe you don't either. But why wait to find out?

The REAL GLASS CEILING

QUESTION: So when does fertility really start to falter? And what age should you start thinking about having a baby?

ANSWER: Sooner rather than later.

Our society makes us believe women can have it all. We deserve it all. We are entitled to it all. Women rarely attended college a century ago. Fifty years ago, few worked outside the home. We've had the vote for less than half this country's history. Today there are female CEOs, astronauts, and senators. We have proven we can work as hard, if not harder, than the guys. This we have earned, and no one can take that away.

However, we not only think we can have it all, but also feel we *should* have it all—that we are entitled to everything because we've worked so hard (or have always gotten what we've wanted). This is fine if you are talking about a college degree, a better paying job, or a flashy new car. The big shocker for some of us (and we include ourselves in this category) is that we never expected we might not be entitled to birth a baby—because of other time-wasting choices (but relevant at the time) we made along the way. But this is the truth. Some of us might not be able to birth a baby.

Our pal Edie, a forty-six-year-old Californian with four kids ages three to sixteen, wonders out loud if perhaps, just perhaps, we women aren't responsible for some of our own problems.

"I think we as women have this huge sense of entitlement surrounding the entire issue of sexuality and reproduction," says the stay-at-home mom. "That sense permeates our culture and sets us up for quite a few personal moments of truth. Sleeping with whomever strikes your fancy, loading up your body with hormone-altering devices, aborting what you aren't prepared to host, getting sexually transmitted diseases that screw up our fertility quotient . . . these have all left real and phantom scar tissue. Then we wonder why we have to take Herculean steps to get the families we have always wanted.

"I mean, it strikes me that we are a generation of women who slept around from our teen years onward," she adds. "Look, we availed ourselves of all kinds of birth control and then amped our hormones up through the roof by having at it with every compelling guy we tripped across. Finally we settle on Mr. Right, calm down, and think, 'Now I'm ready. Let the babies commence!' Then nothing happens . . . for a long time. So then we freak."

Edie knows from whence she speaks. She did it all in her early years—multiple sex partners, birth control, a bout with chlamydia. When she finally settled down, it took Edie almost two years to get pregnant with her oldest son, Peter. She was thirty at the time.

"I was just twenty-eight when I redirected my energies away from recreational to procreational sex," she remembers. "When I didn't get pregnant right away, I blamed Dan's boss. I told everyone he must know my ovulation schedule better than me because he kept sending Daniel out of town at just the moment in my cycle we should have been hitting the sheets.

"Then, I started to get worried. Once a guy I had such a crush on from high school asked why Dan and I didn't have any kids yet. I didn't want to share my sense of desperation and possible failure, so I came back with, 'Is that a rude question, or an offer to remedy my childless state?' Finally, finally, I got pregnant with Peter. Until then, though, I kept worrying—is this my past catching up with me?"

Yes, we've definitely come a long way, baby, but there are some things that we cannot control with our wits, our savvy, our education, and our Palm Pilots. While times have changed, our body's basic biology has not. Women need to make having children a priority and stop thinking we can have everything we want when we want it.

Listen to the wise words of our friend Rachel, who had her children at thirty-five and thirty-nine. "I'm one of the fortunate ones," she says, a reporter for a major Northeast newspaper. "It is easy to live life in the United States without contact with either children or the old, so you can forget where you came from and where you are going. Somehow through that fog of self-centeredness, I heard the voices of two women, an old lady I met at a press conference in D.C. and a midwife who lived across the street from me in Guinea Bissau, a West African country I visited when I was twenty-six.

"The old lady was a fellow reporter. She spoke to me firmly. 'Don't forget to have children,' she said. The midwife, whose roof leaked, felt sorry for me, the daughter of a rich American. She touched my breasts and stomach, telling me they looked all wrong for my age. I was too thin. That soft lumpy tissue that we are in horror of here is the mark of motherhood. It took me a while to hear their words. I had come frighteningly close to waiting too long."

While everyone is different, it's really true that younger women have an easier time getting pregnant and sustaining pregnancies than older women.

The chance of a successful pregnancy plummets in women older than thirty-five years, regardless of their reproductive past. A Danish study researched the combined effects of age and reproductive history and determined that more than 20 percent of all pregnancies in thirty-five-year-old women are unsuccessful due to miscarriage, ectopic pregnancy, or stillbirth. The number increased to 50 percent of pregnancies in forty-two-year-old women. Another study in the February 2000 issue of *Obstetrics and Gynecology* indicated that pregnant women over the age of forty are at a higher risk of experiencing the sudden death of their fetuses than younger women.

But what about all those over-forty celebs we read about and older moms we see at the doctor's office? They're pregnant, right? Well, yes. But while we read about all the older celebrity baby success stories, we rarely read about our favorite actress or singer losing their unborn child to a sudden death. Or the other complications pregnant women over forty face, like gestational diabetes, high blood pressure, bleeding, or an increased chance of having babies born with chromosomal abnormalities like Down syndrome. Only in 2004 did a few actresses finally even admit to having fertility issues and miscarriages.

Of course, there is variability in fertility. Some women do actually conceive easily at age forty. Others, however, have a hard time conceiving at twenty-eight.

How Old Are Your Eggs?

There is a blood test that your fertility doctor can do to measure your "ovarian reserve" or how old your eggs actually are at the time of the test. This test measures the follicle-stimulating hormone (FSH) and estradiol levels in your blood on the third day of your cycle. FSH stimulates egg growth, and each follicle represents a prospective egg. These levels will tell you how hard your pituitary is having to work to actually stimulate your ovaries. If the levels are too high, your pituitary is working too hard, and your chances of getting pregnant on your own are low. If the levels are mid-to-borderline high, it's time to get on the stick and start trying to get pregnant. If your levels are low, don't sit back and relax thinking you've got plenty of time to get pregnant. You may, but you never know when the levels could start rising rapidly, reducing your chances of conception.

Your doctor may also test your levels of inhibin-B, a hormone that inhibits the production of FSH by the pituitary gland. The higher your inhibin-B level, the more eggs you have in your ovarian reserve. The lower your inhibin-B level, the fewer eggs you have. Couple this with the fact that the number of follicles in your ovaries that could be stimulated to release an egg decrease rapidly in the last five to ten years before menopause. Like other hormones, inhibin-B is altered by your stress levels. If you are really stressed out, you will lower the amount of inhibin-B—not good if you are trying to preserve and reserve all the eggs possible.

What an insane hormonal dance. See why we continue to say that normal is a miracle?

The Perils of Early Menopause

Sometimes you need to start making your baby earlier than you want because menopause might start earlier than you planned. Premature menopause (or, as we call it, menopause when you least want it), happens when your ovaries basically take early retirement. They close up shop long before they are "supposed to," leaving you without enough necessary hormones to keep up ovulation and menstruation. The beginning of menopause signals the end of childbearing.

Obviously, if the ovaries aren't working properly, you can't conceive. That's what happened to Lucia, a thirty-two-year-old Midwestern publicist. After having a relatively easy conception and pregnancy with her daughter in her twenties, Lucia figured having another baby would be just as easy. It wasn't.

After a year of trying, she decided to quit her job to stay home with her daughter and focus on getting pregnant. When that didn't work, she began infertility testing, only to discover she was in the throes of early menopause—in her early thirties. Her hair went prematurely gray as well.

"The whole thing just sucks," says Lucia. "You think you have all this time, and you should have all this time, before the start of menopause strikes. Meanie-pause, that's what it is to me."

If you and/or your doctor catch premature menopause at the very beginning, it might still be possible to jump-start everything again with the help of a lot of very strong fertility drugs, but the chances are slim. Ditto the success of high-tech assisted reproduction technology procedures like in vitro fertilization, gamete or zygote intrafallopian transfers (GIFT and ZIFT). Many clinics will not even bother taking a woman who is in premature menopause, whether early-onset like Lucia or when it occurs more naturally in the mid-to-late forties. These women are harder to treat and can skew their statistics with their failures.

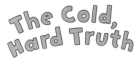

The Cold, Hard Truth

Some hospitals are offering the option of freezing your own eggs for conception later. Talk about the solution for those who want it all. Freeze a few eggs when you're young, build your career, find Mr. Right, and when you're finally ready, if conception is a problem, thaw a couple out, mix with sperm, and insert. It's perfect, also, if you end up being one of the unlucky hit with early menopause or if you suffer from cancer and lose your fertility to chemo and radiation. Of course, since this is a new procedure, freezing eggs for later conception is not a totally reliable process yet—but freezing embryos for storage and use is very commonly practiced with success. To make an embryo, however, you do need some sperm.

To do any of this, you have to have the foresight and money. The trick is to think ahead when your eggs are young. But what if your priorities were like ours when you landed that first job out of college? We sure weren't thinking about a future family. We were wondering if we'd be able to pay for rent, food, the car, and college loans. We barely had money for those things, let alone freezing a few harvested eggs.

If all young women were educated sooner rather than later on the inner aging process, we might think differently. We might consider starting a family sooner or at least planning for one. We've noticed nobody in their twenties and early thirties thinks they will end up alone at forty. But the years pass by pretty quickly, especially after twenty-five.

Our friend, who shall be called Ms. Anonymous, is forty-three and desperately seeking a man. No one was Mr. Right in her twenties. Then she wasted a lot of time choosing men who were not ready. She never thought ahead when it came to men. She never thought she was losing time. She was just living in the moment and dating only hunky, young guys who sure weren't interested in making BABIES!

She is really suffering the consequences of this choice now. She is alone, totally regretting it, and obsessed with finding a man. When we suggested she pass on the men who want to have children because she would not be able to provide them biologically, she responded with "Well, you never know!"

Denial. No one wants to face the possibility that they may be cresting the hill, especially women like our friend—the ones who want it all and are used to getting what they want.

But we are all products of the choices we make. If we had known more about old eggs earlier, we would have considered starting a family sooner or at least planning for one. We know Ms. Anonymous would have, too.

P.S.: THOSE WEREN'T HER EGGS

In 1997, a sixty-three-year-old woman became the oldest woman to give birth in the United States.

Most women having later-in-life babies are doing so with a little (or a lotta) help. Older women who can't get pregnant on their own often turn to in vitro fertilization where the egg and sperm meet up in the lab before being implanted in the woman's uterus. If that doesn't work, then they might engage a surrogate or gestational carrier to carry the baby to term. And most of these women are probably not using their own eggs. (For more on surrogacy, see chapter 23.)

Look at the statistics for getting pregnant post-forty, and it's pretty clear that most women this age who do give birth probably do so with donor eggs harvested from women twenty to thirty years younger. Ditto the fifty-year-plus women who have surrogates carry their babies. Not their eggs! But usually their husbands' sperm because guys with no-problem sperm can spread their seed as long as they can get it out of their bodies. Just look at the late actor Tony Randall. He had two babies with his twentysomething wife when he was in his late seventies. This is more proof that Father Time is a man.

In 2003, former TV personality Joan Lunden chose surrogacy to build her family. The then fifty-two-year-old had three older daughters from a first marriage, a forty-two-year-old second husband who wanted children, and age-related fertility challenges. The couple chose a gestational surrogate to carry the baby. A gestational surrogate, also known as a gestational carrier, has no genetic ties to the child. In fall 2004, Lunden announced that she and her husband were awaiting the birth of their second set of twins with the help of the same gestational surrogate.

Don't Believe Everything You Read

Dad was right: You can't believe everything you read. When it comes to the very public pregnancies of some celebs, the magazines and tabloids have not been getting the real scoop on who's having kids the natural way and who's getting a little help.

Until we went through infertility ourselves, we never thought twice about some celeb in her late forties having a baby. Actually, it made us assume we could get pregnant any time we wanted, too. If you're a reporter and don't know what to ask, you can't ask the question. Any celeb worth her salt knows if the reporter doesn't ask the question, she sure as heck doesn't have to volunteer the answer. Besides, what celeb is going to say anything that might chip the ever-so-perfect world she supposedly lives in? Hardly any.

Frankly, we wish more highly visible women would share the truth and Hollywood wouldn't make midlife motherhood look so effortless. If older celebs would cop to fertility issues and/or donor eggs, other women would feel more comfortable doing it as well. There is nothing wrong with using donor eggs—whether in IVF or with a surrogate. It does not make the child any less precious. Yet these high-profile women having much-later-in-life babies make it seem as if they are doing it all on their own. Then, the media promotes it with all the new baby excitement (which we love) but without asking the tough questions (which we all need to hear.)

We don't want to hear another girlfriend say, "Well, you know I read in the paper that _____ (fill in the blank with the name of a famous celeb) had her first baby at forty-five, so there's no rush. I'm sure it will be easy for me, too."

This is what our friend Maura thinks. She's thirty-nine years old, married sixteen years, and always had protected sex because the time was never right for kids. The house needed to be renovated, the corporate ladder needed to be climbed, and exotic vacation lands needed to be explored. Even her friend's pregnancy problems and multiple miscarriages didn't disturb her. Why? Because look at all the actresses who are pregnant and glowing in their mid-to-late forties! If they can do it, so can Maura! But only time will tell.

Okay, while Oscar-winning actresses seem to be able to birth babies at midlife, the truth is most women trying to get pregnant in their forties won't . . . not without spending money on fertility treatments and/or using donor eggs. And if the Hollywood gals won't tell us the truth about how those pregnancies are coming about, average American women will continue to believe they, too, have all the time in the world to get a guy and get pregnant.

Not fair, Hollywood. Yes, we know everyone wants to have some privacy, but not at the expense of the rest of the women out here. Fess up, please.

Hollywood's Family Values

To be fair, there are several celebrities who have talked about their infertility issues. Some may not have given full disclosure, but that's okay. At least they opened up enough to share with their audiences a portion of their private lives. Brooke Shields conceived her daughter, Rowan, through IVF after several failed IVF attempts and talks about her postpartum depression. Joan Lunden and Deidre Hall are not afraid to share that they are raising children carried for them by surrogates. Courteney Cox suffered several miscarriages before getting pregnant with her daughter, Coco, and ditto for Christie Brinkley.

The Dating (or Waiting?) Game

It's not just men who aren't ready to settle down; it's women. Between the two of us, we know an awful lot of women. Many of these women who are successful and intelligent are also incredibly misinformed, selfish, unaware of how their bodies work, and in denial about age and having babies. Most of them are still holding out for that "perfect" man and think they have all the time in the world to have babies.

"I'll do it after I have the kitchen renovated," one friend told us. When the kitchen was finished, she told us, "I'll do it after we take our cruise to Bermuda." Next it was, "I'll do it after I lose some weight." Then, "Maybe I'll start trying this month because then I won't be pregnant through the summer." (We love that kind of planner!)

But listen to Paula's story. While in Vermont one summer, Julie struck up a conversation with Paula, a thirty-year-old massage therapist who lived in Burlington. When she heard Julie had her kids at thirty-eight and forty-one, Paula said, "You give me hope."

Hope? Seems she had recently ended a three year relationship with a man she really cared for. Why? The guy finally admitted he didn't want kids, and Paula does. While she was sad to lose a boyfriend, she was more concerned about losing the chance to be a mother. Until she met Julie, she thought she was over the hill. Many of her thirtysomething girlfriends were also worried about missing out on motherhood. The men their age weren't in the same place mentally that they were in. The conversations among them had turned to talk about single parenthood, and one of Paula's close friends had recently been inseminated because she was afraid she didn't have time to wait around for Mr. Right to show up.

Good for her for thinking about what she truly wanted in life and figuring out how to get it. So many of us don't.

Work Your (Family Life) Plan

Here's what we think. When you are in high school, college, and in your early twenties, you should "date around" and have fun with different men while trying to determine what you want in a mate or the future father of your child. However, once you hit your mid-twenties, it's time to get a plan for your future family life, particularly if you want to be a mom. It's funny. We spend more time planning a vacation than we do our lives.

If you want to have children, then work your family life plan backward to determine where you currently are in the groove. Begin with where you want to be when you are old. Do you see yourself surrounded with grandchildren visiting for the holidays? Yes? Okay. Put it down: sixty-year-old, supercool grandma (or sixty-five or seventy, whatever works for you).

Next, consider that those future grandcuties will need parents, which you will want to produce sometime before you are forty years old.

Then, you will need a partner to provide the sperm that will create those children and help you parent them, which means you will have to have that partner before you are in your mid-thirties, depending on the number of children you think you may want.

Don't forget to factor in the possibility of fertility challenges, so subtract two years from that must-have-a-partner age, putting you now in your early thirties for securing a committed relationship.

Now back to the dating game. To have grandchildren, you will have to find a man willing to be the father of your children by the time you are in your early thirties. This means that your mid-to-late twenties should be devoted to finding that partner.

While it may sound harsh, don't waste your time with a guy who doesn't want to be a father. You don't have to be overt about it, but the older you are, the more serious your dating should be. Talk about family early on in the relationship. Weed out the guys who are not interested in kids or serious relationships and have fun with them, but don't invest your heart and don't waste your time.

Our friend Elizabeth, a Dallas realtor, dated a guy for eight years before finally asking him when he thought they would get married. He looked at her with a blank stare, shook his head, and said, "Never." He didn't want marriage; he didn't want kids. They had never talked about it, they were having a great time, and he saw no reason to change things. She (finally) saw no reason to stay with him. To date, he is still single, and she is raising two children on her own as a single mother.

Keep your options open while you search for Mr. Ready. You don't have to tell anyone you are looking for the right guy. Think of it as clandestinely interviewing someone for a job—the best job in the world—Daddy.

MAUREEN

You gotta have a plan. When I was twenty-eight, I knew that it was time for me to find a man who was serious, who wanted marriage and children. My clock was ticking. At the time, I was dating a guy I had been with for four years. He was twenty-four, and we were living together. One evening, while we hung out on the couch, I asked him two qualifying questions.

MY QUESTION: What would you do if I got pregnant?
HIS ANSWER: It would ruin my life!
MY QUESTION: Do you ever want to get married?
HIS ANSWER: You don't make enough money for me to marry you.
    Besides, I don't want to get married for another seven years.

These were very wrong answers. Clearly this man was not "ready."

Around the same time, I met Will. At first glance, I thought, I can procreate with this man. He had the genetics that I found desirable: blue eyes, great height, super build, and a great smile. We got along well, and he made me laugh. He was nine years older than me, had lived a full life, and was "ready." How could I go wrong?

To protect my future, I left the not-ready boyfriend and hooked up with Will. Two years later we married. The following year, our son joined us.

You Can Have it All—Just Maybe Not at the Same Time

Here's the truth about kids. They don't care if you live in an apartment or in a house that's paid off. They do not care if the furniture is new, old and ratty, or nonexistent. As long as they are loved by parents who nourish and nurture them, they do not give a darn whether they are wearing this year's designer duds or five-year-old hand-me-downs.

Maureen's mother never decorated a nursery. She bought a crib and put the baby in it when she brought it home. After the third baby, the room sharing began, and after the fifth, everyone shared a room, and no one cared. When Julie brought Amanda home (she was born three weeks early), the nursery was still the guest room with a crib shoved in a corner.

We're sure someone mentioned all this, but neither of us heard it. Or maybe they did, and we weren't listening. We do know for a fact no one ever told us about old eggs. Instead, women have been told they can have it all, and many of us believed that. Well, sister, you can have it all, but you have got to get the priorities right early on, or you may really miss out on the most important part of "all."

JULIE

Robert and I thought we had it all. When we finally decided it was time to add kids to the mix, we were shocked to discover having it all didn't necessarily mean we could have a baby. What?!

Suddenly things like work, travel, and saving the world didn't seem as important as a future with children—our own children. It was an epiphany reached in the dark of night walking home from Christmas Eve service and realizing we may never have a tiny shepherd of our own in the Christmas pageant.

Fast-forward to today. I am a blessed and fortunate older mom with two kids, married to a great guy who is also a fabulous father. I think we're both better parents than we would have been in our twenties: more patient, wiser, and settled. We think we look and act younger than our peers who are doling out college tuition while we're still changing diapers.

But we cannot believe we almost missed our place in the parenthood parade. We often comment that had we known how much fun having kids was, we would have done it earlier. We may even have tried to have more.

We finally understand what having it all is really all about.

To get that career/couple/kids equation that many of us think of as the life plan, Super Woman needs to hang up her cape for a while and focus on family earlier rather than later.

It all gets back to the chick and the egg. You (the chick) may look great, but there's a chance your eggs don't. So why take a chance?

CHAPTER 4
Information Station

Maureen

Once I realized I was having a problem sustaining a pregnancy, I started talking. I asked everyone and anyone if they knew about miscarriages and the reasons behind them. I was desperate to understand my body more and how it worked.

Here's what I learned about infertility: Information is key! Knowing as much as possible helps you properly understand and question your infertility. Being a literary agent, the first thing I did was search for a book, something that would explain to me what I was going through and the journey I was about to embark on. I found nothing that spoke to me—just boring medical text.

I am also not shy about asking questions. I talked to friends and more friends and *more* friends—and even strangers—until I felt I was heading in the right direction. It's amazing how someone you talk to will always know someone who has gone through this. It was through girlfriends that I learned the most important things. I found out about secondary infertility ("what?"), reproductive endocrinologists ("who?"), and the importance of cervical mucus ("why?")—important information for sure.

Lesson learned: Ask questions. Do not be afraid to quiz your doctor, talk to friends, and share your story at your church or club. Ask, ask, ask! You will be surprised at what you find out.

Julie

The innate nosiness necessary to be a reporter served me well when my husband and I discovered we couldn't get pregnant. I became the consummate research fiend, reading every book and article I found on infertility. (Okay, I skimmed some of them.)

Most were, by turn, dry, scientific, confusing, and depressing or didn't address infertility the way girlfriends would. While many books gave me technical insight to the procedures, none prepared me for what I was about to go through physically, mentally, and emotionally. I could read that a hysterosalpingogram (the dreaded dye test to check out the uterus and Fallopian tubes) might be painful, but it didn't describe the sharp, pinching feeling I had or the sock-in-the-gut cramps my girlfriend experienced. It didn't describe the fact that we would endure such dramatically different types of pain. No book talked to me like a friend at a time when a well-informed friend was what I needed most.

Next I checked out the Internet, typing in keywords that would lead me to sites that would provide other keywords. I found chat rooms, support groups, and informative sites. I also found conflicting opinions, misinformation, and horrifying tales of family-making fiascoes. It became mind-numbing to try to sift through what was important and what wasn't. I spent so much time on the computer that my butt assumed the shape of the office chair.

I next wrangled an assignment for the *Dallas Morning News* on infertility, which allowed me to interview some of the top doctors in the business. I even took my reporter's notepad to my doctor appointments and drilled Dr. Cohen, who answered my questions as if we were colleagues, which, in a way, we were.

After surviving the insanity that is infertility, with all the research and testing involved, I think a woman should be given an honorary degree—master's in family planning, a doctorate in procreating—or at least a gold medal for running in the race against time.

Ten Tips for Taking Charge

1. Don't rely solely on your doctor for information. He or she doesn't have time to research every nuance of your problem. You do. Well, you may not have the time if you are really busy, but you should make time!
2. Ask questions . . . of everybody!

3. Become a patient advocate—yours!

4. Your doctor is not God. It's okay to disagree, ask questions, and bring new information to the game.

5. Listen to your body and follow its direction. If you don't know your body very well, reintroduce yourself and learn how it operates.

6. Don't be afraid of infertility. This is something you can beat, a game you can win. You will have a family if you want one.

7. Don't hesitate to bring articles or treatment ideas to your doctor for discussion. Help him to help you.

8. Study and research everything you can.

9. Try to educate your partner, but don't freak if you end up doing all the work. One educated person on the team is better than none.

10. Don't quit.

Once you figure out you're infertile, you become an information sponge soaking up everything you can find about infertility, fertility, getting pregnant, staying pregnant, who's pregnant, and who's trying to get pregnant. What's new in fertility medicine? You want to know. What latest treatments are getting the best results? You want to know. Who are the top doctors in research? You want to know. In your city? You will know. What about alternative medicine? You'll check it out. We did.

If there was an infertility game show on TV, we'd be champions. Hey Wink, we'll take Missed Conceptions for $100!

All kidding aside, we've learned that searching out other infertile couples, clinics, Internet sites, support groups, and information sources can help you take charge. Information is power. Trying to sift through all the information out there, however, can be time-consuming and confusing.

Where Do I Start?

When you can't get pregnant, you swim in a mix of emotions. You feel insecure (how the hell did this happen to me?), inferior (if I can't have a baby, I must not be enough of a woman), scared (how am I going to get out of this mess?), mad (how the hell did this happen to me?), and frustrated (what does *that* mean?). Getting educated is not only necessary for you, but also empowering. Once you know who or what you are up against, you can figure a way around it. Once you understand the tests you are about to undergo, they aren't nearly as scary. Once you learn the lingo of infertility, you can dissect the alphabet soup of acronyms (ZIFT, IVF, LH, FSH, GIFT, and so on) with ease.

As you search for knowledge and investigate the various things that cause infertility, you can begin to play detective and review your past to see if any pieces fit into your particular puzzle. We won't say it's fun, but it is interesting. The more you know, the better and more in control you will feel. With each piece of information, you will become stronger. Promise.

In Good Company

If so many couples are suffering from infertility, how come you don't know any? Well, you probably do, but they just aren't talking. One doctor mentioned that he and his wife had used Maureen's fertility specialist. When we asked if he wanted to share some of his stories, he clammed up. When pressed, he said, "Look, it's my experience that most people don't want to talk about infertility. They don't want others to know what they are going through."

We think he didn't want anyone to know what *he* went through. Gosh, we sure would hate to think some doctors were like some movie stars—afraid we won't like them or respect them if we find out they are just a little like us. It's not like we're going to stop seeing a particular physician just because he and his wife needed some help starting their family. This secrecy is part of the bigger information-gathering problem. When people don't share their wealth of knowledge, it's hard to get the information you crave. The best way to find others like you is to ask around. But if no one is talking honestly, then it becomes a vicious circle—the chick and the egg again. Which came first?

MAUREEN

When I had my first miscarriage, I tried challenging my doctor to make her look deeper into what had just happened to me. But because of my lack of knowledge on infertility, miscarriage, and my own body, I couldn't communicate effectively with her. I know now that I had to understand what my problem was before I could solve it. I knew there was more to it than that, but I was naive and uninformed. Not having the information and not being able to follow through really set me back and caused more heartache than necessary. I don't think I would have had those other two miscarriages if I had been savvier about fertility issues in general and my body specifically.

The interpersonal dynamics of infertility are fascinating. Women who have had success forming their families love to talk, but as new moms or moms of multiples, they don't have much time to spare. Women for whom procedures have failed are also a wealth of knowledge but harder to crack open.

Some of our good girlfriends were hesitant to share their experiences, even when we promised complete anonymity. We sent a few questions to more than forty friends and acquaintances for one chapter and only two responded—two! When we called them on the carpet, we heard things like, "That's in my past!" and "I can't go there anymore." Others changed the conversation when the topic came up. It was fascinating. Once we cajoled them enough, some gave forth the information.

Honest discussion can really bring out the best in all of us. It is your responsibility to open your mouth and ask the questions. When you start the dialogue, you will find someone who has been there or who knows someone who has.

JULIE

Fortunately, not all girlfriends are so secretive. When I was on holiday over the summer, I told everyone I ran into I was writing this book. Women would come to speak with me. "I heard you're writing a book on infertility," they would whisper, crouching beside me as they told me their stories.

Some would say, "Please make sure you tell other women this . . ." and give me the real scoop on a procedure, an alternative treatment, the effects of a drug, or how to keep your marriage intact during the whole insane period. I took lots of notes on napkins and the backs of place mats.

When the dialogue was low-key, they told me everything. When I pressed for more, to e-mail them questions or interview them more in-depth, some squirmed and never came back. Others let me quiz them via phone and e-mail ad nauseam, and made sure I got their stories just right. You girls know who you are. Bless you.

Gal Pals

The best place to find a group of girlfriends who are ready to talk about infertility? A support group. Nationwide, you can find such support groups at organizations like RESOLVE, The National Infertility Association. This nonprofit organization was established in 1974 and focuses on promoting reproductive health. RESOLVE strives to share information on family building options for both men and women and provide support services, education, and physician referral.

Their informative website (www.resolve.org) says, "The mission of RESOLVE is to provide timely, compassionate support and information to people who are experiencing infertility and to increase awareness of infertility issues through public education and advocacy."

Our friend Dorothy found the support she needed at RESOLVE. "I felt very alone with what I was experiencing," says the thirty-nine-year-old mother of twins. "It was difficult for friends, colleagues, and family to truly understand what I was going through and why I felt as I did. They'd say things and do things with good intention that just didn't help. I felt a huge need to be understood, to not feel so alone with this, but I realized that no one could truly understand except others experiencing the same thing."

Dorothy saw a RESOLVE brochure in the office of her RE. Inside, she found ads for RESOLVE's various support groups. "I was looking for women like me whom I could talk with, gripe with, and laugh with about what we were going through . . . and that's exactly what I found. It was a great group of women."

After sharing her story with others, Dorothy felt relief at finding people who understood the whole physical and emotional experience that is infertility.

"They made me feel less alone, less isolated, more normal, and helped clarify my own decision-making process regarding routes I wanted to take toward becoming a parent," she says.

Helen is a member of the same RESOLVE support group. "We started with about twelve women, and there are five of us who have stayed close," says the former schoolteacher and mother of two. "We met for five weeks or so with a social worker, and then some of us continued meeting monthly after that. One of the women I met there is now my best friend."

Helen adds, "Keeping in touch means so much to us all, I think. We all have shared such a life-altering experience; it is very powerful and comforting to be able to talk to them with that shared experience. I mean that experience informs our lives now and in many ways affects our experiences with our own families and other mothers. For me and I think others in the group, the support meant everything to us."

In fact, the gaggle of gals became so close, they still keep in touch now that they have all built their families and support one another in their roles as parents. Of the five chicks who still gather, Dorothy has twins, two others have one adopted child and one biological child, another has an adopted child, and Helen has two biological children.

For many, support groups provide a safe place to voice concerns and hopes and to ask questions and provide answers to others who are going through the same thing. Support groups can also be found at churches, community centers, and hospitals. Your doctor should be able to help you find one in your area. If you live in a rural area or small town, you might even consider starting one yourself. Again, enlist your doctor's help to find other infertile women.

Our informal research shows, however, that many of us don't take that first step to find a group like RESOLVE, which is kind of odd because generally women love to congregate and talk about anything. But with infertility, some women remain in denial, afraid that if they go to a support group, then maybe, just *maybe*, they'll be admitting to a problem they aren't yet willing to face. Others are embarrassed to let anyone—even other women facing the same thing—know what they are going through. Still others are concerned someone they know might see them attending a support group and ask questions. Or, heavens, what if someone they know is there?! (We can't understand that one. What could be *better* than a friend to share the insanity?)

Some women expressed fears of support groups being nothing more than "bitter women angry about not being able to conceive" having chat fests with no positive outcome. "I want to keep negative thoughts out of my life at this point," says Lauren, a thirty-four-year-old who has been trying to conceive for two years and who has not attended a support group. "I don't want to hear other people's problems. I spend enough energy with my own. I think it would be a downer."

We agree that a negative support group would defeat the purpose. If you find yourself in a situation where the group's dynamics don't mesh with your needs, by all means leave. It's okay if it doesn't work out. Find another one.

Neither of us attended support groups, but for a different reason. We each created our own network of infertile friends with whom to talk. Julie had her friend Peggy; Maureen had Carol. Then we found each other, and we never shut up.

We think Dorothy has the best, most honest approach to finding a support group that works for you. "I can only share my experience and hope that something that I say helps in some way," she says. "I figure it's really up to the individual to decide she is ready for and desirous of the benefits a support group provides. For me, the support group was about creating a community of individuals with shared experiences in the context of a situation that made me feel otherwise alone, marginalized, different, and miserable."

Internet Infertility

If you want the sense of community without having to leave your home (or invite others in), the Internet may appeal to you. By using chat rooms and message boards on specific sites, you can communicate with others who are going through exactly the same procedure or emotional upheaval as you. Chat rooms allow you to "talk" (type, really) in real time with others. Message boards are great for grousing or leaving questions to be answered by others perusing the site. Best of all, shy gals (and guys) can do all this anonymously. Simply choose a sign-in name different from the one your parents gave you.

The Internet seems to work well for those with time constraints as well. "I've found FertileThoughts.com to be a great place to vent and get info," says Seth, a guy friend who prefers the anonymity of the Internet to tracking down other men facing infertility. "I visit the husbands' board often. It's a great place for us guys to talk about things. I like it much better than, say, a local support group. With my busy schedule, I can post a question at midnight and check for answers the next morning. It's there for me when I need it, and I don't have to go anywhere or worry about whether I'll embarass myself with a dumb question."

Those who use these chat rooms and message boards often write in acronyms—letters that stand for a word or group of words. It's like a secret code and can be totally confusing if, like us, you lost your Super Infertility Decoder Ring. So here's a quick lesson on infertility lingo. The following is what a message board comment might look like:

DH and I have been TTC for 2 yrs. Every time is BMS. Tiring. 3 MC. Hard. ASA but now moving to ART. Fingers crossed. This BB has been a lifesaver. Gets me ROFL sometimes! BBS.

Translation: Darling husband and I have been trying to conceive for two years. Every time is baby-making sex. Tiring. Three miscarriages. Hard. Anti-sperm antibodies, but now moving to assisted reproductive technology. Fingers crossed. This bulletin board has been a lifesaver. Gets me rolling on the floor laughing sometimes! Be back soon.

See? It's like a foreign language. Fortunately, some sites now have a page dedicated to acronyms. To get you started, we've jotted down some acronyms that will allow you to write while you learn the rest of the online lingo. It's also okay to write everything out and totally avoid acronyms altogether. Frankly, that's how we still do it.

TTC—trying to conceive

DH—darling husband (and its corollary, DW—darling wife)

IF—infertility

2WW—two-week wait

BW—blood work

CD—cycle day

PG—pregnant

MIL—mother-in-law

RPL—recurrent pregnancy loss

SAHM—stay-at-home moms

Dx—diagnosis

E2—estradiol

ED—egg donor

BCP—birth control pills

BBT—basal body temperature

CF—cervical fluid

LSP—low sperm count

SI—secondary infertility

JULIE

I like message boards and have left messages and responded to others on them. It's amazing how totally open and brutally honest we can be if we are totally anonymous. The Web has done that for us. Chat rooms, however, are too hard for me to follow. Everyone types faster than me, so I get frustrated and just leave. And those acronyms made me nuts until I cracked the code. The trickiest part of using the Internet for me is still finding the right keyword to tap into what I really wanted to find.

MAUREEN

Reading other people's stories on a few sites helped me more than I thought. I realized that the honesty of people talking about their experiences helped me to understand my own situation much better. I never found one site that I really liked, but I used all of them as much as I could. Like Julie, I never entered a chat room, and after a while, I would just burn out over the incredible amount of stories online. Sometimes it can be too much.

Computer Sex

Some sites are helpful, some are educational, and some are addicting to read (the message boards). There are even sites that would lead you to believe technology can do everything except have sex with your partner.

Our pal Sally found one that did most of the pre-sex work for her. This dear friend, thirty-nine years old, happily married for ten years, just decided she was going to get pregnant as we were writing this book. "It was time!" she informed us. They were ready! That she is thirty-nine is of no concern to her at this point—even though we have gently tried to prepare her by telling her that things might not be as easy for her as she expected.

Sally told us there should be no problem because she is going to rely on the computer to tell her when her body is ovulating. It is all quite easy, she has informed us. She simply signed up for an ovulation calendar on one Internet site and plugged in her information. Daily, the site sends a message to her computer telling her when it is time to jump on her husband and get to work.

Sally wants a girl, so she paid extra for this site to let her know the best time to make that happen. As a bonus, this site will not only tell her when to have sex, but also the due date and zodiac sign of that little girl she is about to conceive. She loves the convenience of the computer thinking for her. It works conveniently with her hectic schedule because it tells her ahead of time when she should be scheduling those romantic dinners with her husband or getting tickets to hear an old band she and her husband loved while they were dating. She can create a magic moment in which to conceive, schedule it into her BlackBerry, and forget about it. Talk about computer sex! Let's hope her computer never crashes.

While sites like this are fun and helpful if you ovulate "normally"—on the same day of your cycle every month—they are not as easy to use if you ovulate randomly or not at all. If you have uterine issues, plugged Fallopian tubes, or your husband's sperm needs a life preserver to stay afloat, these ovulation calendar sites will not work for you.

Another negative to consider with computerized, Big Brother-helping-you-to-get-pregnant sites, like the ovulation calendar, are the possible head games. Think about it. This site tells you too much information that may never happen—the gender of the child, the date he or she will be born, and the child's astrological sign. We can see how easy it might be to attach to a baby who may never be born. Sure, it's probably fun for a few months, but what happens if you don't get pregnant month after agonizing month? We'd probably boot the computer out the window.

It's also too easy to be influenced with all this technology that it affects what we hear from our own bodies. Couldn't it become a self-fulfilling prophecy that if the computer calendar says today's the day to feel ovulation pain you might convince yourself subconsciously that you are—and miss your body's real signs of ovulation later in the month? We're not saying that you shouldn't dabble in these computer games. Just keep it real.

Before you become a total computer geek, wasting precious months plugging in numbers and waiting for magic, visit a fertility specialist to determine if you have other issues. Then supplement your fertility plan with the computer. If you are thirty-nine years old, like Sally, we *demand* your first stop be the doctor. Honey, the clock is ticking. Of course, you might defy the odds and get pregnant on your first try with the computer. It happens. It didn't happen for Sally, however, and she was crushed.

Online: This Doctor Is Always In

There are thousands of medical Internet sites covering everything from how to find a doctor and whether that doctor has ever been disciplined to definitions of specific diseases, self-diagnoses, and treatment plans. Many sites provide a place for you to ask questions that a doctor will try to address in a posted e-mail a few days later.

Some sites will offer "live chats" with specialists. These are promoted on the site with a specific time to sign on. You e-mail questions or comments in real time to a doctor who is versed in the topic du jour and hope that he or she will answer you. You don't have to e-mail if you don't want to; you can simply read along as if you were listening to a conversation. If you miss the time, often these chats are saved online, and you can scroll through them at your convenience.

We do caution that the Internet doctor does not replace a real live person you can visit in the flesh. You need someone who knows you and what you are going through. There are too many variable in this science and in each woman's body to trust everything to a doctor who only knows you by your sign-in name. He or she can't know what is truly going on with the many facets of your situation and your health. It's okay to use these Internet doctors to run ideas past or get second and third opinions, but they should never replace your fertility specialist.

Medical websites can be dangerous places for self-diagnosis as well. It's all too easy to read these message boards and begin comparing yourself with those online. You can scare yourself with someone else's bad symptoms and situations or convince yourself you're fine when you really aren't based on what some faceless person has shared online. You don't want to catch "cyber-chondria." Unless you have earned an M.D. you probably won't understand everything you are reading or how to put it into proper context.

The Work of Networking

Researching your infertility is time-consuming and confusing at times—and totally necessary if you are going to be informed enough to help your doctor help you. We learned so much about our bodies in our search for understanding our own particularly infertility issues.

Here's what we discovered.

- We couldn't always rely on our bodies to do what we wanted them to do when we wanted them to do it.
- What an incredible miracle it is to conceive a child.
- How much we often take for granted the miracle of conception and birth.
- Doctors don't always know what to do.
- Women actually know more about their bodies than they think because instinct and intuition are strong assets in dealing with infertility.
- There's a big difference between a gynecologist and a reproductive endocrinologist, and it's extremely critical to understand that.
- There are many ways to build your family and always someone who can provide good information because they've been through the same thing.
- Infertility is a game in which everyone really is a winner—because you *will* have a family.

Most of all, we learned about the science of our bodies and the impact that hormones have on the delicate cycle of creating life. Since we are both in our mid-forties now, we've decided we better start studying up on how to deal with our next journey—menopause. Hopefully we won't get there too soon!

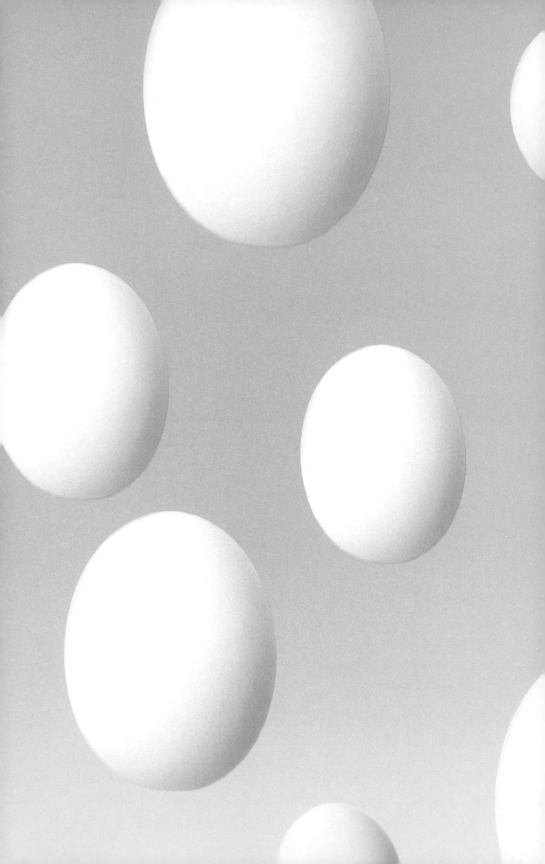

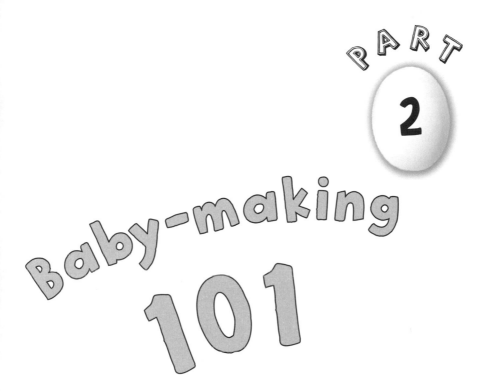

PART 2

Baby-making 101

This section focuses on the basics, the reality of getting pregnant, because making a baby depends on more than just a bottle of wine and a willing man. What happens week after week to a woman's body during her monthly cycle? What is the physical process of conception? When should you use a pregnancy test? How do you use an ovulation predictor kit? How come the chick down the street can get pregnant and you can't?

Julie

Making a baby. That's what women are supposed to do. But sometimes the mind is willing while the body isn't.

You can't always predict *when* you will get pregnant. This is why Maureen and I laugh heartily when some gal pal books a romantic bed-and-breakfast specifically so she and her spouse can make a baby *that* weekend. Not because she knows she's ovulating then, but because it's their anniversary, and they are just ready to have a baby—oh yeah, and they want to have a great conception story.

Here are my conception stories. Since we didn't think we could get pregnant, there was no big buildup to begin with, no need to pay for a romantic rendezvous. I think my son was conceived with little romance during a quickie over the footboard of our king-size bed. My daughter's conception story is a bit more involved. I attribute it to a bad case of poison ivy—so bad the dermatologist prescribed a course of prednisone, a powerful steroid. While taking this medicine, my arms swathed in cutoff tube socks and anti-itch salve, my husband offered me some sympathy sex. Nine months later, there was Amanda. I have not an ounce of proof, but you can't convince me that prednisone didn't somehow help get the old body in balance.

Maureen

You think you know so much as a teenager. I thought I knew how babies were made back then, but I really didn't. I remember when I was still a virgin, and my boyfriend ejaculated on the bed comforter. I was petrified the sperm would jump off the comforter and swim up my birth canal. I was convinced I was pregnant because I had been in the same room as free-ranging sperm.

You can't blame my innocence. I grew up Catholic in the sixties and seventies, and I heard all the stories. I remember my friends telling me about a girl who got pregnant just from kissing a guy, and another who just got naked with a guy and ended up pregnant. This stuff scared the life out of me. Little did I know these were just Catholic urban legends probably created by some nun to scare nice, little Catholic girls like me.

Once they established themselves, my periods were so regular, like clockwork, I could actually determine when I was ovulating, so I didn't use any other form of birth control. I was Miss Day-Fourteen-ovulation, Day-Twenty-eight-here-comes-my-period every month. While making out with my boyfriend, I would be lightly tapping my fingers on his back counting what day it was in my cycle. Is this an okay day or not? For me, counting was part of foreplay. When they replay the movie of my life, I expect to see me during my sexually active years counting on my fingers making sure I was safe to have sex.

Fast-forward to thirtysomething Maureen. When I conceived my son, I knew it was day fourteen of my cycle. It was New Year's Eve; I drank a little too much bubbly, jumped my husband, and presto-bango, created baby Quinn. With my daughter, I tried to follow the day-fourteen routine again. It didn't work. I tried new positions on day fourteen—even lying with my feet up in the air so those little sperms wouldn't have to swim upstream. I still didn't get pregnant. Something wasn't working—and it sure wasn't me!

As much as I feared *getting pregnant* when I *wasn't* trying, that's how much I feared *not getting pregnant* when I *was* trying. Everything about my body I thought I knew was no longer working. The rules had suddenly changed.

CHAPTER 5

Finally . . . UNPROTECTED SEX!

Julie

What did you do during health class—or whatever they called sex ed in your school? What did you *really* do, I mean, because who truly paid attention?

Here's what I did: I read the book at home and looked very closely at all the pictures—particularly the boy parts. Hmm . . . so that's how the penis works! I passed notes during class, made faces with the rest of the class at the appropriate "embarrassing" parts, and answered as few questions as possible. The locker room before track practice was actually the most useful sex ed—like who in high school was going to second and third base and just what that meant.

Oh, and who can forget the movie they showed all the fifth-grade girls back then? The one on menstruation hosted by the school nurse and shown only to the girls? I remember walking out of class rolling my eyes in embarrassment because I was sure the boys knew where we were going (they didn't). Then I watched it with one hand over my eyes and the other hand poking my friend in the arm at all the "gross" parts.

I got Mom's "sex talk" when I was eleven. It consisted of a pack of pastel paperback books on becoming a woman and her availability to answer any questions. Of course, I didn't have any questions.

Dad followed up a few weeks later with, "Do you have any questions about the birds and the bees? No? Good. If you do, you can always come to me or Mom." And off he went out of the room.

I had a lot of biology to catch up on when I started trying to get pregnant.

Maureen

I grew up in a Catholic household where you never mentioned the word "sex"—ever. That was a bad word. You didn't dare discuss it.

When I was in fifth grade, we moved to England for a year when my father, a teacher, was sent on a sabbatical. In England, they don't show that film Julie saw—the one that prepares you for what happens to your body. It wouldn't have mattered, anyway. When my older sister was in fifth grade, my mother wouldn't sign the permission slip to let her see that film. There was no way I'd get to see it.

As a result, I didn't know anything about menstruation—zip, nada, zero. So when I came home one day from playing football in the neighborhood and found blood in my panties, I thought I'd hurt myself playing. I called my mother, who came in, took one look, and told my two older sisters to handle it.

Next thing I know, here come my sisters waving a huge sanitary pad and singing, "Maureen's a woman, Maureen's a woman." I still remember being traumatized, tears streaming down my face, huge pad in my crotch, and saying "I don't want to be a woman." I didn't understand what any of it meant, but somehow I knew my life would never be the same.

When I went to college, my roommate was a hot tamale from Brooklyn whose mother birthed her at age fifteen. This girl ended up teaching me a lot about my body and sex. Our late night talks were the beginning of my sex education.

Ten Things We Bet You Didn't Know About Reproduction

1. Cervical mucus has a purpose—really.
2. Men produce sperm constantly.
3. Conception takes place in the Fallopian tubes.
4. You may not ovulate the same time every month.
5. Ovaries don't necessarily take turns ovulating.
6. An egg has a twenty-four hour life span.
7. Conception doesn't take place the night you have sex.
8. Your Fallopian tubes might be blocked, and you wouldn't know it.
9. Your uterus could be scarred, and you wouldn't know it.
10. Given the right conditions, sperm can live inside you for several days.

Conceptually Speaking

After years of focusing on birth control and doing all you possibly could to prevent pregnancy, you've decided to have a baby. Finally . . . unprotected sex. Free love. Wahoo! Good-bye diaphragm. Adios birth control pill. Ta-ta condoms.

Now is the perfect time to learn about your body and the actual process of conception. You're probably thinking, "I live in this body. I sleep with *that* body. His outie goes in my innie. What else is there to know?" A lot.

We've discovered (shockingly!) that many of our most highly educated and successful female friends do not understand the way their bodies work. They can tell you everything about exercise, nutrition, and why you really do need eight glasses of water daily. But when it comes to reproduction, they're dummies. So were we. We just assumed pregnancy happens, so why try to figure it out? This was until we couldn't get pregnant. Infertility demands a crash course in Body Basics 101.

It's like learning to drive a car. You must have all the information before you insert the key in the ignition. If you don't, you'll probably crash. If you don't understand how reproduction works and why you have fertility challenges, you probably won't get pregnant. We don't want you to be crash dummies for infertility.

So we're going to run through everything you should have learned in health class but missed because you were too busy giggling. If, unlike us, you paid attention in high school, feel free to skim this chapter and move on.

Body Basics 101: This Is Your Body

You live in it, but do you know it? Probably not, and you're not alone. Our reproductive anatomy—the whole part of us that makes us females—is still shrouded in mystery. Funny, we can watch overt reality TV on the networks and hard-core sex shows on cable, listen to shock jocks dissect sex on the radio, and read about whatever kinky stuff you're into in books and magazines, but baby-making basics, the stuff we really should know—our bottom-line biology, for goodness sake—gets buried and whispered about as if it were . . . shall we say, dirty.

If we spent more time educating our kids about the mechanics of their own bodies and less time protesting about how to teach (or if we should teach) sex education in school, we'd all be better off. At least we'd know what the heck was going on each month, and the guys would be more understanding about the hormonal havoc we suffer. Blame society, blame puritanical roots, blame the religious right, blame your parents, or blame your high school—whatever. The fact of the matter is most of us grow up without a clue as to what really happens to our bodies each month. We're keeping it simple here because we are not doctors. But we have pored over a bunch of biology books and have run everything past some top doctors, so we feel pretty secure about our info.

Here's the woman's part in the conception game: We supply the eggs and the home for the growing baby. Unlike guys who manufacture sperm constantly (is that why they're too tired to take out the garbage?), we don't even have to make these eggs—we're born with all we'll supposedly ever need. Now, isn't that typical? Women pack ahead—even before we're born—putting all our eggs into one basket, so to speak, while men have to constantly make their seed. Even at birth, women are prepared for the future.

The Chick or the Egg

As we know now (we knew it before, but just didn't listen, right?), a woman's fertility is at its peak in her twenties. It slowly diminishes until she reaches thirty-five and then plummets rapidly like a stone tossed from a bridge for the rest of her childbearing years. By the time many of us figure out we want kids and how the body really works to create them, we are often on that slippery, downhill slope. As a woman ages, the chances that her reproductive machinery is scarred or marred from past pelvic surgeries or infections increases as well.

Then the question becomes: Is it the chick who has the problem or her eggs?

These Are Your Ovaries

The ovaries are the female's primary sex glands, producing estrogen and progesterone. These glands are about the size and shape of an almond, although they are lumpier. You have two, one on each side of your body, just below your belly button. Every baby girl is born carrying the possibility of her future family with her in the form of one million eggs (give or take) in each of her ovaries.

After a girl reaches puberty—anywhere from ten to sixteen, although the average is twelve to thirteen—one of her ovaries releases one or more mature eggs each month (aka, ovulation). Think of ovulation as the let's-get-pregnant time of your menstrual cycle. Ovulation doesn't necessarily rotate between ovaries—left one month, right the next. There's really no pattern. One ovary may do the ovulating for a couple months, then pass the job over to the other one for a while, or they may actually take turns. Some women (about 20 percent) can actually *feel* ovulation when it occurs. It manifests itself as a slight pain in their lower abdomens. The feeling can range from a little ache to tiny, painful twinges that last a few minutes to as long as a few hours. There's even a name for this: *mittelschmerz*.

The egg is released from the ovary into the pelvic cavity, where it is quickly swept up by the fimbria (those little projections at the end of the Fallopian tubes that look like fingers) and sent south through the Fallopian tube. Once released, the egg has a maximum life span of twenty-four hours.

The problems that may occur with your ovaries can be divided into two groups—physical or hormonal. Physical problems include endometriosis or cysts that fill the inside or cover the outside of the ovaries. Hormonal problems include ovaries that might not ovulate properly or produce too much or too little male sex hormones to be in balance. All of these issues can result in infertility.

These Are Your Fallopian Tubes

Think of your Fallopian tubes as the highways from the ovary to the uterus. These tubes are narrow and delicate, often twisting a bit in little corkscrew turns. Each ovary has its adjoining Fallopian tube in which the egg hopefully meets the sperm and is fertilized. Whether fertilized or not, the egg travels down this narrow, four- to five-inch tube toward the uterus. These stringy tubes are lined with cilia, which look like tiny hairs or fingers and act to push the egg along en route to possible fertilization. Fertilization, when it occurs, happens inside the Fallopian tube. The united egg and sperm spend their five- to seven-day honeymoon there, moving toward the uterus. If the egg is not fertilized, it will disintegrate at the end of its twenty-four-hour life span and either be reabsorbed by your body or expelled as part of your period.

These tubes can also become partially or completely blocked over the course of a woman's lifetime. The culprit may be scar tissue from endometriosis, pelvic inflammatory disease (PID), or a birth defect. This blockage acts like a wreck on the highway and prevents the egg from traveling south or the sperm from traveling north. If egg and sperm don't meet, you don't conceive.

You can still conceive if only one Fallopian tube is blocked, although, of course, you cut your chances of conception in half since you're in effect operating on one cylinder. The doctor will determine if your tubes are blocked with a special test called a hysterosalpingogram (HSG). Tests are discussed in-depth in chapter 9.

Also, clear Fallopian tubes are crucial to assisted reproductive technologies such as GIFT and ZIFT. With gamete intrafallopian transfer (GIFT), the egg and sperm are put into the Fallopian tube by the doctor with hopes that fertilization will take place. Zygote intrafallopian transfer (ZIFT) is similar to IVF in that the eggs are fertilized in a petri dish by the doctor, but the resulting embryos are put into your Fallopian tube to continue their journey, rather than your uterus.

This Is Your Uterus

Consider this muscular, pear-shaped organ to be the mother ship. The uterus is where it all happens—the final resting spot for the united egg and sperm, now called the fertilized egg. The typical, nonpregnant uterus is about the size of a small pear and hollow, but has the capacity to expand to fit a growing fetus—amazing.

The fertilized egg implants itself in the uterine wall, which (hopefully, in a perfect world) has prepared a lush lining, called the endometrium, to nourish it. The uterus then acts as the incubator for the developing embryo and subsequent baby. If the lining is not conducive to support the fertilized egg, or if there is no fertilized egg that month, then this endometrium is discharged during menstruation. This lining is the blood you see each month.

If your uterus is too small, tipped the wrong way, divided by a thin layer of tissue into two chambers (called a bicornuate uterus), partially divided (called septate uterus), inhabited by fibroid tumors, or overgrown with polyps, you will have fertility issues that need to be solved.

This Is Your Cervix

The cervix is the bottom opening of your uterus; the front door to the vagina. If you use tampons and push one in as far as it can go, you may bump into your cervix. This is also what your doctor is looking at during your annual exam,

JULIE

I guess I really took my uterus for granted, never realizing all the things that could go wrong with it. Actually, until I wanted to get pregnant and couldn't, I never bothered to think about it at all. Here's this organ, tucked inside your pelvis, about the size of your fist, that only bothers you once a month when it discharges its contents. What could go wrong with a uterus?

Apparently, a lot. In my case, uterine sonograms showed a skimpy endometrial lining that was too thin to support life. Additionally, white patches of scar tissue (?!) showed up on parts of my uterus as well. Scar tissue is also not conducive to an egg attaching or a placenta forming.

To find out what was going on, my doctor had to go in. Dr. Cohen suggested a hysteroscopy. After knocking me out with general anesthesia, he dilated my cervix and inserted a thin fiber-optic "flashlight" called a hysteroscope, which let him view my womb (womb with a view?).

During the hysteroscopy, Dr. Cohen removed the white patches of tissue with a tiny instrument that scraped the inside of my uterus. This is called ploughing. The idea, as I gather, is similar to a farmer tilling up the soil in a field. If you try to plant a seed on hard, compacted soil, it can't lay down its roots and grow—same with patchy white scar tissue on a uterus. It's not good for a fertilized egg to attach roots and grow, either. So Dr. Cohen literally scraped up those patchy areas of my uterus. I like to picture him wearing farmer overalls rather than a lab coat, hoe in hand, roughing up the dirt to create more fallow ground—soft crumbly soil full of nutrients as opposed to hard, clay-like soil unable to be penetrated—the perfect environment for a seed (or fertilized egg) to snuggle down in and grow.

Dr. Cohen must have also had some type of microscopic camera inside my uterus as well because when I came to and was again coherent, I saw some interior uterine pictures I don't think you can take with a regular 35-millimeter.

when your feet are in the stirrups, the sheet is over your knees, and the speculum is in place. Besides standing sentry to the womb, the cervix also produces cervical mucus—that slippery clear fluid sperm love. The cervix also dilates, or opens, when your baby is ready to be born.

When you get close to ovulation, your cervix will pull up a little higher, soften and widen its opening slightly to allow the sperm entrance. After ovulation, the cervix sinks back down and starts to harden. Right before your period, your cervix should be very low and hard. You can feel these changes with your fingers throughout the month if you want.

This Is Your Vagina

All of us know where the vagina is located and what its basic purpose is, but to be consistent, let's go through the basics. The vagina is a four-to-six-inch muscular tunnel with smooth, slippery-when-you're-aroused walls located between the cervix and the vulva (the name given to the external female genitalia). The vaginal lips are the folds of skin outside the vagina, that close off the opening. When you're turned on, the vagina expands so it can fit most penises; the vaginal lips fill with blood and plump up as big as those on the mouth of a certain lead singer for the Rolling Stones. The vagina also expands again to become the birth canal when your baby is ready to enter the world.

Don't cringe or freak out, but you should familiarize yourself with your vagina. Get a mirror and check it out. Put your fingers inside and feel around. It should feel smooth. It shouldn't hurt to do this, nor feel dry. If you feel something odd, like bumps or a burning sensation, call your doctor.

Cervical Mucus: What Is It, and Why Should You Care?

It's amazing the number of women—our former uneducated selves included—who don't know about cervical fluid, aka cervical mucus. You probably recognize this fluid—it's the wet stain in your panties midmonth and the white or yellow discharge you find there on other days. But do you know what it does? We didn't, but all of us should.

Our friend Linda, pregnant at forty-two with twin girls after seven AIs (artificial inseminations) and three IVFs, had no clue about cervical mucus until she was well into her infertility odyssey in her late thirties. "I just thought I had this gross discharge once a month—I thought I was unclean. It grossed me out, and I would just stick a tampon in midmonth. It didn't dawn on me that it was part of my cycle! You know, they never talked about cervical mucus in health class."

Another girlfriend Shea, a forty-three-year-old mother of two tykes, didn't discover her cervical juices until she was being fitted for a diaphragm in her late twenties. "I asked my doctor how this would work, and he told me it covered the cervix. When I quizzed him further about placement, he looked at me like I was an idiot and said, 'Do you mean to tell me you've never touched your cervix before?' Well, I went home and looked this all up, and that's how I found out about cervical mucus. My mom didn't tell me. I doubt she knew any more about it than I did . . . certainly not enough to fill me in."

Here's the scoop. Cervical mucus is produced by the cervix and is crucial for helping sperm slip up the vagina easily because it creates an environment in which they can live for days. Its unofficial title should be "Nourisher, Protector, and Mover of Sperm."

As you progress through your monthly cycle, your cervical mucus increases in volume and changes texture, based on increasing levels of estrogen in your body. This mucus transitions throughout the month from sticky like school paste to thinner like Elmer's glue to slippery-stretchy like uncooked egg white back to thick, sticky, and possibly even yellowish. You are considered most fertile when the mucus becomes clear, slippery, and stretchy—the raw egg-white stage. At this stage of the month, there is more cervical mucus produced in hopes that some sperm will come your way.

MAUREEN

It wasn't until I was thirty-six and having a Pap test that I heard about cervical mucus. My doctor happened to mention I was ovulating as she looked up at my cervix. I asked how she knew, and she told me about the egg white consistency of the mucus and how they carry the sperm upward. It's insane to think it took thirty-six years to learn that information—until I remember sex was a bad word in our house. Imagine what my mother would have done if I'd asked about cervical mucus!

It's nice to know I'm not alone in my late-blooming status—Julie didn't know either. And I was on the phone recently with a good friend, a very successful Manhattan career woman. She's forty-one, not married, never had children. She had been suffering from a cold and, as we were on the phone, happened to sit down on her toilet to take a pee (oh, come on, we all do that!). She let out a shriek and exclaimed, "Oh my God, I have a cold in my vagina!" She was looking at a wad of good old phlegmy cervical mucus. I think she called it vagina snot. The result of her cold, she thought. I had to educate her. She was completely shocked. She had no idea . . . none. She told me she never understood that "whole ovulation thing." Most of us don't.

JULIE

Just to add on here—I didn't really get into the groove on cervical mucus until I met Maureen, which means after I had my two kids! How did I miss this? I mean I had noticed it, but never paid attention to the changes, never tried to figure it out. I wish I had taken the time to study it before.

Anyhow, since I can't take the Pill anymore because of the clotting problem I have, the monthly changes in this mucus now serve as a supplemental form of natural birth control for us. Just reverse the whole procedure and avoid your partner when the mucus is sperm-attractive and heralding the arrival of ovulation.

Multipurpose, that cervical mucus. The sooner you know about this, the better off you will be.

Fertile cervical mucus even looks special under a microscope. If you were to smear some cervical mucus on a glass slide during your most fertile time and pop it under the scope, it would look like frosty fern patterns. You don't have to be a scientist to see this. You could borrow a simple microscope and take a look if you really want to.

You should learn to read your cervical mucus to figure out when you are ovulating. It's easy, and you can chart it, if you like that kind of thing. Here's what you need to do: Once a day, wash your hands and check your mucus. Stick a finger into your vagina and pull out a bit of the stuff. If you can't find any, push your finger further up toward the cervix until you do. This works best if you are sitting down on the toilet. Look at this mucus under the light, checking its color and consistency. Try to pull it apart between your thumb and forefinger. Write down what you find on the calendar. When it gets clear, stretchy, and stringy between your fingers, you are producing mucus optimum for sperm to swim through. This means ovulation should occur in the next day or so. Go have sex with your partner. After ovulation, increased progesterone helps create mucus that is thick, sticky, and more opaque. There will also be less of it.

After a month or two, you should be able to immediately "read" your cervical mucus and know where you are in your cycle—even if your cycle is irregular. Do keep in mind a few things: Those antihistamines you take for allergies may dry up not only your sinuses, but also your cervial mucus, which might make it confusing when you test. There are theories out there that some women may ovulate twice during one cycle, so to be safe, if you find any mucus present, you need to consider ovulation is near or occurring. Finally, you can get pregnant during your period—if you have a short cycle that month, have sex toward the end of your period, and right before an early ovulation or if you have cervical mucus but can't tell because you are also bleeding. So many things to consider!

Basal Temperature and How to Take It

Want another easy ovulation predictor? Take your temperature every morning and chart it for a few months. Immediately following ovulation, your basal body temperature (BBT) can bounce up anywhere from 0.5 to 1.6 degrees Fahrenheit. This bounce isn't dramatic or long-lasting like a fever. If you were to chart it daily, it would be more like a spike. This spike occurs because releasing an egg through ovulation signals your body to produce more progesterone. An increase in progesterone increases the body temperature.

To detect this, you will need to buy a basal body temperature (BBT) thermometer, which measures smaller increments of temperature than a regular thermometer. These nifty thermometers are available at just about any drugstore. Take your BBT each morning before you even get out of bed. Chart your temperature for a few months to see if there's a pattern. If you are one of those lucky ones who ovulates the same time every month, you'll see a pattern you can actually use when planning conception. If you ovulate irregularly, you will see spikes at different times of the month.

What will you do with this information? Use it to plan intercourse. Women are the most fertile in the two to three days prior to ovulation (and the temperature spike). It can take a day or two after ovulation for the progesterone to build up enough to spike your body temperature. Remember, sperm can live a couple of days in cervical mucus, but the egg only has a twenty-four-hour window of opportunity. If the sperm show up ahead of time and hang out waiting for ovulation, all the better opportunity to meet up with that egg.

Combine the temperature chart with your cervical mucus chart, and you should really start to see a picture of what's happening with your body—and when you should be having baby-making sex!

MAUREEN

When I realized unprotected sex alone was not going to be enough to get me pregnant, I pulled out my tattered copy of *The Joy of Sex* to reread what I thought I already knew. Guess what? Even after conceiving and birthing one baby, I discovered just how much I had forgotten.

After studying the basal body temperature (BBT), I started taking my temperature every morning. My particular brand of thermometer beeped many times to let me know it had captured my temperature, and I could take it out of my mouth. My son, seven years old at the time, stumbled into my bed one morning bleary-eyed. "Mom, what is that loud, beeping alarm clock? It keeps waking me up." Quinn obviously has great hearing since he could hear those beeps coming down the hall all the way from my bedroom. I chuckled to myself that this was more like an *alarmed* clock—an alarmed biological clock.

Funny how that alarmed clock woke my son but never my husband.

Ovulation Predictor Kits

Don't want to chart your temperature? Think playing with your cervical mucus is icky? Okay, go to the drugstore and pick up an ovulation predictor kit. You don't need a prescription, you won't need a thermometer, and you won't need to touch your vagina. You'll find these kits on the same aisle as pregnancy tests, tampons, sanitary pads, and condoms. We'll warn you, however: They're pretty pricey, ranging from twenty to fifty-five dollars each.

These kits work by pinpointing a surge in luteinizing hormone (LH) produced by your body just prior to ovulation. They're actually pretty easy to use (you pee on the stick or pee in a cup and put the stick in) and promise to predict ovulation twenty-four to thirty-six hours before it happens, which is helpful for coordinating sex.

Here's the downside: While they measure LH, they don't tell you if you actually ovulate after a positive surge. They also don't tell you the quantity of the LH surge, either. Unfortunately, LH can surge with or *without* the actual release of an egg. Another problem—false-positive LH surges may occur before the real one. This can happen if your urine becomes too concentrated overnight, and you test with first urine (which some packages tell you to do). You also have to use these tests for several days in a row, depending on the length of your monthly cycle. Most kits have enough tests for five to nine days. But if your cycle is irregular, you'll actually have to buy a couple of kits to use over an even longer period of time. This adds up to *mucho* money. Our suggestion if you're irregular? Save your money and chart your temperature and cervical mucus first to see how that works.

By the way, if you have a fertility problem such as a blocked Fallopian tube, hormone imbalance, and so on, you may use these tests perfectly every month, have sex at the right time, and not become pregnant. If you monitor ovulation and it's regular, but you don't get pregnant, go see a fertility specialist. Something else is probably wrong.

Ultimately, you have to listen to your body. It will tell you when you are ovulating. It will give you all the signs. Just pay attention.

We learned about ovulation kits from a friend in California who said, "I went to the drugstore, bought this kit, peed on it, and it said I was ovulating. So I had sex with my husband and got pregnant." This is the same type of woman who comes out of the hospital after having a baby skinnier than when she got pregnant, claiming labor didn't hurt at all, and ready to have sex again with her husband as soon as possible. So, we should have known she was not like us.

Maureen went to the drugstore, and after refinancing her house to pay for a couple of these predictor tests, peed on them, had sex with Will at the right time, and waited. Nothing happened. She did this for a couple of months and then gave up, investing the money in Starbucks instead. Julie didn't even bother trying to use an ovulation predictor kit because her periods were so irregular.

This Is His Body

You live with it, but you don't know it. Sure, you're on very friendly terms with the penis, and while this is your guy's big player in the conception game, it has an astonishingly large support team. We'll meet all of them in a minute, but first let's highlight a couple of key players.

Like you, your guy has a pituitary gland, the brain's hormone control center. And like you, men also produce LH and FSH, which are important in the hormonal baby dance. His main male hormone, however, is testosterone. Testosterone is in charge of sperm production. Sperm is the male counterpart to your egg, necessary for conception to occur. Semen is the fluid in which sperm rides into your reproductive system. Semen is actually a combination of fluids from a couple different glands in your guy's body.

While most men have the ability to be fertile every day of their postpubescent lives, there are a few problems that can prevent them from fathering children. These include producing too few or no sperm, malfunctioning or misshapen sperm, blockage along the normal exit path sperm follows during ejaculation, and damage caused by disease.

This Is His Penis

The penis is a multitasking organ. The penis not only transports semen into a woman's vagina, but also is the path through which urine is eliminated. This operates with an on/off *SEX* switch. When the switch (your man) is turned on, the penis is erect and hard, full of blood (the erection) and ready to help make a baby. Urine cannot pass through the penis at this time. When the switch is off and there's no chance of sex occurring, the penis is soft. Urine can pass if he has to go to the bathroom.

There are three basic phases to a guy's baby-making process—get an erection, have an orgasm, and ejaculate semen into a woman's vagina. Surely, even if you have had sex with only your husband, it is no secret that all penises are *not* created equal. Some are big, some are small, some are thick, some are thin, some are circumcised, and some are not. No matter what they look like, unless there is some underlying plumbing problem, any penis can get the three main phases of this job done.

Maureen has a great analogy about the penis. It's like a puppy, always in need of a pat, always ready and willing to please, and more than happy to go out and play. Unfortunately, like a puppy, it can demand a lot of attention.

This Is His Urethra

The urethra is that skinny tube in the middle of the penis through which either urine or semen flows out. Actually, urine flows while semen sort of explodes out the urethra's opening at the tip of the penis, but that's all semantics.

These Are His Testicles

The testicles, also known as the testes, hang out below the penis and are often referred to as the "crown jewels" or more crudely as the "balls." Packaged together, the penis and testicles form the exterior male reproductive organs— what Julie's son Graham calls "the teapot."

These oval-shaped glands house both the testosterone production facility and sperm factory. Testosterone is the hormone largely responsible for a man's masculine characteristics and sex drive.

The sperm is produced in the microscopic seminiferous tubules inside the testicles, where they develop to near maturity before being passed along to the epididymis, a long, coiled tube at the back of the testicles.

If you were impressed that women are born with about two million eggs in their ovaries, you'll be blown away to discover that the testicles produce up to 200 million sperm every day. Boys develop sperm when they reach puberty and then produce it daily for the rest of their lives—meaning a guy is fertile every single day from adolescence on.

The testicles hang out in a skin pouch called the scrotum. The scrotum is like the temperature keeper, pulling the testicles (and thus sperm) closer to the body when it's too cold and letting them hang over to cool off in hot situations. A varicose vein in the testicle, called a varicocele, can cause problems by heating the testicles to a temperature that's not conducive to producing and maintaining healthy sperm.

JULIE

This reminds me of a joke my college roommate, Barb, once told in the dining hall back at Cornell University. Here it is.

> **QUESTION:** If you had a six-inch penis growing out of the middle of your forehead, how much of it would you see?
> **ANSWER:** None, because your balls would be in your eyes.

Barb would always demonstrate this joke using a banana and two oranges from the fruit bowl on the salad bar. It's one of the few I always remember, and it's good for a laugh. Try it.

This Is His Epididymis

The epididymis stores the young sperm cells. This ultrathin tube is tightly coiled, which is good because pulled straight it is about twenty feet long. Think of the epididymis as prep school for sperm. This is where sperm hone their swimming skills and fertilization abilities. Once they are capable (about fifteen

MAUREEN

I had a long and stressful labor with my son. I didn't know his gender, and I had been looking forward to that moment in my life when they would hold my baby up and say, "It's a . . . !"

After twenty-six grueling hours of labor, the baby was born only to be whisked away because he had ingested meconium and needed immediate attention. Nobody bothered to tell me if the baby was a he or a she. I missed that Hollywood movie moment—the sight of your little newborn baby being held up between your legs.

As I lay there, my husband went over to where the nurses were tending to the baby. All of sudden, I heard Will gasp, "Oh my God, look at those *cojones*!" That was the instant I knew I had a boy.

Of course, neither of us realized at the time that babies are born with swollen sex organs, so my husband was really proud. His little man had big balls.

It's still difficult for me to believe my body created a penis—not to mention *cojones*.

days), they are ready for sex to occur and ejaculation to happen. At that point, they rush out through the vas deferens like wild-eyed surfers in search of a wave of fluid on which to ride into the vagina.

The epididymis is not immune to problems. It can be infected or damaged by a disease called epididymitis.

This Is His Vas Deferens

Saying "vas deferens" always makes us feel like we are speaking with a foreign accent—sort of Arnold Schwarzenegger-ish. An easier, more descriptive name for the vas deferens is sperm ducts. There are two of these long (about fifteen inches), narrow tubes that carry sperm from the testicles to the seminal vesicles. Think of these as you do Fallopian tubes in a woman—highways transporting golden seed.

This Is His Prostate Gland

What? The prostate? What's the prostate doing in a section on reproduction? It surprised us, too, given the prostate gets more play today for the cancer that can occur there later in life. But here's what it's supposed to do before it enlarges later on and keeps your partner up all night peeing.

This little gland, when normal, is walnut-size and sits snugly around the junction of the vas deferens and urethra. The prostate also produces a thin, milky fluid that is part of the semen. This fluid nourishes the sperm. During ejaculation, this fluid joins the sperm and other fluids to create the resulting mix called semen.

This Is His Cowper's Gland

These are two tiny glands (about the size of peas) located just below the prostate and off the urethra. Cowper's glands produce a clear fluid that also nourishes the sperm and it helps neutralize the acidity of any urine that may remain in the urethra.

During ejaculation, this fluid joins the sperm and other fluids to create the resulting mix called semen. The fluid from the Cowper's gland, however, is the first out the gate. You would recognize this as the clear, slippery "pre-ejaculate" fluid that arrives first, neutralizing the acidity of the urethra and paving the way for the sperm. By the way, sometimes a few sperm could arrive in this pre-ejaculate fluid, too.

This Is His Seminal Vesicle

These look like little sacs tucked up around the back of the bladder. Their job? To produce a nutritive substance for sperm that makes up about 65 percent of the semen (seminal fluid). During ejaculation, this fluid joins the sperm and other fluids to create the resulting mix called semen.

What Happens Next

When the sperm-laden semen is ejaculated into a woman's vagina, it finds one of the following two things:

1. If she's ovulating, the vagina's a great place to be, full of sperm-friendly cervical mucus and a pathway to an open cervix.
2. If she's not ovulating, sperm find the vagina to be hostile territory laden with hazards like thick mucus they can't swim through and a

cervix that is shut tight. In this case, the sperm won't survive more than a few hours.

More on Sperm

Most women know that sperm look like little tadpoles—rounded bodies, long squiggly tails. Here are a few more compelling stats on the life and times of our fertilization friends.

- From start to finish, it takes about seventy-two days for primitive cells to form and evolve into mature sperm cells that are ready, willing, and hopefully able to penetrate an egg and cause fertilization.
- At any given time, there are about 700 million sperm stored in the epididymis and vas deferens.
- During ejaculation, 50 to 200 million sperm are in the semen mix.
- Only a small portion of all the sperm in semen survive long enough to make it to an egg in the Fallopian tube.
- Healthy sperm can live up to seventy-two hours in a friendly environment—warm, wet, and with the proper pH balance.
- Healthy sperm can live only a few hours in a hostile environment.
- Actual sperm (and testicular fluid) only make up about 5 percent of the semen mix. Seminal vesicle fluid accounts for 65 percent, and prostate gland fluid accounts for 30 percent.
- Once they find the egg, those weary sperm use the rest of their energy to beat against its outer layer in an effort to be the one to penetrate it and start conception. Perhaps this is where the cliché "beating one's head against the wall" comes from?

CHAPTER 6
BABY Production: The WEEKLY REPORT

Maureen

My cycles were so regular—twenty-eight days to the hour—I could rely on the rhythm method, which, given my birth control history, is lucky.

Since breast cancer runs in my family, doctors suggested I stay away from the Pill. I had an IUD expel itself the day I was supposed to take my Shakespeare final in college. (I'm one of the small percentage of women who has a uterus that screams "get the hell out of here" to foreign objects like IUDs.) Out went the IUD, and in went the diaphragm, which came with numerous bladder infections and one nasty kidney infection. Next—condoms. My partner hated them and so did I.

On to the infamous sponge—the form of birth control memorialized in that *Seinfeld* episode in which Elaine hoards sponges, wondering if potential suitors are "sponge-worthy." I am one of the rare women who is not sponge-worthy. I am allergic to the sponge, and ended up lying in my bathtub having convulsion-like shivers and hot flashes. I was told never to use them again.

After all these birth control fiascos, I ended up using the rhythm method. Once I figured out the basics of that, I'd go into hibernation on the week I was most fertile. My life revolved around my cycle.

When I got married, I turned to David Letterman as my birth control. The week I was most fertile, my husband would go to bed and I would hang out with the television. Honey, just going to watch a little Letterman. Who knew that watching Letterman wasted precious fertility time? Thanks, Dave!

Julie

I don't really remember when I got my period. I do remember my friend Mary telling me about tampons in junior high, so I must have been about thirteen or fourteen years old.

What I also remember is that my periods were never heavy, and I never had cramps. My cycle was never regular. I never went psycho or had crying jags brought on by PMS. I never experienced hormone upheaval each month like many of my girlfriends did, and I never thought this was a problem.

In retrospect, this probably was a problem—one that would manifest itself two decades later when I first tried to get pregnant. I now wonder if my periods never hit their groove because I started running track in seventh grade—the advent of Title IX, the debut of women's school sports, and right when my body crashed into puberty. I ran track all through junior high and high school and did cheerleading in the fall and winter. I was in excellent shape.

When I was nineteen and in college, I went to Planned Parenthood and got a prescription for the Pill. For the first time, I had a twenty-eight-day cycle. Wow. Sure made planning for my period that much easier. I stayed on the Pill for the next sixteen years.

Sixteen years spent with hormones suppressing my body's ability to ovulate. Hmm. Was that a problem? Doctors say no, but I wonder. Would I do it again? No. Not because I think the Pill messed up my cycles, but because I think my cycles were out of whack before and being on the Pill just masked all that. I might have realized that I had a problem sooner if I had noticed my period was irregular over those sixteen years.

Ten Monthly Mistakes Women Make

1. Women go on the Pill to regulate their cycles without first determining why they are irregular.
2. They disregard heavy periods.
3. They ignore breakthrough bleeding mid-month.
4. They consider light periods a blessing.
5. They have productive baby-making sex at the wrong times of their monthly cycles.
6. They think that every woman has a twenty-eight-day cycle and every woman ovulates on day fourteen.

7. They spend lots of time in hot tubs while trying to conceive.

8. They have sex every other day in an effort to get pregnant.

9. They do not take time to study their bodies' rhythms and compare that with what is considered "normal."

10. They dismiss a period that is shorter than twenty-four days or longer than thirty-five days apart.

Getting pregnant is more complicated than just sperm banging into an egg. It's actually a high drama with a possible fairy tale ending—all rolled into one incredible monthly feature presentation. Egg and Sperm are born, grow up, and leave home in search of true love. Although they've never met, they sense one day they will meet the One just for them. Sperm overcomes many obstacles to reach Egg, who is meandering along waiting for true love to change her destiny. Sometimes they pass each other like two ships in the night, and both die unrequited. When they do meet, it's love at first sight, and they join together, never to be parted. If you just insert the names Meg Ryan and Tom Hanks in place of Egg and Sperm, you've got a blockbuster romantic comedy.

Frankly, so many variables must coincide in such a synchronized fashion for conception to occur that it's amazing it happens at all. Then, for our bodies to successfully carry a pregnancy to term . . . well, to repeat ourselves, normal is a miracle.

The most common cause of infertility in about 60 percent of cases involves ovulation and sperm problems. During ovulation, a woman's brain, pituitary gland (the brain hormone control center), ovaries, and hormones all work together in a pretty intricate manner. Problems emerge when there's a hormone imbalance messing up communication among the brain, pituitary gland, and ovaries.

The most common red flags for ovulatory problems? A period lasting longer than six days or monthly cycles shorter than twenty-four days or longer than thirty-five days apart. Irregular and/or unpredictable monthly cycles, no periods (and thus no eggs waiting to be fertilized), odd breakthrough bleeding, minimal bleeding during a period, or very heavy periods should all trigger concern.

A Woman's Cycle

Obviously, having a regular period is pretty important for conception. If your monthly cycles are regular, it's easier to predict when ovulation will occur—and sex should take place. Understanding how your body works will also help you know what your doctor is up to with all the tests, drugs, and surgeries that infertility may involve.

Let's look at what happens to our bodies week by week through this cycle.

Week One: What Happens?

This is the week of our period—that time in our cycle when we bleed and perhaps experience cramps or feel a little bloated and tired. We may feel depressed if we start bleeding if we would rather be pregnant instead.

The first day of our period is considered Day 1 of our monthly cycle. While we tend to consider it the end of the process, our body considers it the beginning (kind of like spring cleaning each month we don't achieve pregnancy). Out with the old uterine lining, and in with the new. Time to dust off the eggs and get ready to start trying to make a baby again.

The blood we see each month is the uterine lining, also called the endometrium, leaving our bodies. This lining had the rich nutrients that would have nourished a fertilized egg had one made it to the uterus. If we get pregnant, the endometrium will also support the placenta. Most menstrual cycles last between four and five days, although some women can go as long as seven days and that is considered normal for them.

At this point, our progesterone and estrogen levels are low while the follicle-stimulating hormone (FSH) is rising. This is known as the preovulatory or follicular phase of our cycle—the time the egg (ovum) is maturing and getting ready for ovulation. During this point, while we finish bleeding, our pituitary gland is secreting lots of FSH, which works to stimulate the follicle to do its job. Think of the follicle as a bubble of fluid that envelopes and protects the maturing egg as it readies itself for ovulation. These growing follicles also produce the hormone

MAUREEN

On the occasions I would stay home from school with menstrual cramps, my father would invariably ask me what was wrong. I would tell him I had terrible cramps. His reply? "Yeah, I've been feeling the same way. I think there's a stomach virus going around." God bless him.

My mother would hand me a heating pad and tell me to go lie down. We didn't use Midol in my house. My sister's remedy for cramps? A few swigs of blackberry brandy. That actually worked.

estrogen. This estrogen, in turn, will begin to deliver a message to our uterus to begin creating a new lining.

Week Two: What Happens?

The egg in the follicle continues to mature. As we discussed in chapter 5, only one ovary produces the "winning" egg(s) each month, and the ovaries do not necessarily alternate. Fortunately, you have two ovaries. If something happens to one, you have another to pick up the slack.

The estrogen produced by the follicle signals the uterus to build up the endometrium, and it begins to put the brakes on FSH, which lets the cervix know it's time to start producing that cervical mucus. We will start to notice more mucus showing up in our panties, thinning out to egg white consistency the closer we get to ovulation.

As the week progresses, the egg ripens and makes its way toward the surface of our ovary. By the end of this week (if we operate on the "normal" twenty-eight-day cycle), the egg should have popped through the surface of the ovary waiting to be swept into the Fallopian tube by the fimbria—those things that look like little fingers at the top of the tubes. Drum roll, please. It's time for ovulation!

But since everyone is different, some of us will ovulate early—during the first part of this week. Those who ovulate "normally" (and who does, besides Maureen, that is?) will release their egg(s) on day fourteen—the last day of week two. And those who ovulate late will make it happen sometime the following week—or if under extreme stress like that caused by illness, moving, divorce, or the death of a loved one, even later. Watch the cervical mucus and chart, chart, chart.

The release of the egg from the ovary is prompted by a rush of estrogen that triggers a surge of luteinizing hormone (LH), which in turn stimulates enzymes to soften the surface of the ovary, allowing the follicle to rupture and the egg to "pop" out. This would be the ideal time in our cycles to use a home ovulation test to detect the LH surge—it will turn the test stick a bright color on the day when the LH is most concentrated in our urine.

This increase in estrogen in our bodies around the time of ovulation works to increase our sex drives. This is Mother Nature's way to be sure we have sex with someone (preferably our partner!) at this point of our cycles and with luck become pregnant. If we take the time to notice, along with increased cervical mucus, our breasts are usually fuller around ovulation, we feel sexier, and we are more eager to jump our spouses. This is the ideal time in our cycles to have sex, sex, sex. Once the egg is released, it has a twelve to twenty-four-hour window in which to meet and mate with the sperm.

Week Three: What Happens?

If you are charting your basal body temperature (BBT), sometime this week your temperature will spike. It always spikes after you've ovulated thanks to a surge in progesterone. As estrogen levels go down and progesterone levels go up, your temperature goes up. There's a lot of surging going on around here.

Again, what's important here? Charting both your mucus and your temperature. We aren't normally nags, but we do feel checking these two bodily functions out will help you immensely as you get to know what's normal for your body.

Meanwhile, inside our Fallopian tube this week, the egg is being moved south to the uterus by the cilia. To give perspective, an egg is the largest cell in our bodies, about the size of a teeny grain of sand, or a little speck of sugar, or the period at the end of a sentence. The egg may take this whole week to cruise the four to five inches of Fallopian tube. Well, to a speck of sugar, five inches is a long, long way.

During this post-ovulatory week, we move into what is called the luteal phase. This is the point between ovulation and the start of our periods when the uterine lining builds a lush, nourishing environment for the fertilized egg.

At this point in the week, luteinizing hormone stimulates the follicle that just released our egg last week to take on a new role—corpus luteum. Corpus luteum is the name given to the follicle after ovulation because it has turned yellow (corpus luteum is Latin for "yellow body"). The corpus luteum (aka post-ovulatory follicle) in turn begins producing progesterone, which it will secrete for up to two weeks after you ovulate.

Progesterone alerts the glands in our endometrium to create a nutrient-rich lining to nourish the fertilized egg when and if it arrives. Without nourishment upon arrival, the fertilized egg will not live. If your doctor thinks you have luteal phase defect, this means that the time between when you ovulate and menstruate is not long enough—or your hormone levels are not adequate enough—to create this nutritive lining onto which an egg can implant.

Progesterone also signals your ovaries not to ovulate again before you bleed, and it causes the cervical mucus to get thick and eventually disappear as you get closer to your cycle's end. In other words, you're closing up the fertilization factory this week, as most of us do . . . although it will be a little later for late ovulators.

Week Four: What Happens?

Now that the corpus luteum is manufacturing progesterone, the pituitary gland backs off its LH production. If you are not pregnant, this decrease in LH signals corpus luteum to begin breaking down. When this occurs, progesterone begins decreasing, as does our estrogen and our basal body temperature. At this point in our cycles, if we aren't pregnant, our BBT will continue to drop, and our periods will arrive soon afterward. But if we are pregnant, the BBT stays high. This sounds confusing, but if you are charting your cycle, this will make more sense.

So, if you're not pregnant, this can be hell week for some women as the symptoms of PMS (premenstrual syndrome) set in—usually seven to ten days prior to our period starting. PMS can manifest itself in painful, tender breasts, bloating, puffiness, and pimples. Oh, and need we mention the manic mood swings so many of us suffer?

JULIE

Here's my reproductive biology 101: Listen to your body. It may be trying to tell you something.

For years I was smug because I had light periods, no cramps, and no PMS. I couldn't understand my girlfriends who complained about all these monthly problems. My only problem was irregularity, which I solved by going on the Pill. While on the Pill, I didn't gain weight or suffer any other side effects other pals warned me about.

In retrospect, all of this could have been a sign to me that something in my body may have been out of balance. I say that because after having been pregnant five times, birthed and nursed two babies, my body suddenly jumped into a very regular cycle pattern. At the ripe age of forty-three, I finally had it all—tender breasts, cramps, hormonal shifts so bad I'd weep over a sappy commercial on TV one minute, and be ready to rip my hair out because the trash man left the recycling bin on the wrong side of the driveway the next. Every month on the eighteenth or nineteenth, my cervical mucus would get stretchy, and I'd get horny. On the twenty-ninth, thirtieth, or thirty-first, I'd get my period. After three decades of being irregular, I can now predict my cycle almost to the day every month.

How convenient. Just in time for menopause!

MAUREEN

Unlike Julie, after thirty years of being regular and counting the days every month, I am pleased to tell you that my periods have now gotten lighter. The cramps are gone, the mood swings history, and the bloating minimal. I can't even tell you what day I had my period this month. This is a milestone for me, given the fact that my life has revolved around my cycle. I have never not been aware of exactly when my period was due. I didn't have a clue this past month. It was so liberating. It made me realize just how consuming the entire thing has been throughout my life.

Although I'm bad at math, I have spent my life counting—always counting the days until my next period. What about getting pregnant again, you may ask? Please. We have a toddler and a preteen. Who has time for sex? I figure this method of birth control is good until Quinn goes to college.

Conclusion: Being a woman is just exhausting.

This is also hell week for those of us who wanted to get pregnant this cycle and feel our period coming on instead—such a bummer. Or for those of us who remain PMS-free and wonder or worry about whether we are pregnant. Or not. Or pregnant. Or not. It's insane.

The end of week four marks day twenty-eight—the last day of a "normal" cycle. This is when we "average" women will get cramps as we start our periods. Some doctors refer to menstruation as "progesterone-withdrawal bleeding" because that is exactly what is happening: Progesterone levels are dropping as the corpus luteum breaks up.

The minute your period arrives, you are back to day one of week one . . . and the whole process starts over again.

Week Five: What Happens?

When it comes to reproductive math, there are always some slight variables with each person. For those of us who don't have those nice, neat, normal twenty-eight-day cycles, we move into week five . . . and that's okay. For us, ovulation may occur in week three or even week four instead of on day fourteen. Following ovulation, our bodies still have all the same things to do to get us to conception or menstruation. By the way, you can have a twenty-eight-day cycle one month and a thirty-four-day cycle the next. However, extremely erratic periods can be signs of problems.

The fact that each woman's cycle can vary is why it is so important that we chart our cervical mucus and temperature in an effort to figure out what's going on inside our bodies. If ovulation is delayed for any reason—stress, poor diet, illness, or the fact that it's just normal for you to ovulate later—then this and maybe part of next week as well is your catch-up week.

Why Should We Care?

No two periods are the same—unless you're talking about the one at the end of a sentence. That's important to note. Understanding your particular cycle will help you and your doctor design a plan of attack on infertility: what tests to do and what drugs to prescribe. Here are some other things that studying your monthly cycle might showcase.

- Abnormalities in your uterus, Fallopian tubes, and ovaries
- Whether or not you are ovulating and/or ovulating adequately
- If you can't/don't ovulate adequately and therefore can't/won't build up a lush lining
- If your ovaries are out of eggs
- If your ovaries don't produce enough estrogen and therefore uterine lining may be too thin to support the fertilized egg
- Whether your hormones are screwed up—for example, maybe your pituitary gland is not producing that oh-so-important-for-egg-release spike in LH

When our girlfriend Leigh first decided to get serious about getting pregnant, a few questions concerning her monthly cycle troubled her OB/GYN and helped her begin to pinpoint possible fertility issues.

"My doctor told me to have sex on days ten, twelve, fourteen, sixteen, and eighteen if I wanted to get pregnant," says the Maryland-based mother of two. "I asked her what I should consider day one—the day I first started spotting or a few days later when my menstruation really got going. And she said, "Hmm, there may be a problem here."

Leigh had always assumed it was normal to spot for a few days before her period really kicked in. Apparently, it had been normal for her. After studying up on women's reproductive health, Leigh thinks the spotting may have been a sign of luteal phase defect—her body not spending enough time creating that lush endometrium before it began expelling it. Maybe there wasn't enough progesterone being produced. Leigh doesn't really know. All she does know is that with her OB/GYN's approval, three months later she was seeing a reproductive endocrinologist

MAUREEN

Before I studied all this, I had two monthly cycle breakdowns. One was for getting pregnant; one for not getting pregnant. These are not scientific. The Trying-Not-to-Get-Pregnant chart worked swell for me. The Trying-to-Get-Pregnant chart . . . well, let's just say I wish I'd had this book around back then.

Maureen's Old Let's-Not-Get-Pregnant Plan

WEEK ONE: Day one to seven: Have my period.

WEEK TWO: Day seven to ten: Lose bloat and have three days of free sex (yeah).

Day 10—14: Wear chastity belt because I'm off limits. Watch lots of David Letterman as birth control—as in "I'll come to bed after Letterman, honey."

WEEK THREE: Day fourteen to sixteen: Still off limits just to be safe.

Day 16—21: Have fun post-ovulation! Best days in the cycle. The only time in the month I feel like a whole human being. My clothes fit, I can think straight, and I'm not afraid I'll get pregnant. (Sounds like the life of a man every day.)

WEEK FOUR: Day twenty-one to twenty-seven: Start getting bloated and irritated. Head fog appears. Okay for sex, but who wants it when your stomach looks pregnant from the bloating.

Day 28: Ding! Period arrives. Cramps and the works. Oh, what fun. Let's start all over again.

Maureen's Old Trying-to-Get-Pregnant Chart

WEEK ONE: Day one to seven: Have sex. Husband very happy to oblige.

WEEK TWO: Day seven to fourteen: Have lots of sex. Constantly. Husband very happy to oblige.

WEEK THREE: Day fourteen to twenty-one: Keep having sex. Husband very happy to oblige.

WEEK FOUR: Day twenty-one to twenty-seven: Have sex only in the dark because I'm bloated. Husband still happy to oblige.

DAY 28: Buy pregnancy test and pray.

and getting the workup. Her period was the key that prompted Leigh's OB/GYN to waive her normal procedure: She sent Leigh to the RE after three months of unprotected sex, not her usual twelve-month wait. If you are aware of your cycle, you may help your doctors speed along your diagnosis and save precious time.

Your period might be wacky for a few months from stress or illness or when you first come off the Pill. Birth control pills work by actually controlling your fertility hormones, raising some while suppressing others or keeping them at a consistent level. When you stop taking them, your body might have trouble trying to do the work itself. It takes some women several cycles to get their hormones back in proper balance and their periods regular again. And because everybody is different, other women, like our girlfriend Ann-Marie, come off the Pill and get pregnant the following month with no problems.

When Do You Actually Conceive?

It's not when you think and certainly not during sex. If you have sex on Saturday night and ovulate Sunday morning, there's a good chance you are actually conceiving in the produce section of your local grocery store when you're shopping for dinner Sunday evening.

Here's the low-down: To get pregnant, you must have sex a few days before, during, or a day after ovulation. Sperm can live inside us for up to five days—providing the conditions are just right. If our ovulated eggs have a twelve to twenty-four-hour life span, then we could conceivably have sex five days before ovulation and get pregnant or maybe even the day after ovulation, although that is more iffy.

If you have sex near the time of ovulation, it stands to reason that you'll increase your chances of getting pregnant. Some doctors recommend days fourteen or fifteen of a twenty-eight-day cycle as the best days to have productive sex. But that's if you have a "normal" cycle. Who is normal? Remember, not all women ovulate within the normal ovulation window of their menstrual cycle.

As we mentioned before, "normal" fertile couples have a 25 percent chance of getting pregnant each month. So, using this statistic, you can figure that about 75 percent of those who have unprotected sex should get pregnant within one year. The theory with spending all this time learning about ovulation is that you can increase your chances of making a baby if you become so familiar with your cycle and the hormonal and physical changes that occur within your body each month that you can figure out exactly when you ovulate.

If you actually had a normal cycle and weren't fighting infertility, you could also use this information as a method of birth control. It's the old inverse theory. Don't want to get pregnant? Avoid your partner like the plague when you're ovulating. Of course, that's not our problem, is it? By the way, women can and sometimes do get pregnant if they have sex while having their periods. The key is connecting egg with sperm, and sometimes that happens even if they are menstruating—they ovulate early at the end of their periods, or they didn't lose all of the endometrium and if everything lines up just right, and there's a lining to which the egg can attach, they are preggers.

Here's some more basic fertility math that helps determine how women with a "normal" cycle can tell when they are ovulating and most fertile. Figure out when your next period is due to begin and count back twelve to sixteen days. This will give you a range of days when you will probably be ovulating—about day fourteen for all those twenty-eight-dayers out there. Or course, for this to work, you have to know how long your cycle usually lasts

Get the Juices Flowing

The best way to get pregnant is to have sex. Sounds simple enough, doesn't it? Except that we don't think women are having enough sex. In quizzing all our friends and most of our acquaintances (even those who have no trouble pro-creating), we have stumbled upon a startling trend: the lack-of-lovemaking. It seems many couples who should be boinking like bunnies are not having much sex—at all. Why? Too tired. Too stressed. Working too late. And these are the ones without kids! Those of us with little kids, well, forget it. We'll tell you straight up we're not having sex. Okay, maybe once or twice a month when we feel like we really need to do it just because. We're too exhausted otherwise.

So how much sex does or should the average child-free couple have? Who really knows? Sure, there are statistics out there—once a week, twice a week, twice a day. But what is the truth? That is the question. Our culture is overstressed and overworked. We highly doubt we have ever met a couple who really has sex the number of times a week they say they do.

Think about it. Who wants to admit they have sex only twice a month, maybe? That doesn't sound so good. But if we say we jump our husbands three nights a week, who can prove us wrong? No one. So we can get away with saying whatever we want.

When you are young, responsibility-free, and really frisky, you have sex constantly because you can. Then life starts to kick in: career pressures, family pressures, and relationship pressures. You get married, and life becomes more predictable. You take things (like your partner) for granted. You're too tired.

We've had doctors tell us about businesswomen with tight schedules and high-powered careers who have come into the office complaining they can't get pregnant. When quizzed about their sex lives, it turns out they were having sex only once or twice a month, usually *not* when they were ovulating. And they were surprised. They had thought they needed IVF *right now* when in actuality, they needed more time in bed with their husbands.

The point is that all of us have to make more time to have sex—those who want kids and those who have kids (and want to keep their spouses). Sex is fun, and sex is necessary if you want to get pregnant no matter how overworked, overstressed, and exhausted you are.

More Math

We've already established that the average "normal" couple with no fertility problems and who is not using birth control has about a 20 to 25 percent chance of getting pregnant in any given month. We've also established that women begin to lose fertility in their mid-thirties. Let's take a look—based on your age and optimum conditions—at how many opportunities you have left to conceive.

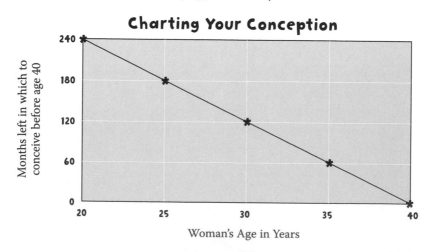

Charting Your Conception

Y-axis: Months left in which to conceive before age 40
X-axis: Woman's Age in Years

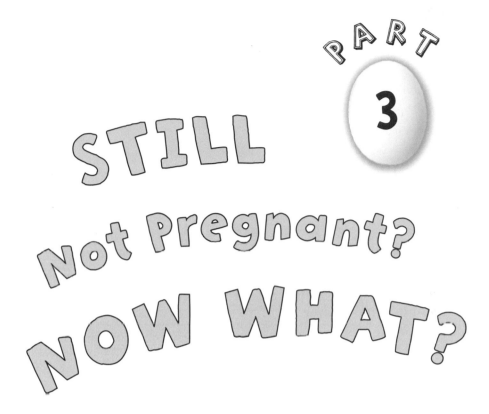

STILL Not Pregnant? NOW WHAT?

PART 3

Not everyone conceives according to plan. Now it's time to deal with your new reality. In addition to facing the fact that you really are having fertility issues, you will need to make some changes in your diet, in your exercise program, and maybe even in your attitude. You'll also need to find the right doctor and clinic, go through an alphabet soup of tests, and evaluate the impact of all this on your body and psyche as you try to complete your family.

Julie

Infertility is real-world angst in what becomes a surreal world. Infertility is more than just a medical experience. Its an all-consuming physical, emotional, social, and psychological journey. Its a messy combination of hope and heartache with a little pain and PMS tossed in. In addition, infertility treatment is expensive and time-consuming and has the potential to overwhelm you entirely.

And maybe, just maybe, at the end of it all, if you are lucky, you will walk out of the hospital with a precious, sweet baby.

Or maybe you won't.

You see, unlike a normal pregnancy with a nine-month timetable and a predetermined result, infertility sets its own pace dotted with surprises from beginning to end.

Even my doctors, all of whom I consider almost family at this point, didn't prepare me for everything I encountered along the way. It was my newfound friends who assured me that the overwhelming guilt I felt at not being able to conceive was normal and who helped me quit blaming myself for a medical condition over which I had no control. They told me the tests could take forever and some would hurt, and I would give more blood than I thought I even possessed. These women were also there to lament the hormone-induced weight gain I went through and to share tips on how to keep the romance alive when making love had been reduced to optimum days circled in red on the calendar.

A doctor can tell you to put your feet up after sex. A friend will get on the floor and show you how to do a gravity-defying headstand guaranteed to propel sperm to their destination without breaking your neck.

Thank God for girlfriends.

Maureen

One of the life lessons I've learned is that people don't tell the truth about their experiences. Childbirth is one of them. No one seemed to have had a difficult delivery, as I did with Quinn. It seems that all my friends labored for an hour, pushed for five minutes, and popped out their babies. Then, they left the hospital a size six. I, however, labored for twenty-six hours, pushed for six hours, and popped a blood vessel in my vocal cords, stripping me of my singing career. I left the hospital a size twelve or fourteen, depending on the designer. Postpartum, I had to have one surgery to repair my vocal cords and one to repair the damage to my vagina (that's another story). I felt so alone in my reality.

When I began to struggle with secondary infertility, I found the same cone of silence. No one wanted to give up too much information or tell the whole truth. One close friend who I knew had been through infertility was so cryptic, it was difficult to tell what she'd been through. Again, I felt alone in my reality. It wasn't until I met a fellow chick (Julie) that I was able to dish. Julie was the first person to be straight with me about infertility. This changed my entire experience. She understood the real deal, and she shared. The truth is not fun, but, as they say, it ultimately sets you free.

Reliving infertility has been cathartic for me. We've heard the same from many women and men we have interviewed. Courageous couples have chosen to relive their experiences for this book, to tell the whole truth, in the hopes that others will benefit from their pain and suffering and be inspired by their success stories.

CHAPTER 7
The REAL DEAL

Julie

Fertility, like most things in life, is all about balance. It wasn't until after my bout with infertility, however, that I finally realized the importance of balance in making your body work right.

For years, I lived a life out of whack. I was compulsive about work, obsessive about exercise, and addicted to travel and fun. No time for relaxing. Always on deadline. Rush, rush, rush.

For years, I didn't bother balancing my personal checkbook consistently, either. I did it once a year. Then it was a huge procedure. Took days with paper strewn all over the spare bedroom: logging checks into the computer, using a calculator and a pen, and referencing and cross-referencing. After discovering a costly mistake involving two large checks I didn't write in the register (oops), I got into the habit of balancing the checkbook every month.

Not balancing my daily life almost caused a costly mistake, too—the loss of my fertility. That's a bigger "oops" than a few measly misplaced dollars. I guess I could say I have no regrets about my past lifestyle, but only because I lucked out. I'm a midlife mom with redirected priorities who slid into the world of diapers, playgroups, and PTA just before the door slammed shut.

Maureen

I had always known I wanted a family, but I wanted lots of other things first. I never wanted to feel that children prevented me from doing and accomplishing the things I so desired in my life. My mother gave up a great deal of herself and her dreams for her children. I always appreciated it but felt bad because she never had a chance to really accomplish all the things she wanted.

So I never wanted to let go of me. After having Quinn, I chose to wait for my second, never thinking I wouldn't get what I wanted—how naive and pompous. I almost missed the boat, but fortunately for me, I grabbed control of the rudder, turned my ship around, and, by the grace of God, sailed it home, with my two children aboard.

I wouldn't call it lucky. I would call it being humbled, educated, and blessed.

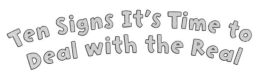

Ten Signs It's Time to Deal with the Real

1. You won't give up your gym membership and 15 percent body fat ratio, even to get pregnant.
2. A balanced diet means you try to hit all the food groups sometime during the week.
3. Breakfast is three cups of black coffee, lunch is a diet soda and a bag of chips, and dinner is a toss-up.
4. You're morbidly obese.
5. You don't want to get "fat."
6. You don't make enough money yet, are waiting to make partner next year, want the kitchen redone first, and really need to see Europe as a couple. Oh, and you're thirty-seven years old.
7. You haven't met Mr. Right yet.
8. You've been on the Pill for eighteen years and wonder if it's time to get off. (It is.)
9. You drink Red Bull all day and work out for two hours every night.
10. You tell everyone you want children, but secretly the thought of a big lifestyle change really scares you, so you keep putting it off.

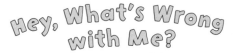

Hey, What's Wrong with Me?

Faulty fertility can be caused by everything from premature menopause to pollution, and from old eggs to slow sperm. But denial and self-sabotage are often the biggest challenges to overcome. Translation: Women can unwittingly sabotage their chances of getting pregnant and sustaining that pregnancy successfully.

Denial is quick to cure. Once you and your doctors determine your fertility problem(s), you simply come to grips quickly and completely educate yourself about everything. We tried to be one step ahead at all times—prepared with questions and knowledgeable (as best we could) about the procedures we might have to undergo. And don't be afraid to look stupid. Ask questions that you think are dumb. Deal with what is real—the Real Deal, as we like to call it. Handle infertility the way you would any large challenge—with your eyes wide open and your mind sharp. If you do, you're on the right path.

Denial is one thing; self-sabotage is another matter. Our pal Jenn, a thirty-seven-year-old orthodontist in Oklahoma, is engaged to be married in ten months and desperately wants children. She had been trying to conceive for seven months prior, hoping to get pregnant and deliver before the wedding so as not to be fat in her gown. (We know we have some shallow friends. Who doesn't?)

At our urging, Jenn went to a fertility specialist, where she discovered both her Fallopian tubes were totally blocked, glued together from a past infection. The fertility specialist told her IVF was her only option—the sooner the better, given her age. But with her wedding ten months away, Jenn couldn't stomach the idea of being "too pregnant" then and "ruining" the pictures. But waiting ten months put her closer to thirty-nine years old. We are sad to say Jenn opted to go with the formfitting dress and nice pictures and was unsuccessful with her first IVF. She is now forty and getting ready for IVF number two.

The real deal? Time is precious. Don't waste it. The biological clock waits for no one.

Facing the Fact

To steal a line from an old pop tune, "You can't always get want you want, but you get what you need." Or in many of our cases, we get what we deserve when it comes to our fertility quotient.

How so?

Well, we fill our prime procreation years with career-climbing, job-juggling, thrill-seeking, and serial dating. We tone our body fat away, eat crappy food, and get as few hours of sleep as possible. Some of us smoke, do illicit drugs occasionally, and/or drink more than we should. We're not really sure we want to change our lifestyles, but we do want kids . . . eventually. Then we wonder why we can't conceive on command when we finally settle down at thirty-six or thirty-seven years old. Because we feel entitled to be parents, we get angry when we realize it isn't happening as quickly as we'd like. This causes us to waste more precious time being pissed off, before we finally admit something might be wrong and seek some help.

What's all this got to with our fertility? A lot.

Faulty fertility is caused by a bevy of things, including irregularities in ovulation and menstruation. These irregularities increase with age, excess exercise, and weight that fluctuates more than the stock market, among other things. Stress also screws things up—excess stress has the ability to change hormone levels and cause irregular ovulation. High stress levels can also cause spasm of the Fallopian tubes and decreased sperm production. None of this is good for making a baby.

Yes, we've all heard this stuff, but we really haven't listened. It's difficult to live a balanced life, but when it comes to fertility and reproduction, it's more important than we ever thought.

We found an article in an October 2004 issue of *New York* magazine that blew us away. The cover pictured the silhouette of a very slender pregnant woman. The article was about women's obsession with being thin and pregnant—a toothpick with a basketball belly. After reading this, Maureen's comments were dead-on: "My God, have we as women lost touch with the idea of nurture?"

To successfully nurture a baby, women have got to get their priorities straight. It takes a great deal of selflessness to raise a child, starting with before they are even born. If staying thin is more important than getting pregnant or staying that way, perhaps you should reconsider. Women starving themselves before and during pregnancy, as well as overexercising those nine months away, is criminal. Regardless of scientific findings that attempt to deny this, we can't imagine there aren't some sort of repercussions. In fact, certain nutritional deficiencies in the mother do negatively affect the growing baby's brain development. These are things that show up down the road.

God created women's bodies to blossom and procreate. If we are choosing to go against that, perhaps we are not ready to nurture a new life. If we are not nurturing ourselves through nourishment of our bodies and souls, then how could we possibly nurture a new baby? How could our bodies be safe, warm havens for babies if we are abusing ourselves—and then we expect our bodies to perform on demand? It's selfish and self-centered.

Here's the real deal: You can't always get what you want, without paying some price.

Age Matters . . . Again

At the risk of sounding like broken records—particularly in light of all the media attention on midlife mommies and famous celebs getting knocked up in their late forties and fifties—there really is a prime time for getting pregnant. It's when we are young—the younger, the better.

For those of us who didn't get pregnant in our twenties, here's the deal. Women who get pregnant in their late thirties and forties run the risk of more complications like abruptio placentae, placenta previa, gestational diabetes, preterm delivery, and miscarriage. Older women also have more chances of having endometriosis and of delivering babies with genetic defects. But because we hear all the media stories about women in their late forties and even mid-fifties having babies via IVF, we think only about the positives, not the negatives.

A woman reaches her peak fertility sometime in her mid-twenties, when her chance of conceiving each month is about 25 percent. After that, the odds drop. By her mid-to-late thirties, a woman's chances of conceiving is about 30 percent less or 17.5 percent each month. By forty, the chances drop to a conception rate of about 12.5 percent per monthly cycle. Now, couple those odds with plummeting egg quality—important not only for "normal" conception, but also for any assisted reproductive technology like IVF, which depends on several good-quality eggs.

But it's not just your fertility you have to worry about as you age. Birth defects are also associated with older mothers. If you are twenty, the chance of having a baby with Down syndrome is about one in 1,667, and the chances of other birth defects are about one in 526. At age thirty-five, those chances increase to one in about 378 for Down syndrome and one in 192 for other birth defects or abnormalities. When you are forty, the chances are about one in 100 for Down syndrome and one in sixty-six for all other birth defects. Finally, at age forty-five, there is a one in thirty chance of having a Down's baby and a one in twenty chance of having a baby with any other birth defect.

It doesn't take a rocket scientist or even a good calculator to figure out the best odds.

To determine if you have a baby with Down syndrome or spina bifida or any of several other genetic abnormalities, your doctor will suggest that you undergo special tests called amniocentesis (amnio) or chorionic villus sampling (CVS). It should be noted, however, that CVS only checks for genetic problems, not neural tube defects.

An amnio is performed around week sixteen to eighteen and involves the longest needle you have undoubtedly ever seen inserted through your abdomen and into the amniotic sac around your baby. The fluid, which is actually your child's waste product and contains fetal cells, is withdrawn and sent to the lab to be tested for abnormal chromosomes. CVS is usually done sooner than an amnio, around week nine to twelve. The doctor inserts a tiny needle through your cervix in an effort to extract a bit of placenta for chromosomal testing. The same test can be done abdominally, which we personally think sounds safer, at eleven to fifteen weeks. By the way, both amnio and CVS tests run a slight risk of causing miscarriage.

Dads also bring some age-related issues to the table, according to various studies. We read one that concluded that children born to older dads (over age thirty) may have a higher risk of developing schizophrenia. Schizophrenics suffer paranoia, hear nonexistent voices, and are generally fearful. The first signs of schizophrenia show up at adolescence and early adulthood. The link was stronger in fathers with no family history of schizophrenia, and it remained important even after taking into account other factors that might increase the risk of schizophrenia. The researchers found that for every ten-year increase in paternal age, there was an almost 50 percent increased risk of schizophrenia in the children.

These are studies. Studies don't mean it *will* happen to you, but they do provide food for thought.

The real deal? Age matters.

Fat Cats and Skinny Minnies

Can you be too fat or too thin and have it affect your fertility? Yes to both. Infertility can be a result of a scale that tips too dramatically on either side of your ideal weight.

If You Are Too Fat

If you are overweight and facing fertility issues, extra poundage may be your greatest problem. Being too fat can affect the hormone signals to your ovaries.

Overweight women can also suffer increased insulin levels, which in turn can cause the ovaries to produce too much male hormones and stop releasing eggs. Women with polycystic ovary syndrome (PCOS) often have this problem and are often overweight. Obesity can also influence menstrual irregularity.

Sometimes, simply losing weight by dieting and exercising can balance the body and return fertility. "Miracles can happen," says Cheryl, a stay-at-home mother of daughter Ainsley. Cheryl and her husband did three years of fertility treatments before finding a doctor who focused on her weight.

"After all these years of trying to get pregnant and having a miscarriage, doing fertility drugs, and timing everything just right, we changed doctors," says thirty-six-year-old Cheryl. "My new doctor suggested, since I have PCOS, that I lose some weight. I took a six-month break from fertility treatment and did just that. I was one pound over my ideal weight when I found out I was pregnant."

If You're Too Thin

Maybe you can't be too rich, but you can be too thin, if you want to get pregnant, that is. While normal exercise won't affect most couples, extensive exercising can reduce sperm production in men and stop ovulation in women. Obviously, neither is too good for conception.

Exercise-obsessed women lower their levels of estrogen—the hormone that makes us female. Studies are finding that skinny women obsessed with low body fat are surrendering their periods, essentially tossing themselves into menopause, and losing a larger number of their eggs prematurely each month. (Those eggs are jumping ship. We can almost hear them screaming, "Hostile environment! Every egg for itself!"). This loss of precious eggs means a diminished ovarian reserve. Additionally, these estrogen-starved women place themselves at a higher risk for osteoporosis.

Even those who are not really underweight but have a low percentage of body fat can have menstrual irregularities. Olympic or competitive athletes are at extreme risk for messing up ovulation and suffering from infertility and so are women who run marathons and participate in triathlons.

Tell your doctor your exercise regimen—and don't lie. If you bike ten miles a day, run eight miles a day, take a spin class in the morning, and swim a mile every night, your exercise routine could be an infertility factor. We have a friend, a forty-year-old magazine editor in Chicago, who has been trying to get pregnant for two years. Rhea has been married for eight years, but spent the first six years convinced she and her husband were a great family with just her two stepdaughters visiting every other weekend. In the meantime, she and her husband participated in marathons and triathlons nationwide. It was their hobby. It was actually how they met—running together in San Francisco.

After two IVFs, Rhea has given up. "I'm not meant to be a mother, I guess," she told us.

Further discussion discovered she never bothered to quit exercising strenuously during the two years of fertility treatments. She didn't want to stop. She didn't think it mattered.

"I told my doctor I worked out, and he said it was no problem," she said.

Well, she didn't tell him she was a triathlete, although he frankly should have guessed something was up since she ripples with muscles. Every week during her treatment, Rhea would run up to 40 miles, bike between 50 and 100 miles, and swim 1 mile every other night. She was excessive.

"My eggs are shot. I guess I just have old, tired eggs," Rhea told us.

We don't know about that, but what we do know is that Rhea's doctor was diagnosing her without having all the facts. Had he done a thorough history on her, he would have known she and her husband were both exercise fiends. He could have explained to her the importance of estrogen, weight, and fat when it comes to fertility.

When we told Rhea she should have cut back her exercise regimen if she really wanted to get pregnant, she was stunned. It never occurred to her that she would have to change her lifestyle if she wanted to conceive. But it wouldn't have mattered. Rhea didn't want to stop working out—even to create a baby.

"Exercise is my life," she said. "I was fat as a kid. I'm not going back there."

Creating a life is about compromising our own lives. A baby's brain needs fat to develop. That should be enough right there to get you off the treadmill for a few minutes. Research shows that almost 75 percent of "normal" patients who were below their ideal body weight due to dieting and had trouble getting pregnant conceived spontaneously when they got their weight back in balance.

If you are doing fertility treatments, your figure is going to round out by virtue of the drug regimen alone. You will have big boobs, a big tummy, and big hips. Don't be afraid of them.

Weight gain can reverse the ovulatory defects of the ultrathin. A balanced diet under the supervision of a doctor is a good first step in fertility treatment. Do a friend a favor and share this information at the gym, especially with skinny

MAUREEN

Since I have a showbiz background, I always exercised a lot and ate light. When I got pregnant with Quinn, I swam miles every day, which I believe ultimately hindered my delivery. My muscles were just too tight, not allowing the elasticity necessary for delivery.

When I discovered I had secondary infertility, I finally realized the difference between being fertile and fat. I wasn't fat, I was trying to get back my fertility. I resigned myself that my body was going to be round. My husband didn't mind it either. Makes sense. If you look at the simple biology of procreation, padding in the appropriate areas signals fertility in a female and attracts males.

In order to plant a seed successfully, the soil must be plump and rich. If you would choose having a flat stomach and small boobs over having a baby, then you can put this book down right now. It's close to impossible to have both. More power to the women who can actually pull it off.

I have to question the sexuality of men attracted to women built like thirteen-year-old boys. I know a couple in which the woman looks like Peter Pan. She's skinny as a rail, no breasts, hips, or stomach to speak of. They had two children together, and I would often wonder what it was like for that man to make love to this skinny woman. What was he grabbing onto? Well, I guess ultimately it was someone else because he eventually left her for a young, skinny male.

minnies who have reproductive problems and no clue as to why. What good is it to be gym-trim, fat-free, and fertility impaired? We're pretty sure there's no free lunch out there. If you find one, however, and you're trying to get pregnant, we suggest you consider eating it.

The real deal? Get your weight to a healthy normal place and keep it there.

A Peek at Your Past

Let's do an informal background check. The way you live your life—what you eat, how you sleep, and who you sleep with—can all affect your fertility. Catching a sexually transmitted disease, particularly if it attacks your Fallopian tubes, can wreck your fertility. Doctors estimate that 20 percent of women who get pelvic inflammatory disease (PID), the by-product of sexually transmitted disease (STD), become infertile. Problem is, most of the people who get an

STD are in their teens and twenties—those years we are attracted to high-risk behavior like moths to a flame. Who thinks about STDs and their whole impact on future fertility when you are hot in the moment?

One of the most insidious and most common sexually transmitted diseases (STD) is chlamydia. Julie once had a doctor tell her he figured more than 50 percent of the single twentysomethings in Dallas had chlamydia. Most don't even know it because chlamydia causes very few symptoms, so it is often spread unwittingly. Forty percent of untreated chlamydial infections will result in PID. Gonorrhea, our country's second most common STD, can also cause PID and infertility.

So, let's see . . . one night of condom-free pleasure in your twenties versus thousands of dollars of fertility treatments in your thirties. This is a no-brainer and makes wearing a condom seem like less of a hassle. If your past is littered with multiple sex partners, few condoms, and never getting checked for STDs, share this with your doctor. It may be a crucial piece to your fertility puzzle.

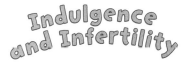

Indulgence and Infertility

We shouldn't drink or smoke too much. Who doesn't know this? Too much alcohol, caffeine, and tobacco has the potential to harm a woman's reproductive health. The same big three can damage sperm. That may be new information for you.

Consistently drinking too much alcohol can alter estrogen and progesterone levels and cause menstrual irregularities. Abusive drinking can result in ovulatory abnormalities and early menopause. Consuming too much caffeine has been associated with an increase in spontaneous abortions. Other studies indicate that women who drink at least 300 milligrams of caffeine daily, the amount found in two to three cups of coffee, may reduce their chances of becoming pregnant by about 25 percent. Women who smoke have much lower levels of estrogen during their monthly cycles. Smokers tend to enter menopause earlier than nonsmokers.

Is any of this really surprising? Of course not. So if you want to increase your chances of getting pregnant during fertility treatments, cut back on these indulgences drastically. We'll allow you one cup of coffee, tea, or cola a day, but we draw the line on the cigarettes. Ask your doctor about an occasional glass of wine or a beer. You may need it to survive the fertility shots.

Eating Disorders

Eating disorders like starve-yourself-skinny anorexia nervosa and its binge-and-purge cousin bulimia nervosa do not make baby making easier. Women with eating disorders usually have very irregular or no menstruation and/or impaired ovulation. Eating disorders can also alter endocrine function.

Any doctor worth his or her salt will be brutally honest about the importance of normal body weight and eating patterns on reproductive functions when a woman presents herself with ovulatory dysfunction and obvious eating disorders. But you can't depend on this. Anorexics, because of their extreme thinness, are easy to spot. Bulimics are trickier. Women who binge eat and then throw up to stay skinny may appear to be normal weight. So, embarrassed or in denial about their disease, they never tell their doctors—who, by the way, are not mind readers.

If you have an eating disorder, get help before you try to get pregnant. No sense wasting the time and money on infertility treatments, if you aren't going to eat properly. Besides, women who have eating disorders that continue should they get pregnant, often end up gaining less weight than they should, and have more complicated pregnancies, smaller babies, and problems breast-feeding, not to mention postpartum problems.

The real deal? Eat, eat right, get up to normal weight, and quit barfing if you want to have a baby.

Food for Thought

You need to feed your body to keep it healthy—protein, fat, carbs, fiber, and lots of water. You need to bypass the latest fad diet—particularly the high-protein ones—and concentrate on eating balanced meals. Why? Because recent research, like the stuff presented at the European Society of Human Reproduction and Embryology in 2004, shows that a moderately high-protein diet could reduce your chances of becoming pregnant.

Researchers in Colorado discovered that a diet containing 25 percent protein messed up the normal genetic imprinting pattern in early-stage mice embryos, as well as the embryos' implantation in the uteruses and the subsequent fetal development. Fifteen percent fewer embryos from mice on the high-protein diet developed further when implanted compared with the control group. At day fifteen, embryos that stuck it out were behind in development compared with the control group.

This investigation was done with mice, but the data may have implications for us. Until further research is done, we wouldn't eat more than 20 percent of our daily diet in protein if we're trying to conceive. In our own unscientific test, Maureen noticed that when she eats a diet rich in vegetables, fruits, grains, and olive oil, she seems to produce more cervical mucus. If she eats a great deal of meat, she produces less.

A diet rich in junk food or packed with preservatives is not good if you're trying to conceive because poor nutrition can be a cause of infertility and so can preservatives, additives, and all the other crap in our food. Diet sodas? Don't even go there with us.

If you insist on eating crap, at least take a multivitamin.

The real deal? Your mother was right; a balanced diet is important.

Environmental Issues

Pollution, pesticides, and pregnancy. Not a great combination. We know the planet is in an environmental mess. The air is dirty, the rain is full of acid, and the landfills are overflowing with nonbiodegradable junk. We often can't swim in the water or eat the mercury- and PCB-laced fish. It follows pollution would affect infertility. Doubt it? Consider some of the scary research.

Sperm counts have dropped by half in the past fifty years. Semen volume is also down compared with the past. Culprits include persistent environmental toxins like chemicals from ordinary plastics in your house and pesticides in your food.

Studies have also shown pesticides, plastics, and other environmental pollutants can bind to estrogen receptors in the body and depress both male and female fertility. Think about this the next time you go grocery shopping or hesitate at recycling.

Then there's noise—a biological stressor that affects the whole body, raises blood pressure, transforms blood chemistry, and impairs hearing. According to studies, continued, consistent exposure to noise pollution over seventy-five decibels (the sound of city traffic) can contribute to insomnia, anxiety, irritability, and emotional stress, as well as infertility.

There is an ever-increasing body of evidence that chemical pollutants can affect the gender of your baby. Consuming fish laden with polychlorinated biphenyl or PCB, the man-made chemicals formerly used as coolants and lubricants, may affect the gender of newborns, according to research outlined in a 2003 issue of the journal *Environmental Health: a Global Access Science Source.* Women exposed to PCBs are less likely to give birth to boys. Although no longer in use, PCBs are stored in the fatty tissues of fish. Investigators from the Harvard School of Public Health and the Wisconsin Department of Health and Family Services studied the PCB levels in the blood of parents living around the Great Lakes who ate large quantities of fish. Eating contaminated fish caught in the Great Lakes has been associated with lower birth weights, shortened menstrual cycles, and reduced fertility of women, as well as neurological disorders. By comparing the PCB levels of their volunteers with the genders of their children, they found a connection between high levels of PCBs in the blood of the women and reduced chances of bearing boys.

And did you hear the one about the fish in Texas that can't get pregnant because of the water? It's fascinating. There was a news blurb on Dallas TV a few years ago that caused Julie to pick up the phone immediately to call Maureen. It seems scientists were worried because fish in a local lake were not reproducing properly. Why? Too much residue from birth control pills in their water. Just by being in the water, this contraceptive was working on the fish.

How does that happen, you might ask? Well, if you take birth control pills, some of that chemical is released when you urinate. Where did you think that water went when you flushed the toilet? Now, add into that all the pills folks dump in the potty, as well as whatever else they are actually taking that they excrete, mix in a little pesticide runoff, and so on. Well, you get the picture. It's a wonder the fish survive at all. But what about us? Sure water is treated before it comes back into your house, so it is safe to drink. But it does make us wonder.

The real deal? We're not scientists, but there sure seems to be some connection here.

Unexplained Infertility

What you can do when they really don't know? If unexplained infertility is your diagnosis, it is what it is. But before you accept this, be sure your doctor has done everything possible to come to that conclusion.

"If some doc could just say 'Gail and Jim, here's why you can't get pregnant,' we would be disappointed, but we could then deal with it and move on," says our friend Jimmy, a West Coast insurance agent. "Maybe we'd be foster parents; maybe we would adopt. But without knowing if we can have our own children, the whole rest of our life is uncertain."

Unexplained infertility accounts for anywhere from less than 5 percent to as much as 20 percent of infertility cases. The wide range of difference is directly dependent on how much work and history on you your doctor has done. A truly committed physician will work until he or she exhausts every possibility before tossing in the towel with an unexplained infertility diagnosis.

So our first line of defense is to suggest you keep trying until you are convinced you have unexplained infertility. At that point, it is time to do some soul-searching. Are you ready, for example, to move on to adoption or the big high-tech guns like IVF?

The real deal? Make your doctor work, and be sure you have the right doctor working for you!

JULIE

I won't let my husband, Robert, or our son, Graham, wear those wrinkle-resistant, stain-repellent khakis or trousers. I would prefer no men wear them, but I can only control the clothing choices of two. My good girlfriend, who works for a major pants manufacturer, described all the chemicals involved in creating those easy-care bottoms. She won't let her own husband wear the pants her employer produces.

"It's like walking around all day in a wrinkle-free, chemical-dipped sack," she said.

Chemicals caressing your men's private parts. That's good enough for me to stick with old-fashion cotton and ironing. Or wrinkled. The wrinkled look is big in our house.

CHAPTER 8
INFERTILITY
IS a
TEAM SPORT

Maureen

I found my fertility doctor through the pages of my insurance book. I chose him because he was the closest to me and was affiliated with a prominent university.

Dr. Bronson was a character, wearing bow ties and long lab coats during each visit. He was very clinical and scientific in his approach. He did have a wonderful sense of humor, but was far from the touchy-feely, sensitive type. His mission was to get me pregnant, and I couldn't argue with that. His clinic was busy but ran on time. The waits were minimal, and his staff was warm. He had an extensive background in the field and really knew his stuff. His examination of me was extensive. He did not indulge me in my sadness during our failures but rather encouraged me to keep moving forward. This I liked.

His clinical approach worked for me. It kept me focused and forced me not to dwell. His dedication to his patients and to his work was tenfold. But he was a doctor, not God—something I always remembered.

Julie

My sister-in-law recommended my reproductive endocrinologist, and our experience with him was incredible. I can't say enough good things about Dr. Cohen—or the OB/GYN to whom he subsequently referred me. This doctor was not only competent, well-educated, and successful, but also compassionate, kind, and respectful. It's too bad we can't clone him . . . although with technology now, it's probably not such a stretch.

Anyhow, he also had a great staff and supportive office environment. They made sure I understood everything going on right from the start. Before my first appointment, they provided me with a booklet of general information on the clinic, which explained their goals and objectives; procedures and protocols; a listing of their staff, office, and phone hours; and their financial and insurance policies. More importantly, they seemed attuned to the emotional needs of couples on the baby quest. They asked that couples not bring any other children to the office. They kept boxes of tissues in all the rooms. They encouraged you to cry and didn't make you feel stupid or lousy when you actually did. Sometimes, they cried with you.

My husband even enjoyed coming with me to the clinic. They encouraged us to ask questions, never kept us waiting long, and always spent plenty of time with us. We felt as if everyone really cared about us. Dr. Cohen discussed all the procedures and formulated a plan with us. We always felt as if we were in control, which was always important to me, albeit guided by someone with credentials, certifications, expertise, and track record.

Ten Unscientific Signs of a Good Clinic

1. It has top notch doctors who have appropriate board credentials, membership to medical societies, and hospital privileges.
2. It is open on the weekends and willing to stay open late or open early if that works best with your body.
3. It has a compassionate staff.
4. It does not allow children and babies in the waiting room.
5. It keeps plenty of tissues in convenient places.
6. It makes an effort to know and remember you and your partner's names.
7. It updates the sexy magazines in the men's bathroom (deposit room) occasionally so that they don't look so bedraggled and "used."
8. It doesn't reveal personal information when doctors or staff leave messages at your home or office.
9. It is discreet and understanding when accepting your partner's "deposits."
10. It has someone to hold your hand, whisper a prayer, or give a thumbs-up when you are undergoing procedures . . . just so you know they understand.

"Oh my God, where do I begin?"

While there is no statistical data to prove we're right, we think this is the universal first question asked aloud by all of us who have decided to seek help in the baby-making process. Figuring out where to start can be daunting, but facing infertility is all about managing your own care, doing more research than a Ph.D. candidate, and surrounding yourself with the right people.

Getting in the Game: Team Building

Think of your infertility as a big sports event—your own personal Super Bowl with you starring as the quarterback. Your goal is to create a family. The first thing you need is a team to help you attain that goal—a team that includes your partner and medical staff. You also need a great coach, your doctor, to help create a winning game plan. Finally, you need cheerleaders—friends and/or family members you can count on for support.

Got your head in the game? Good. Let's go.

Taking Charge

Consider yourself the captain of the team, captain of your destiny, quarterback in the fertility finals, coordinator of your future family.

Your partner, while involved, will most likely defer to your plans. We women have to do most of the work here—from coordinating the team at the start to physically birthing the child at the end. Frankly, it surprises us how much of this the women actually shoulder.

When it comes to making babies, the woman works closely with the coach, calls the plays, and synchronizes her team. Unless your husband has a sperm problem or physical defect that will need to be corrected by surgery (more on that later), *your* body will be the physical testing ground. *Your* emotions are the ones that get to run haywire. *You* get to ride the hormonal roller coaster, gain weight, get shots, endure surgeries, and travel to and from the doctor's office so often you'll be tempted to ask about a mileage rewards program.

You will probably need a playbook, so buy a loose-leaf binder in which to keep all the information you are going to gather during this process.

Finding the right fertility specialist (your coach) is one of the most difficult and most important things infertile couples do. To start, you need to know what type of doctor treats infertility so that you don't waste precious months in the wrong place. A general practitioner or family doctor may be where you start, but it definitely is not where you should end up.

Finding a Doctor

Your doctor is your coach. This person creates the offensive, comes up with the game plan—with your input, of course—and maps out strategies. During infertility treatment, you will see this person and his staff as much or more than you see your friends. The relationship is intense.

DEFINITIONS

OB/GYN: Obstetrician-gynecologist: A doctor who specializes treating female diseases, caring for pregnant women, and delivering babies.

Reproductive endocrinologist: In addition to their OB/GYN training, these doctors specialize in treating female hormonal disorders.

General practitioner: This is your family doctor.

Urologist: The guy's version of a gyn doctor, the urologist specializes in the kidneys, bladder, and male reproductive organs.

A Gynecologist Is Not an Infertility Expert

Women who are having problems getting pregnant usually start off talking to their OB/GYN doctors. This is because for many the OB/GYN is the primary care doctor and specializes in treating women's diseases.

The biggest mistake many women initially make—including us—is to think a gynecologist can treat infertility. This can rank as a major oops and a huge waste of precious time. While in general, these doctors can do the basics in fertility workups—pelvic exams, tracking basal body temperature charts, checking baseline hormone levels, diagnostic laparoscopies—most are not trained as infertility specialists. Many, however, do like to dabble in it, to the detriment of your progress. Some will even tell you that they have "learned on the job" by helping other patients get pregnant. *Do not buy this. Treating infertility is a science, not a sideline.*

This is also no time for misplaced loyalty. You can love your gyn doctor and still be a good person if you get another opinion on your fertility. You are not being unfair or disloyal to your regular doctor. In fact, they should encourage you to seek another opinion. We have friends who stuck with their OB/GYN doctors for years while trying to get pregnant, or their husbands who stuck with their urologists. They went through tests, treatments, and tons of money, but still didn't get pregnant. It wasn't because these doctors weren't good in their particular specialty—it's just that they didn't particularly specialize in infertility.

When you don't get pregnant right away, you'll likely go into denial and assume that it will happen next month. But within two or three months, you no doubt ask your gynecologist what could be going wrong.

Most OB/GYNs will get right to work on basic fertility testing and then move you and your files to a specialist. This is what you want them to do. However, some OB/GYNs will continue to try to treat you past the basics. This is not good. Women can waste precious time in the wrong places because they don't know any better or figure their gyn doctor knows all about infertility, too. But sometimes they don't.

JULIE

When I initially expressed my infertility fears to my former gynecologist, he put me on Clomid immediately, without even testing me. "Let's try this," he said, and off I went to the pharmacy to fill the prescription.

I trusted him. I had been going to this doctor for several years and had good experiences with him as a gynecologist, so I figured he knew what he was doing. After three months on Clomid with no results, no mid-month consultations, no pelvic exams or ultrasound each cycle to determine if there were any ovarian or uterine abnormalities, and no follow-up by this gynecologist, a friend asked me why I wasn't seeing a fertility specialist.

Specialist? I thought I was! Who knew?

So I changed doctors and went to a reproductive endocrinologist. When he did my workup, we discovered that, for whatever reason, Clomid actually acts like birth control for me. There was no way I would ever get pregnant while taking Clomid. I sure wasn't expecting a fertility drug to prevent me from getting pregnant!

Needless to say, I quit going to that gynecologist and had my files sent to another—an OB/GYN recommended by my fertility doctor, an OB/GYN who specialized in high-risk pregnancies and left infertility to the experts, as it should be.

MAUREEN

My California gynecologist had a policy that she wouldn't refer you to a specialist until you had suffered three miscarriages. She felt after three, "something must be wrong." As far as I was concerned, after one miscarriage in a thirtysomething-year-old woman, something *can* be wrong, and a specialist should be called immediately.

At my age, I didn't have time to kill (no pun intended) messing around having three miscarriages. They should have at the very least started working with me after my second miscarriage. To me, this was sadistic and unacceptable behavior.

Gynecologists should be more attuned to fertility issues and more willing to pass patients on to the experts in that field. Period.

"It is worse than ever with OB/GYNs keeping infertility patients too long," says a Southwest fertility specialist we'll call Dr. A. for Anonymous. "They need to realize and accept what they don't know and send these women to us sooner rather than later. Let us reproductive endocrinologists do our job—and then we'll get these women back to them as soon as possible for them to do their OB work. These doctors don't realize the damage they are doing and the time they are wasting for these poor women. They'll put a woman on Clomid for two years before she finally comes to us, and when we get her, thanks to the overuse of Clomid by her gynecologist, her uterus is shrunk to the size of our thumb. We then have to pump her full of estrogen just to get her back to square one. It's a shame. A lot of women just don't know any better, but the doctors do."

We both spent way too long with our gyn doctors before we found out we needed fertility experts. We aren't out to ruffle medical feathers, but to alert our sisters. Our stories are not unique, and it's difficult not to feel bitter when you learn the hard way that you have wasted precious time. Like most of you, when we started this journey, we didn't know what questions to ask or the times to push for more information.

Remember, you are the quarterback. The quarterback never goes into the game without understanding the play or what the coach is doing.

All Docs Are Not Created Equal

General consensus here is that depending solely on a gynecologist to help get you pregnant—unless he's your husband and actually having sex with you—is a big, fat, time-wasting boo-boo. While most medical professionals are great, not all accept their limits or recognize when a problem is beyond their scope of knowledge. Having the words "fertility specialist" under a name in the phone book or taking one postgraduate course in infertility does not make a fertility specialist.

Who You Gonna Call?

If you are experiencing a problem getting pregnant, have discussed this with your gyn doctor, and are still child-free, it's time to run, not walk, to a reproductive endocrinologist.

Let's look at the difference.

Gynecologist: Gyn docs, like all doctors with an M.D. following their names, have completed four years of medical school. After this, the student does an internship, choosing to either stay in a specific field of medicine or to do a rotating internship that introduces him or her to a variety of medical fields. If the doctor then decides to specialize in a specific field like obstetrics and gynecology, he or she completes a residency program with a few months dedicated to the intricate aspects that contribute to female and male infertility.

To become board certified in obstetrics and gynecology, the doctor must graduate from college and medical school and complete a four-year residency training in OB/GYN. In addition, he or she must pass a written examination in OB/GYN, complete a two-year practice experience, and pass an oral examination in OB/GYN.

Reproductive Endocrinologist: Doctors who are board-certified in reproductive endocrinology must complete all the requirements for board certification in OB/GYN. They also have to complete a two-year fellowship in reproductive endocrinology and pass a written and oral exam on the topic. When they complete everything, they are considered board certified. Doctors who have done everything except take the oral examination and who are still in their practice experience are considered "board eligible" in reproductive endocrinology.

The Other Guys

As you begin your fertility workups, your doctor may refer your partner to yet another doctor—one who specializes in male body parts. Here's who they are.

Urologist: These doctors have completed an additional three-year residency training in evaluating and treating kidneys, urinary tracts, bladders, and male reproductive organs as well as a minimum of two years' training in general surgery. To become board certified, these doctors must practice for at least eighteen months, including a year of urological surgery. When it comes to fertility issues, urologists deal with the wannabe dads, checking out the penis and related parts, doing semen analysis, checking for varicose veins in the scrotum, and checking the sperm quality.

Andrologist: The most highly qualified physicians to deal with the hormonal aspect of male infertility, andrologists can almost be considered scientists rather than doctors. You rarely see them as they spend most of their time working in the lab, usually with sperm. In addition to studying all the stuff a urologist has to know, andrologists also complete an additional two-year fellowship in andrology and have to pass an examination to become board certified.

Point to Ponder

If a gynecologist has a few months educational experience in infertility and a reproductive endocrinologist has three years intensive training, who do you want helping you? It's a no-brainer, isn't it? You want the one who has the most knowledge and experience of helping women get pregnant.

So don't let any gynecologist practice his or her infertility techniques on you. Let him or her go take advanced medical classes and become board certified. You immediately get yourself to a reproductive endocrinologist, preferably board certified, who is current on all advancements in this rapidly expanding industry.

Hiring Your Help

We want the best—best haircut, best education, best wine with dinner, and best infertility specialist. If we're playing a game, we want to win. We want the coach everyone knows can get the job done.

Common sense tells us that 50 percent of the doctors out there graduated in the bottom halves of their classes. Call us crazy, but we don't want the guy who barely scraped by in med school. We want that gentle, caring Marcus Welby type with good study skills, good experience, and a global perspective. The doctor who keeps abreast on what's new. Hey, if they like to keep medical journals as bedside reading, all the better. We don't care if they're male or female, although that makes a difference to some women.

We approach our medical team the way we do just about everything from buying a dishwasher to a digital camera to a car—research the heck out of it. So should you. Ask your doctors, their nurses, and your friends who they suggest and why. Read those "Top Doctor" stories in the city magazines. (Julie even reads the ones that aren't in her city!) Look potential doctors up on the Internet, and check out the diplomas hanging on their walls. Ask lots and lots of questions.

When our friend Leigh decided to move immediately to IVF after suffering miserably through nine months on a variety of fertility drugs, she also decided to find the clinic with the best national success rate and go there. "I figured if I had to go through such drug-induced misery, I at least wanted all the best resources behind me. I wanted to maximize all my chances into one month. Put all my eggs in one basket, so to speak. In making this decision, I went against the advice of two very respected reproductive endocrinologists who wanted me to try a bunch of other things first—things that my insurance would cover. I didn't listen. I went to the clinic with the best success rate—and got pregnant with our twins on my first IVF."

While Leigh opted to go straight to one of this industry's top shops with great results, not all women think bigger and "best" is better.

Our friend Sydney went to *the* top Manhattan medical center and *the* top doctor in the world—the biggest and the best! Dr. Big (as he shall be known) helped Sydney achieve a pregnancy through blastocyst (her hubby's sperm couldn't swim worth a darn and had to be injected directly into the egg) and IVF. Needless to say, our pal was overjoyed at her good fortune and happy with her caring doctor.

When Sydney returned a few years later to try to provide her daughter with a sibling, she found a different situation. Dr. Big had been written up in so many magazines and was so in demand that the kind doctor she had known had become an arrogant sot! The cozy waiting room and comforting staff had changed. Now in the mornings, she joined as many as seventy women waiting to see this doctor for a "miracle cure" to their infertility. Sometimes Sydney sat in this waiting room for five hours before she saw the doctor. (This is beyond rude. We start charging our hourly rate if we wait this long.)

After six cycles and hundreds of thousands of dollars spent on more "experimental" procedures (she never asked exactly what he was doing, so shame on her for simply trusting him), she left his practice for another doctor. After another blastocyst procedure and IVF, she birthed a son. By the way, her second doctor was not listed in any magazine as the best, but he did get results.

The moral of Sydney's story? The biggest and best may not be right for you. Trust your instincts with this one. Don't just stay because your doctor is considered the greatest because if he's not there for you, all of his greatness is worth nothing to you.

The bottom line is that we've learned to take charge of our health care. You should, too. You wouldn't buy a car without asking questions, would you? Just curious.

When looking for an infertility specialist, a good place to check first is with your insurance. If your insurance dictates which doctors you can see, then the choices are limited already, and you'll know where to start. If you have a PPO that pays a percentage of the cost of doctors out-of-network or good old-fashioned insurance that doesn't dictate a doctor, you will have more flexibility.

If you have an HMO or PPO, don't panic if your insurance company representative can't find any reproductive endocrinologists in their list of approved doctors. Sometimes they don't break them out like that—they just lump them together with gynecologists in their lists. If that's the case, try asking your regular OB/GYN for a list of reproductive endocrinologists he or she knows or can recommend. Every OB/GYN will know at least one they can suggest. You can also check the phone book, call your local department of health, or contact local hospitals.

One of the best ways to find a doctor is to ask friends, colleagues, and family members who have gone through infertility themselves. They will know who has the best track record, nicest staff, and latest technology.

Nurses are another great source. All nurses, whether they work in the emergency room or the delivery room, know which doctors are good, which ones are bad, which ones wash their hands each time they visit a patient, and which ones eat garlic for lunch. You know what we mean. Collect all the names you can find, then check with your insurance company for those specific doctors.

You can also use the online search engines. RESOLVE, a nationwide support group for couples having problems trying to conceive, and will provide a list of all the fertility specialists in your state if you are a member. These lists also feature some information on each doctor's credentials, so you can see how much training each doctor has had. The fee to join RESOLVE is nominal.

Experience Counts

We cannot stress enough how important it is to find a doctor with a broad spectrum of experience. Julie's doctor was a board-certified reproductive endocrinologist originally from South Africa who went to school in Capetown, Rhodesia, as well as London. He has worked and taught extensively all over the world, including the University of Tennessee, Mt. Sinai Medical Center in Cleveland, and the University of Texas Southwest Medical School in Dallas. He attends global conferences and keeps in touch with other doctors around the world, even though his clinic is located in Dallas. This gives him access to vast amounts of knowledge, insight into what other doctors outside the Dallas Metroplex are doing and succeeding at, and new technologies that are working even though they are not part of the typical protocol.

You want a doctor with credentials and experiences—not just credentials and not just experience. You want someone who is either aware of or open to listening about the latest developments in fertility studies. You want someone who leaves town occasionally to meet and share experiences with other doctors at conferences. This is how he or she will discover what is going on in the fertility world outside their little corner of it. This is where your doctor might discover other reproductive endocrinologists working off experiences (theirs and others), helping hundreds of women conceive by doing things they hadn't thought of or hadn't read about in scientific journals. A doctor who did it all in the same place—went to college, medical school, and did his or her residency in the same city, then stayed there to practice may not have been exposed to a wide variety of experiences.

A doctor who does only research offers one perspective. One who only sees patients has another. A reproductive endocrinologist who only teaches has yet another. A doctor who does it all brings more to the table. You can check out doctors in the *Directory of Medical Specialists*, published by Who's Who and available at most public libraries. Hit the computer to check a physician's credentials on the Internet.

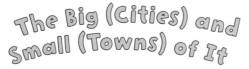

The Big (Cities) and Small (Towns) of It

We live near big cities—Dallas and New York. Big cities offer more options simply because of their size. This makes it easier to find a great doctor who has compassion and credentials. But not all women have those options. Some live in small towns in remote or rural areas. The nearest specialist might be two or three hours away, and there may only be one choice. In these situations, we must work with what we have and create an environment that works for us.

If you're in this situation, determine how far you can or are willing to travel because fighting infertility means frequent trips to the doctor for tests, shots, blood work, ultrasounds, and so on. Once you find a specialist you like, you might ask how to coordinate with your local doctors, labs, and pharmacy to administer shots, compound (physically make) special drugs, or help with the easy-to-monitor procedures. This may help eliminate travel time, stress, and strain on the pocketbook.

Clinically Speaking . . . Now What?

Once you find a doctor, make an appointment. These folks are busy with the current boom in baby making, so you may have to wait a few weeks to get in. That's fine. It will give you time to research the doctor further and get your medical records shipped from your OB/GYN over to his office.

Ask your gynecologist to send all the test results you have had to the specialist. Call to be sure they have arrived before your appointment. If a hysterosalpingogram has been done, call the X-ray department or radiologist's office directly for the X-ray films and go pick them up. A written summary report of X-ray or lab findings is not as helpful as the real thing. Take them to the appointment with you, so the doctor can review them with you there.

When you make an appointment, ask about fees and insurance coverage. You can also ask about the doctor's training and success rate. When our friend Louise called to make her appointment at the clinic, she actually asked the receptionist which of the doctors was the nicest. "Without hesitating, she told me they both were very nice and well liked by their patients," says Louise. "I could tell by her tone that she meant it and wasn't forced to say that, and it gave me more hope and confidence when my appointment did arrive—and she was right!"

While you are on the phone, ask about the office policy concerning children. Julie's doctor asked women who had other children not to bring them to the clinic out of respect for patients who were still trying. We never realized how important that small gesture was until we compared our own clinic notes. One of the nurses at a clinic Maureen attended was pregnant while she took blood and assessed other patients. Now, you can't begrudge this woman her pregnancy, but as a patient trying to conceive, it's frustrating to watch another woman's belly swell while yours isn't. It's emotionally draining. So, ask what, if any, policy your clinic has about small children in the waiting room.

Also quiz them about messages. When Julie's clinic had to leave messages for her, whether at home or the office, they never identified themselves as part of the fertility clinic. This is great—especially if you haven't shared your baby-making story with your coworkers. You may not want your secretary or office mate to take a message from "Rosemary at the fertility clinic" calling to tell you, "Your FSH level is X, and your progesterone level is Y. Oh, and by the way, your husband's sperm looks real good. Call us!"

To avoid embarrassing situations or having to share your situation with people not on the holiday card list, ask how the clinic will communicate with you. Establish your own ground rules. Provide specific numbers. If you want them to call you only on your cell phone or at home, tell them. Help them help you.

What Do You Mean You're Closed on the Weekends?

It's also important to ask about the clinic's days and hours of operation up front. This is a biggie. This is so huge, you should probably underline it.

Here's why: Women don't ovulate only between 9:00 A.M. and 5:00 P.M. Monday through Friday. We ovulate at different times during the month, and that time may change from month to month, so we need a fertility clinic that responds to those needs. Many fertility procedures, shots, and surgeries depend on precise timing with your cycle. What good is a clinic that is closed on the weekend if you happen to ovulate on Saturday or Sunday?

"I've seen patients who, before they came to me, had cycles canceled because the fertility office they were going to was closed on the weekends," says Dr. Cohen, whose office is available 24/7 for his patients. "That is not something a fertility office does. If you are really treating infertility, you don't close on the weekends. Period."

Now you can see why it's important to ask this question.

Here's what you want: a clinic that is open when you're ovulating, need to get a shot, or need to do a procedure at a specific point in your cycle. You want a doctor and clinic with flexibility, who will be there when you need them—depending on what your body is up to that month. They should be willing to

MAUREEN

One month when we were doing an insemination, I ovulated on a Sunday. Unfortunately, the clinic was closed on Sundays, which meant I had to push this insemination to Monday. Huge issue for me, since timing is everything in this conception game. However, the rules of the clinic bound my doctor to this calendar.

When I brought it up, the nurse told me, "Don't worry, it'll be fine. There's always a little window of opportunity." So I went on Monday, had the insemination a day late, and didn't get pregnant that month. Does it really matter if you don't hit the day exactly? I know this is not an exact science; I would have been happier with the result if we had done the insemination on Sunday. Then there wouldn't be any doubt in the back of my mind.

I want a doctor who will fight for me and tell me we will have success, then try everything possible to help me succeed. I hate that sense of "what if?" What if we'd tried X? What if I'd done more research? What if the clinic had been open on Sunday?

The only way you will eliminate the "what-ifs" is by taking charge of your infertility.

open early, stay late, and come in on the weekend if that is what it takes. (And that *is* what it takes.)

Find out if procedures like inseminations can be done on weekends if needed. Be sure your clinic can serve you before you sign up. Clinics with a 24/7 mentality really do exist, so don't be deterred by doctors who disagree. Just make a point to find one.

What to Expect at Your First Appointment

Once you meet the doctor, interview him. It never ceases to amaze us that women will spend more time agonizing over a new outfit than they will talking—really talking—with their doctors. A fabulous new Prada suit with just the right Manolos won't prescribe hormone shots, perform surgery, or provide you with with the chance to have a baby. But a doctor will. Don't you want to know everything about this person before you sign up to bare your soul? Of course you do.

When you meet the doctor, feel free to ask about his or her training, education, postgraduate work, and continuing education. Ask why he or she chose this line of medicine.

Bring your partner to your first appointment. Most doctors want to meet with you initially as a couple. Be prepared to answer questions about your health and family history. Many doctors will send you a work sheet to fill out before you come in. For all you shy gals, this topic does not lend itself to modesty, so don't be surprised at the personal nature of some of the questions. We're talking about making a baby here and that includes all the bodily functions and parts associated with that process.

The physician/patient component of your infertility team is important. You need to be informed about what treatments are available and why your doctor is choosing one course of treatment over another. If you read something in a magazine, share it with your doctor. But remember, what is right for one couple may not be right for another, either physically, financially, or emotionally. Bottom line: Don't be afraid to question your doctor.

Here are few questions to get you started.

Ten Questions to Ask Your Doctor on Your First Appointment

1. How do you like working with patients?
2. What is involved in the initial fertility exam?
3. What is your personal availability to patients?
4. How do we get our questions answered?
5. Are your labs and sonogram facilities here in the office, or do I have to go somewhere else?
6. What are your days and hours of operation, and how do you coordinate those with my body's schedule?
7. What is the office's ability to do and success rate of assisted reproductive technologies, IVF, and GIFT? (Some doctors and/or clinics favor one procedure or drug therapy. Others have great success with in vitro fertilization or surrogate pregnancies. Find out what your RE does.)
8. Are procedures done at the clinic or another location, and at what hospitals do you have privileges?

9. Based on my age, health, and heredity, what are my statistical chances of getting pregnant, and what are my best options?

10. How can my partner and I best help you help us?

Playing to Win

As with any good relationship, communication is key. Let's reiterate—don't be shy. Your doctor is the one person who knows, needs to know, or will soon know some of the most intimate details of your life, like when you ovulate, how fast your partner's sperm can swim, and when and how often you have sex. When you put it in perspective, asking about the effects of a hormone drug or just how much weight you will gain on it doesn't seem like such a big deal, does it?

Don't worry about being labeled a troublemaker if you ask too many questions. It's your body. It's your future family. It's your time, commitment, and money. You need to know what is going on, and you need to take responsibility for finding out. You are also responsible for making sure your doctor has a clear picture of you. Doctors do not magically know everything about you just because they are doctors. They are not mind readers. You are not their only patient, so it is your job to keep them informed.

If you are too embarrassed to ask about something (and there are always a few questions that make even the boldest of us cringe or turn our partner's cheeks a bright shade of pink), simply jot down what you want to ask on a notepad and hand the page to the doctor during your next visit. Keep the pen and pad ready, so you can write down the answers. Even if you can remember them without taking notes, having something to do with your hands and eyes can help ease any discomfort the most modest of us may have.

Let us repeat that, as you are probably beginning to discover, fighting for your fertility is not for the modest. You are going to be stripped down to your reproductive core. It might not make you feel any better, but we do promise you'll be surprised how quickly the modesty fades. Women who never thought they could say "penis" without blushing will find themselves not only using the word "penis" multiple times in a conversation, but will also eventually discuss with strangers whether standing on your head after having sex really does make a difference or if just tossing your legs over your shoulders for ten minutes is good enough.

Don't believe us? Just wait.

It's Just Not Working Out: When to Find a New Doctor

Occasionally, you will run into a doctor who simply doesn't—and won't—get your problem. That's fine, as long as you understand you don't have to put up with that.

The relationship between you and your doctor definitely should be a partnership. It should also be courteous, not patriarchal or "doctor knows best." Insist that your doctors share the information. This isn't Latin here. Well, maybe some of the fancy medical terms have Latin roots, but they can give them to you in average-Joe language. It's your body. You need to be informed about what's going to happen to it.

Our friend Louise left her first reproductive endocrinologist for talking down to her and chastising her mercilessly when she forgot to take her injectables with her when she flew to her father-in-law's unexpected funeral. The guy had no compassion, so she left.

She then talked to several women friends at work who referred her to her new gynecologist—a woman who had experienced infertility herself before having two children. That doctor then referred her to an RE who took Louise and her husband to the next step.

Even the best, most credentialed doctor may not have the personality or "fit" or be as aggressive as you want. Some doctors excel at technique, but don't handle the emotional side of things very well. We've all heard the cracks about bad bedside manner. People joke about it for a reason; it exists. Personally, we can handle bad bedside manner if the doctor boasts the utmost competence and is surrounded by a bunch of fabulous, compassionate nurses. If the doctor has a stellar track record of bringing the joy of motherhood to infertile women, we'll deal with a cold, robotic personality. But we don't *want* to, and neither should you if you don't have to.

If you don't like the doctor's behavior or approach to your situation, leave. Trust your gut instinct and get out. You are paying good money, and you deserve to be treated with dignity and respect. Your questions should be answered and your concerns addressed. Everyone has a bad day now and then, so you have to evaluate the situation. If it's a rare occurrence to be rebuffed, that's one thing. If it's commonplace, fire the doctor and get a new one.

For some reason, people feel this sense of loyalty to a doctor, even if they are being treated poorly. Guess it goes back to the medical degree. They have one, and we don't. It's common to be deferential to someone who is supposed to be the expert. But doctors are just people like us—perhaps with more schooling. They have good days and bad ones, and some have crummy personalities while others epitomize the Hippocratic oath. If you stick with a doctor with whom you don't click, it can certainly sour the experience for even the most serene patient.

Fear of Failure Factor

Here's a shocker. There are a few doctors out there who may actually see *your* infertility as *their* failures. They view getting you pregnant as a goal to increase their statistics, prestige, or whatever. When you don't get pregnant, you become the brunt of their frustration. Fortunately, these doctors don't make up the majority. They don't even make up the minority. Like we said, they are few in number, but it is always best to be prepared.

Of course, all doctors want success for different reasons. Most truly want to help their patients create families. But success makes them look good, too. It increases their statistics, which in turn increases their ability to get more patients.

One of Maureen's doctors brought up the possibility that they were coming to the end of his course of treatments for her as his "throwing in the towel." He made it sound as if he were quitting on her! This was after Maureen spent eight months of her life driving forty-five minutes each way to and from his clinic several times a month. This is his idea of compassionately sharing the possibility that he can't help her achieve a child? What woman wouldn't feel like she'd been dumped into the "old hen" category?

After rushing to his office for an unplanned sonogram and leaving her ten-year-old son to arrive at an empty home after school, Maureen was told the third insemination didn't work and that they were at a place where she and the doctor had to make some choices. It was at that point, with her feet in the stirrups, that her doctor informed her that their success rate for IVF, her next option, was zero for women her age. Maureen was stunned. She hadn't thought to ask him about his treatment plans and success rates when she first began seeing him almost a year earlier! She was worried about her son, had just been told she wasn't pregnant, and now, legs still in the air, was trying to understand her doctor's comments about her future fertility while he was busy washing his hands.

He then proceeded to tell her they had one last shot before "throwing in the towel." They could do injectable drugs and insemination. Fortunately, she had the presence of mind to ask him what his success rate was for this last course of action. He never answered her question. She never went back.

The moral of this story: You may feel shocked, betrayed, or angry by a doctor's words or actions, but don't feel guilty. The doctor's problem is not yours. Just recognize it sooner rather than later, grab your file, and move on.

Ten Signs It's Time to Look for a New Doctor

1. He or she is insensitive to your needs and desires.

2. He or she seems to be working without a solid treatment plan.

3. He or she is offended when you bring in treatment information you've found on the Internet, read in a magazine or newspaper, or heard about on TV.

4. He or she wants to keep trying the same treatment that has been unsuccessful for several cycles.

5. He or she dismisses your questions and concerns.

6. He or she is foggy about your case, forgets what's already been done, and has to be reminded about tests and treatments that have already been done.

7. He or she rushes through your appointments and doesn't seem to have time for you.

8. He or she is not carefully monitoring your drug treatments and procedures.

9. He or she can't or won't tell you the reasons for choosing a specific course of action for your case.

10. No one from the office calls you back in a timely fashion.

MAUREEN

If I hadn't met Julie, I don't know what would have happened. Most of my girlfriends didn't get what I was going through. Julie, however, guided me. She was a cheerleader. She informed me about things I wasn't aware of and was a great source of support during my most trying infertile times. Her knowledge and support played a monumental role in the conception and birth of my daughter and for that I am eternally grateful. I only hope this book can serve as a support to those of you who are not as lucky as I was to find someone like Julie.

JULIE

I made the mistake of thinking my husband could shoulder all my emotional baggage on this journey. When Robert and I started on this road, I was embarrassed about being infertile. I kept thinking it was a mistake; I could fix it or find someone else to fix it before family or friends found out. My husband and I decided to keep it to ourselves, so we did for about eight months. I didn't even tell my mother, best friend, or college roommates. It was awful. I would never do that again.

Don't Forget the Cheerleaders

Once you've found a doctor and had your first appointment, you can fill in the sidelines with your cheerleaders—your support team. Your support system is crucial to your emotional well-being during the whole infertility process. These people can and should be friends, relatives, other women who have experienced infertility . . . anyone who is compassionate and willing to listen. More on how to pick them later.

Husbands Can't Do It All

You cannot expect or demand your husband or partner to be your sole support.

There are three reasons why you shouldn't expect to lean only on your partner.

1. He's going through it, too.
2. He's a guy.
3. He really doesn't get it.

That last one might sound harsh, but it's reality. Boys are simply wired differently from us girls. Even if they are our partners and best friends, they are still men. We've interviewed enough guys to know they really don't know what to say to us during this whole thing, so let's help them out by finding someone else with whom to discuss this topic ad nauseam.

Can You Help Me?

So what to do? Find a friend who understands the situation. Fertile friends don't always make the best buddies for infertility talk. They can't relate. If they haven't had problems conceiving, it's difficult to be empathetic. If they don't have kids yet, they might not want to discuss your situation because they are in denial that infertility could happen to them. Instead, find another woman who has faced or is facing the same thing. There are a lot of us out there. Ask your clinic if they can recommend any support groups or if there is another patient with a situation similar to yours who might want to talk. Check out chat sites on the Internet. Call the RESOLVE office in your town.

Try to avoid negative people. We're big believers of getting negativity out of your life because the stress can hinder fertility. Hanging out with angry, bitter people or listening repeatedly to others' sad stories can be counterproductive. Instead, find a girlfriend who understands what you are going through, and set up a buddy system with her. If you can't find that person right away, get a journal and start writing. Trust us, you'll be glad you did.

CHAPTER 9

TESTING, TESTING, 1-2-3,

Julie

Infertility treatments are quick and painless. Ha! As opposed to ha-ha!

Rare is the infertility patient who conceives with just a few painless pills. For me, conversations with my doctor ranked as the most painless part of infertility therapy. I had tests. I had shots. I had surgeries. I gave so much blood, it's a wonder I didn't become anemic. Of course, a lot depends on your pain threshold. I have friends who can stick themselves with a needle and not think twice. I have to look away and hum loudly when a nurse draws someone else's blood.

Robert was involved, too. He did a semen test, which means he stepped into a restroom, ejaculated into a cup, came out, and handed it to a nurse. It didn't hurt a bit, unless you count a bruised ego.

Maureen

My husband is nothing short of Superman. I know because the doctor told me.

Will brought his sperm sample to the andrology lab on his fiftieth birthday. He was not a happy man that day, definitely not thrilled to be fifty. Then, he arrived only to discover he was supposed to make an appointment to deliver his specimen. The simple instruction to make one appointment, and he blew it. I can't even count the number of appointments I had to make, and I never missed one.

But he gave the woman those puppy dog eyes, and she caved and took his cup to test it. He came downstairs into my appointment with my RE and announced he didn't think that cup of semen had his best shot. He was tired and taking aspirin. My doctor told him to call the lab and cancel the test, if he didn't think it was best. He could try again another time.

"We need your best shot," my doctor declared. With this, my weary husband picked up the phone and called the lab to cancel the test. Suddenly, his face changed.

"What?" he exclaimed. "Really? Oh. Okay. Fine. Thanks. Thank you."

His eyes lit up. His face turned rosy and bright. Apparently the lab had already tested his specimen and declared it the best sperm in the history of the lab. He was nothing short of Superman! Will, the Superman of Sperm!

What an unexpected birthday present and right on time. Will smiled for weeks.

Ten Things No One Tells You About Fertility Testing

1. There are a lot of tests.
2. You will provide more blood in a year than most Red Cross blood donors, but without the doughnuts and juice.
3. Your insurance may not cover some/part/all of these tests.
4. You may not need all the tests.
5. These tests are not quick and painless.
6. All this testing is time-consuming for women.
7. You will be confused.
8. Your doctor will not tell you everything about these tests unless you ask.
9. You will feel like a lab rat.
10. You should not let anyone do anything to your body that you don't fully understand.

What Is an Infertility Evaluation?

An infertility evaluation is the first step to treatment. Think of it as a fertility physical on your and your husband's reproductive systems. Everything should be scrutinized—from your hypothalamus and pituitary gland to your ovaries, Fallopian tubes, uterus, and vagina. The same goes for your partner—the hypothalamus, pituitary gland, and reproductive plumbing should be investigated as your doctor begins the search for what's wrong with your fertility.

On your first visit, you and your partner will have a long consultation with the doctor, followed by a physical for you, possible semen analysis for him, and blood work for both of you. Other tests you may have to endure include ovulatory function tests, a hysterosalpingogram (HSG), and a laparoscopy. For your man, the first steps will probably include a medical history, physical exam, semen analysis, hormonal testing, and tests to see if his sperm can fertilize.

For all you overachievers out there, expect to fail at least one of the fertility tests. The older you are, the more negative results there will be. These "failures," however, should be considered blessings. Why? Well, now you know what you need to fix.

Also, we want to emphasize that it's *your* body. Don't let anyone do anything to it that you don't fully understand. Ask questions about drugs, procedures, schedules, results, options, and success rates. Be honest in your responses to your doctor's questions and demand the same from your medical staff. Fully informed is fully empowered.

Now, let's take a look at what you should expect.

History Lesson

For your first scheduled appointment, you will (should) be asked to fill out a rather long questionnaire/history about your medical, surgical, and gynecological past, as well as family history and lifestyle issues. This will help them determine potential past problems that might be hindering your fertility.

Fill out all the forms you are given before you go to your appointment. Julie's doctor sent it to her ahead of time. Maureen's doctor had her fill it out online and return it prior to her appointment as well. We suggest you ask for this questionaire ahead of time as well. Send it back or drop it off ahead of time so that the doctor has an opportunity to review it before you go. Bring your copy along to the visit. Covering all your bases will speed things along.

In addition to quizzing you to death, your doctor will also want to see any other fertility or reproductive records you might have from other doctors. To avoid delays, bring or have your OB/GYN or family doctor send a copy of your files, including X-rays, ahead of time.

Take your time filling out any forms. It is pretty crucial. Do it with your partner, since there will be historical questions for him as well. Historical questions? What could come up? Well, there's a laundry list of things that could raise a red flag. We've broken down a list of questions your doctor should ask you and your partner and why he or she should ask them. These are also questions you should ask yourself and be ready to expound on at the first appointment.

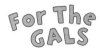

Overall health

Have you ever had a serious disease?

What about kidney or liver problems?

Have you ever been diagnosed with thyroid problems?

Ever suffer from anorexia nervosa or bulimia?

Do you have a history of blood clots?

Do you smoke? If so, how much?

Do you drink alcohol? If so, how much and how often?

Do you do illicit drugs? If so, how much and how often?

Have you ever been diagnosed with any heart problems?

To Pinpoint Potential Hypothalamus Problems

Have you ever had a severe head trauma? (Fall down the stairs or receive a blow to head?)

What about extreme weight loss or gain?

Are you under stress?

How often and how much do you exercise? What do you do?

To Pinpoint Potential Pituitary Gland Problems

Have you had any tumors?

Have you had radiation in the past to treat tumors?

Can you detect certain scents or have you noticed a deficiency in your sense of smell?

Have you ever suffered severe head trauma?

Do you take or have you ever taken antidepressants?

To Pinpoint Potential Ovarian Problems

Do you have painless or painful periods?

Do you know if you suffer from polycystic ovary syndrome?

Have you had any surgery on your reproductive organs in the past?

Have you ever had radiation?

Have you ever had chemotherapy?

What is the frequency, duration, and regularity—or irregularity—of your periods?

To Pinpoint Potential Fallopian Tube Problems

Have you ever suffered an ectopic pregnancy?

Have you ever had a ruptured appendix?

What about endometriosis?

Have you ever contracted a sexually transmitted disease or suffered from pelvic inflammatory disease?

Have you ever had surgery involving your pelvis?

Have you ever used an IUD, which can cause scarring and be tough on the tubes?

To Pinpoint Potential Uterine Problems

Has anyone ever told you that you have a tipped uterus? A malformed uterus?

Has anyone ever said you suffer luteal phase defect?

Have you ever had hormonal injections? If so, for how long?

Have you ever had endometriosis?

Have you ever used an IUD, which can cause uterine scarring?

Has anyone ever said you have Asherman's syndrome or fibroids?

Have you ever been on birth control pills?

To Pinpoint Potential Cervical Problems

Did your mother use DES (diethylstilbestrol) while she was pregnant with you?

Have you ever had cervical surgery?

If you have been pregnant before, did you suffer cervical incompetence that caused premature delivery or required a stitch?

Is intercourse ever painful for you?

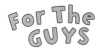

To Pinpoint Potential Testicular Problems

Did you have mumps as a child?

Did you have mumps as an adult?

Have you ever suffered testicular injury? (Been kicked in the nuts really hard?)

Have you ever contracted a sexually transmitted disease? If so, which ones?

Do you have any odd varicose veins (aka varicocele) on your scrotum?

Do you do a lot of bike riding?

Do you smoke? If so, how much?

Do you drink alcohol? If so, how much and how often?

Do you do illicit drugs? If so, how much and how often?

Do you spend a lot of time in a hot tub?

To Pinpoint Potential Penis Problems

Have you ever suffered impotence?

What about any other sexual dysfunction?

Have you ever had a problem with or injury to your penis?

Have you ever suffered a spinal cord injury?

When you ejaculate, how much seminal fluid do you produce?

At the Office

Your initial visit will begin with an appointment with your doctor who will go over your history and review his office procedures. This is your chance to ask questions and set out your game plan and treatment goals. Your new doctor will then share with you the tests you will/may need to undergo. Hopefully, he or she has handouts, like Julie's doctor, that explain every procedure in average-Joe language. It is totally fair, and to our minds advisable, to ask your doctor what he or she is testing you for and why, how the procedure is done, who will do it, and where. And, once you know the test results, ask how he or she will fix what's wrong. We even think you should ask point-blank if the tests will hurt. We have friends who balked at certain tests because girlfriends told them they hurt. Here's the truth as we know it—nothing in fertility testing is more painful than labor, and you will survive that, too.

Physical Exam

The next step will be a physical exam for you. This should include a pelvic ultrasound—usually performed trans-vaginally by sticking a rod-shape wand called a transducer into your vagina and using sound waves to showcase your reproductive plumbing on a screen. It's actually very cool to see—more fun when the sonogram features a baby, but that's down the road. The ultrasound helps the doctor check for any problems or abnormalities in your uterus, ovaries, and Fallopian tubes. The doctor can also observe your endometrial lining and your ovarian follicles. Think of it as a mechanic looking under the hood—trying to ascertain what he has to work with. Most doctors like to do this initial test just after your period to get an idea of what everything looks like at rest. The ultrasound will be repeated at different times in your cycle throughout your fertility treatment when your doctor wants to see how your reproductive system is responding to ovulation or drug stimulation.

Testing

Here's the unfair part. The woman has about a zillion tests. The man has two for sure (semen analysis and blood work), maybe three (a test for STDs like chlamydia). Get used to it. It continues when you get pregnant. The woman carries the kid for nine months and goes through labor. The man ejaculates once, brags for nine months, then hands out cigars after his partner births the baby. Such is the circle of life.

Her Tests

While you are doing these tests, your partner will have finished his blood or semen test and will be sitting in the waiting room reading a magazine or be back at work.

By the way, be sure your husband at least knows your doctor's name and the clinic's location. We were talking to a friend's husband—we'll call him Joe—and when asked the name of his wife's fertility doctor, he drew a total blank. His reply?

"How can you expect me to know that? I only had to go there twice to drop off my full cup. My wife did the rest."

We'd like to say he's unusual, that most guys are involved with every aspect of their partners' infertility treatments. But unfortunately, he's an average Joe, just like many, many men out there. However, most do seem to recall the names of their wives' fertility doctors, so don't let your husband get away with that.

The Blood Hormone Levels Tests

Many vials of blood are drawn by a nurse to be used for a multitude of tests. The blood is sent to a lab to be checked for your levels of a variety of hormones necessary for reproduction—estradiol (estrogen in the blood), prolactin, luteinizing hormone (LH), follicle-stimulating hormone (FSH), progesterone—as well as antiphospholipid antibodies, anti-sperm antibodies, and thyroid tests (like a TSH) when indicated. You will probably also be tested for hepatitis and AIDS as well, since this is the law just about everywhere, so don't be freaked out.

By the way, this is not the last time you will be giving blood. Get used to it.

Ovulatory Function Test

This is the test that measures your ovarian reserve, or remaining egg supply. The doctor will draw blood to check FSH, estradiol, and inhibin-B levels, as well as do an ultrasound to check your ovaries and count follicles—usually on day three of your cycle. High inhibin-B levels indicate lots of eggs. If the levels are low, it indicates a decreased ovarian reserve.

Other Tests

Once you have finished your first visit and set of tests, the groundwork will be laid for the next series of exams. Here are some other tests your doctor may suggest you have.

Hysterosalpingogram (HSG)

This is an X-ray dye test performed in a radiology department to assess the inner lining of the uterus and to ensure the Fallopian tubes aren't blocked. Here's what happens: You lie on an X-ray table while your cervix is opened enough to accommodate an instrument or catheter through which a liquid dye is inserted. The dye fills up the uterine cavity and Fallopian tubes while the radiologist takes a few X-ray pictures. The HSG takes only a few minutes to complete. You can look on the video screen at the pictures being taken.

Afterward, the instruments will be removed, and you will remain on the X-ray table for a few more minutes. The HSG can be a little painful—a pinch with slight or major cramping like menstrual cramps, depending on the woman. We didn't have a lot of pain with this one. But if you do, remember that it's a quick test.

Endometrial Biopsy

This test checks the quality of the uterine lining and consists of the doctor taking a scraping of tissue from the endometrium. This helps determine if your lining is thickening at the right rate during your monthly cycle in conjunction with the hormones your body is secreting. If it is, then your uterus is considered "in phase." If the endometrium is not at the right thickness, you are "out of phase," and your doctor will use this tissue to determine how many days you are off.

This test is done while you are lying on the examination table with your feet in the stirrups. Your doctor will dilate your cervix and insert a thin, pointed instrument with which he or she will scrape a bit of uterine lining. It is a very short test—like a minute or two, max. Pain-wise, this test hurt Maureen more than the HSG did. Some women don't like the little tool being inserted, while others don't mind, but get cramps later. Julie is no help here because she has repressed the whole darn thing.

While currently controversial, an endometrial biopsy late in the cycle (day twenty-six) read by a pathologist well-versed in reading them remains one of the cornerstones of uterine functional assessment.

Postcoital/Cervical Mucus Test

Also known as the PCT, this post-sex test checks the compatibility of your man's sperm with your cervical mucus.

Here's what you have to do: Have sex (at home, not at the doc's office!). A few hours later, while your husband is back at work, you go to the clinic to have some of your cervical mucus scooped out and studied. The exam will help the doctor determine whether the mucus is hospitable to your partner's sperm. If there are lots of dead sperm in the sample, your doctor will want to do more testing to check for anti-sperm antibodies and analyze the pH of your mucus. None of this hurts.

Hysteroscopy

The hysteroscopy allows your doctor to glance around inside your uterus using a thin, lighted fiber-optic scope. Getting the inside view on your uterus helps pinpoint any growths, adhesions, scarring, or abnormalities in the organ's shape.

The scope is inserted through your dilated cervix. Most likely, your uterus will be expanded with a sterile liquid solution or gas—all the better to see you with, my dear. Some doctors will perform an endometrial biopsy at the same time as the hysteroscopy. Some will also try to fix any problems in the uterus—like removing scar tissue—while they are in there.

This procedure can be done with either general or local anesthesia. Julie had it done and highly recommends the general anesthesia, unless you have an incredibly high pain tolerance or just want to be semi-aware of your surroundings at all times.

Perch your partner in the waiting room because you will need him to drive you home and pick up your pain medication.

Laparoscopy

Not really part of the basic testing, laparoscopies are outpatient surgeries that allow the doctor to check for endometriosis or pelvic scarring that don't show up in any other tests. We discuss it here because many, many women undergoing fertility treatment will get this done at one time or another.

During a laparoscopy, the doctor views your internal reproductive organs by way of a lighted fiber-optic scope inserted through your belly button. If any abnormalities are found, such as endometriosis, the doctor can fix the damage right then by making another small incision two to three inches lower in the abdomen and inserting some small tools. Most fertility or reconstructive pelvic procedures are done through the laparoscope nowadays, which is great. It means fewer women need a major cut to correct their tubal and ovarian abnormalities and can continue to wear skimpy bikinis if they want. On occasion, it may be essential for your surgeon to make a larger cut, but any reasons for this are usually clearly explained in the consent form, so be sure you read that document—don't just skim it for the good parts.

A laparoscopy is an all-day procedure, since it is done in the day-surgery division of a hospital and requires general anesthesia. If you need this surgical procedure—and it really is not something that should be done prior to getting all the basic testing done—you will be knocked out and woozy when you wake up.

Again, if you are looking for your partner, he should be in the waiting room reading magazines because you will need him to drive you home and pick up your pain medication. This is a must for laparoscopy patients. Julie was not only too groggy to drive after a laparoscopy, but also ended up spewing fluorescent green vomit (courtesy of the anesthesia) all over the floor of Eckerd Pharmacy while waiting for them to fill her pain meds. Robert hustled her out pretty quickly after that.

His Tests

While we go through dozens of tests, men give some blood and have a semen analysis. That's about it at the start—even though, as we mentioned earlier, the male is either the sole or a contributing cause of infertility in about 40 percent of infertile couples.

Semen Analysis

The semen analysis is an easy, painless procedure that tells the doctor everything he or she needs to know about your guy's juice. It involves a favorite male pastime: ejaculating. He goes into a bathroom or private room, ejaculates into a sterile cup, and hands it either to you or directly to the nurse if the sample is collected at the clinic. If the sample is harvested at home, you will have to rush it to the hospital. It has to be there within one hour of leaving his body and will have to kept warm snuggled next to a body part—yours or his. Seriously.

The lab will then measure things like the time it takes for the semen to liquefy and its volume, consistency, and acidity. Inspection under a microscope will determine the sperm count, percent of moving sperm (called motility), shape (called morphology), and how many sperm are alive and how many are dead, as well as whether there are white blood cells or bacteria present that might indicate an infection.

What's considered "normal" semen? Samples that contain more than 20 million sperm per milliliter with more than half of them swimming forward and 30 percent or more shaped correctly.

By the way, there are two semen analyses that check out sperm. One uses a computer and makes a basic guesstimate based on statistical data. It's okay, but you really want the other, called the Kruger Morphology Test, which is based strictly on physical appearance. A person actually stares at slides of your guy's sperm, checking, counting, and making notes on 200 sperm from the sample he provided. They look at the head, neck, and tail of each of these 200 sperm. When the test is done like this, 14 percent normal is considered great! Go buy the guy a present! He's a super sperm producer! If fewer than 4 percent are normal, pregnancy might be difficult. If fewer than 1 percent are normal, you are going to have a difficult time.

If the analysis comes back okay, your guy is pretty much done with the testing—although your doctor may want two semen samples collected on separate days for comparison.

His Blood Hormone Test

This is your partner's needle-induced workup to measure blood levels of hormones involved in sperm production, such as LH, FSH, testosterone, liver function, and thyroid when necessary. Basic blood work today usually also includes a hepatitis and an AIDS test, required by law. Like your blood tests, a vial or so of blood is drawn from his arm and sent off to the lab with instructions from your doctor that say what he or she wants to know—couldn't be easier.

With the completion of these two tests, providing they come back normal, your man is done with his medical testing. He can now devote the rest of his time to taking care of you.

Let the Games Begin

A few caveats before you begin your journey. If you're still hiding the fact you are going through infertility treatments from coworkers and friends, you will have to continue functioning like a normal person, despite the emotional and physical upheaval you will endure.

Here's what you can expect: You will go to the doctor's office multiple times a month and pretend everything is fine. Because of all the tests and blood work, you will have to come into work late, leave early, take long lunches, and convince your boss you are still getting all your work done. You will give so much blood that, unless you wear long sleeves, your friends might think you've become a heroin addict. Eventually, all this will wear you out, and you will tell your boss and coworkers you are infertile in an effort to evoke some sympathy and peace of mind—or you will quit your job.

Time is also money. If you need your company insurance to help pay for fertility treatments (and who doesn't?), you will have to be sure you can juggle both your office and personal responsibilities. We have been lucky in that we are both self-employed, so we have flexible schedules. Who cares that we have to work all night to make up for the time committed to clinics during the day? If we'd had any boss other than ourselves, we probably wouldn't have lasted.

After going through it ourselves, we believe there should be a paid leave of absence granted to woman undergoing infertility treatments. It is outrageous that we have to take on this physical and mental stress while continuing to function at a high level at our jobs. It won't happen, but it sure would be great. All we're asking for is six months. Well, thank God women have that multitasking gene.

So, how do you keep score in this game? By forgetting all the win or lose rules. By remembering that infertility treatment does not always lead to biological babies. Look, it's called the *practice* of medicine for a reason. Like many aspects of medicine, infertility treatment is an inexact science. It's important to keep this in mind. Have a positive outlook, but don't be a Pollyanna. Be wary of promises to "cure" you. Between 25 and 30 percent of women facing infertility will walk away from the procedures without a biological child, but that doesn't make you a loser. You have gained the knowledge necessary to make the next step: donor eggs, surrogacy, adoption, whatever. If you want a family, you will have one. In that regard, no one totally loses at infertility.

MAUREEN

The first time Quinn ever came home to an empty house was because of infertility. Generally, I scheduled appointments in the morning to be home when he arrived from school. This time the doctor was delayed more than two hours and therefore so was I. The hospital was an hour from home, and I had no choice but to stay because I needed to be seen. My heart raced; my anxiety level went up. I was so concerned for my little boy, who was nine at the time, coming home to a locked and empty house. I called my new neighbors (we had just moved to town) who assured me they would pick him up from the bus and take him to their house. He was fine, but I was tied up in knots being over an hour away from him. I am grateful for the support of friends and neighbors who had no idea why I was really at the doctor. When they say it takes a village to raise a child, it also takes a village to have one when you are going through infertility.

CHAPTER 10

Be-(A)-Ware!

Maureen

Here's what I know now: Infertility is wrought with deep emotional issues, as well as medical, moral, and ethical ones. Until we are faced with them, we don't realize they exist. Being aware of the risks and situations that may come our way may not make the decision process any easier, but at least it may help us to brave the tidal wave when it hits us and keep us from drowning.

I didn't know any of that ahead of time. I wasn't prepared for the issues I faced with infertility. If I could advise my younger self, I would say, "Maureen, don't make any hasty decisions about procedures and drugs. There is always more than meets the eye when you are entering into any kind of complicated situation, especially when it comes to your health.

"Stop, Maureen," I would say. "You must stop . . . think . . . research . . . discuss . . . then decide."

The words I wish someone had told me.

Julie

There is so much about infertility you can't know until you have been through it. I often go into big projects on blind faith, gut instinct, and perseverance. Sometimes, a little knowledge ahead of time would have been helpful.

Here's an example. Robert and I live in a house that was originally built 100 years ago and thirty miles away from where it sits today. This big, historic home was slated for demolition in a swanky part of Dallas, and the church that owned it said we could have it if we would move it off-site. Sure, we said. How hard could it be? And we plunged in, dismantling the house and physically moving it north to its new home. Today, you can't tell it wasn't built on the land it commands.

It was a lot of work. No one can believe what we went through with this house. We can't believe all we did to succeed, but we did it. We never thought we couldn't do it. We didn't know what to be aware of or what to fear. We just trusted our contractors and our instincts and did the work necessary to achieve the results we wanted. Sure, there were problems along the way, but we figured them out and stood by our decisions.

It was the same with building our family. We knew what we wanted—children—and figured out what we needed to do to achieve the results. Just like with the house, we jumped in without a lot of research. Along the way, just like with the house, things cropped up that we didn't expect. We had to make decisions, then stand by them as a couple. Some were easy. Some were hard. Some still haunt me.

The biggest difference? With moving a house, it's okay to be unaware of all the details—or you wouldn't do the project. With infertility, it's better to know up front what might happen, so you can survive the process.

Ten Things to Keep in Mind

1. Fertility treatments, like all medical treatments, entail risks.
2. Fertility drugs are very powerful.
3. Some aspects of fertility treatments are still considered investigational.
4. You may be faced with some tough moral, ethical, and physical decisions during infertility treatment.
5. Listen to your doctor, read everything you can on a treatment or procedure, weigh the risks, then make your decision.
6. Trust your gut instinct.
7. Fools rush in where angels fear to tread.
8. Remember that normal is a miracle.
9. You don't always get what you want.
10. There are many ways to build a family.

To the uninformed, infertility can seem pretty benign. Couples go in for treatments and come out the other end with a baby. If it's the Hollywood version, you don't even know the celeb went through twelve IVFs and postpartum depression to create Junior, unless her publicist thinks a tell-all could help promote her next movie.

But the truth is, infertility treatments and the many decisions involved are not benign. There are tough decisions to be made almost every step of the way. The drugs used are powerful and able to alter your body both physically and emotionally. The long-term ramifications of pumping your body full of fertility drugs are not totally understood. There is an element of chance involved in family building through better science. Older women face different issues carrying a child than do younger moms-to-be. To preserve the life of the mother and/or babies, a couple may have to abort some embryos. Depending on where you live and who your doctors are, you may have to deliver a miscarriage and recuperate on the maternity floor. How do you decide what to do if an amnio comes back with a bad result? What if you have to deliver that baby you want to terminate? What do you do if you are advised to selectively abort some embryos? How do you decide what to do with all the frozen embryos you no longer wish to implant?

We're not trying to scare you. But infertility has a serious side we were unaware of until we were smack-dab in the middle of treatment trying to make decisions. Obviously, it didn't stop either of us. Some issues mentioned weren't even on our radars (how fortunate we were). But other women did face challenges they never dreamed existed. We know women who have seen the gates of hell with their infertility treatments and survived with great courage and amazing fortitude. Their stories need to be told so that you walk this journey with your eyes wide open.

What Are the Long-term Effects of Fertility Drugs and Treatments?

Honestly? No one really knows.

There is speculation that there may be some consequences. Actress/comedienne Gilda Radner died of ovarian cancer in 1989 just shy of her forty-fourth birthday. High-profile fashion journalist and *Harper's Bazaar* editor Liz Tilberis also died from ovarian cancer in 1999 at age fifty-one. Both women had gone through years of unsuccessful infertility treatments. Tilberis, who also wrote the book *No Time to Die,* made reference to the possible connection between her nine IVF attempts and her cancer. Radner, who also did extensive infertility treatment, did not. Articles in popular magazines dissect this topic regularly, but there is no conclusive proof one way or the other at this time. Most studies have shown that the long-term follow-ups of women who have had fertility treatment had no significant increased incidence of ovarian cancers, particularly if they got pregnant. This is pretty reassuring. However the jury is still not out 100 percent, so once again we are talking moderation here. Few treatment cycles may minimize the risks, as does actually conceiving during one of them.

In November 2004, a study came out saying women who drink milk are more prone to ovarian cancer. Hmm, could it be due to all the hormones our cows are pumped up with, hormones that come to us through the milk? We wonder.

"It did occur to me while I was taking the medications that this whole procedure could be a time bomb," says Linda, a forty-three-old year mother of twin boys resulting from IVF—her fourth IVF. "I guess we'll never know, but it didn't stop me. If I do get something like cancer sometime down the road and if it is because of the drugs I took to get my babies, it's a moot point. I'm glad I did it. I figure as long as I remain healthy, and have sense of humor, and pray my body is strong enough to overcome anything that attacks my immune system down the line, I'll be fine."

Our friend Cate was thirty-nine years old when she did six cycles of multiple fertility drugs to stimulate her egg production for IVF with a surrogate. Surprisingly, unless she has totally blanked out on the memory, Cate suffered no side effects from the hormone drug cocktail her fertility specialist prescribed.

While Cate produced a large cache of eggs each time, none of them took when they were implanted in the surrogate. Cate and her husband then began the adoption process. Two years later, Cate was the mother of a newborn boy. Right after the adoption finalized, Cate began suffering a strange string of ailments. Sinus infections so severe as to require an operation and more infections following the operation. Then, her hair began falling out. Arthritis attacked her joints. Her immune system was in collapse. This was odd for a forty-one-year-old woman who had always been the picture of health.

Cate went to several doctors, but no one could figure out what was wrong. Finally, she went to a wellness center in Massachussetes for a week. "They ran every test known to mankind on me and discovered I have hypothyroidism," says Cate.

Hypothyroidism can be caused by hormone imbalance. Fertility drugs mess with your hormones. Is there a connection? Who knows? The doctors are not saying there is any relation, but who's to say there isn't?

So, do fertility drugs cause cancer or anything else? We don't know. We do know there are women out there who think there may be some correlations of their health problems and the fertility drugs they ingested, but no scientific data says definitely yes. Much literature addressing this issue actually says the opposite—fertility drugs that spur on ovulation don't increase the cancer risk, either ovarian or breast. Most are like a 2004 study from the University of Pittsburgh that found no association between cancer and fertility drugs. To be fair, other studies have established that women who have never been pregnant at all are most at risk for ovarian cancer. If you suffer infertility and thus have never been pregnant . . . well, then it makes sense: that infertile women may be more prone to get ovarian cancer. As for breast cancer, excessive exposure to high estrogen levels may increase the risk of this disease. What is excessive? A month? A year? A lifetime? What's long-term? What's short-term? Where's the definition of excessive? We couldn't find it.

Here's our thought. If you have a risk of ovarian, breast, or any kind of cancer in your family, tell your doctor before you start treatment. Discuss the options and ramifications of drug therapy. Ask for literature. Read it. Then make a decision that's best for you.

The More, the Merrier?

Some fertility drugs, such as Clomid and Pergonal (discussed in-depth in chapter 11), increase the number of eggs released each month. This means that fertility patients may conceive more than one baby—a lot more. Between 1980 and 1997, the number of births for triplet or more pregnancies increased more than 400 percent—rising dramatically from 1,377 to 6,737, according to a 1999 report from the Center for Disease Control (CDC). It makes sense: The number of fertility patients increased dramatically in that time period as well.

The biggest problem with carrying multiple babies is that they don't cook in utero as long as your conventional single baby. While normal gestation for a singleton is forty weeks, that time frame shrinks with more babies on board, creating the risks associated with being born premature. Triplets tend to arrive on average at about thirty-four to thirty-seven weeks, quadruplets at around thirty-one weeks, and quintuplets at about twenty-eight to twenty-nine weeks. (Much of these early deliveries, however, should be preventable with extensive bed rest and the use of drugs that suppress uterine contractions.) Premature babies in general, and multiple births in particular, tend to result in lower birth weights. Premature multiples are really tiny. The CDC report also noted that rates of low and very low birth weights, as well as infant mortality, were four to thirty-three times higher for multiples as compared with one baby. The rates increased as the number of babies increased from twins to triplets to higher. Most babies born in triplets weigh in at less than 5.5 pounds. All babies born in multiples greater than three (like quads, quints, and so on) come into the world weighing less than 5.5 pounds. Super low birth weights bother doctors because of the potential problems posed for these children as they grow. Fortunately, many of these teeny babies grow out of the risks when they begin to pack on the pounds. However, even fertility doctors, who understand how precious each pregnancy is to their patients, are now urging couples to avoid massive multiples in one pregnancy. Some even go so far as to call multiples the one negative aspect of fertility treatment.

Since we never had a multiples pregnancy, we don't have a dog in this fight. But we do suggest you be aware of the possibilities in your pregnancy.

Selective Reduction

For some people, twins, triplets, quadruplets, or even more seem like a joyful bonus. For others, this many children at one time is an overwhelming burden. Four, five, or six babies might not be financially feasible if all were born healthy. Pregnancies of this magnitude can endanger a mother's health as well.

Multiple babies is an issue you and your partner need to consider *before* you swallow even one pill or receive one fertility shot. If you know you would never be able to abort even one embryo, let alone two or three, you might not want to take the powerful drugs that make multiples more likely. Selective reduction is the term for causing a few of the developing embryos to abort, while the remaining twins, triplets, or singleton remain to flourish. While becoming more common, selective reduction is still a tricky procedure that involves inserting a needle into one of the fetuses to inject a chemical solution like potassium chloride. An ultrasound is then performed to ensure that the selected fetus's heart has stopped beating. The "reduced" fetus is then normally reabsorbed by the mother's body. Reductions are normally done at between nine and eleven weeks. Not all doctors or hospitals can or will do this procedure. If you go this route, be sure your doctor can handle it.

There's something else you need to know—just because you make the hard choice to reduce to a smaller number of fetuses doesn't mean the remaining babies will make it. Sandy's didn't.

Sandy, a forty-six-year-old New Yorker, suffered unexplained infertility in the early nineties. She became pregnant with IVF quintuplets in 1992. She was overjoyed to be pregnant, but concerned to be carrying so many babies. Her doctor suggested she selectively reduce to twins. Because she had signed on to be an experimental case study for this clinic, she agreed. When she got to the clinic for the procedure, one of the five embryos had already expired.

"I wanted to jump off the table," says Sandy. "I didn't want to go forward with the selective reduction, which was relatively new back then. I was afraid I would lose more naturally and didn't want to take any chances with the embryos remaining."

However, since Sandy had signed paperwork as a case study, she felt intimidated. Two of the four embryos were aborted. But four weeks later, the remaining two died as well.

"I had nothing," says Sandy, who went on to have two children on her own a few years later. "But my husband and I learned a lot from this process, most importantly to trust your instincts, be informed, and know when enough is enough."

When it comes to carrying multiples, be sure you don't end up in an undesirable (for you) situation. Determine how many children work for you. Talk turkey with your doctor and partner. Be sure everyone is on the same page before ingesting any drugs. Be aware.

Unused Embryos

Here's the scenario: You take fertility drugs, and your eggs are harvested for whichever assisted reproductive technology your doctor has determined will work best for you. You produce a bumper crop of eggs—more than you can use. You use what you need, have all the children you want, and still have some frozen embryos left. Now what? What do you do with unused embryos? This is Alison's dilemma.

"What do I do?" our friend Alison, mother of one daughter and twin boys, asked us. "I have eleven unused embryos on ice at the clinic. I'm done. But who is going to want the embryos of a forty-two-year-old woman? I can't give them away, and I can't just have them destroyed either. I don't know what to do."

Here are the choices we have found for unused embryos. You can destroy them, or you can put them up for "adoption."

Some organizations, such as Nightlight Christian Adoption in Fullerton, California, offer cryo-preserved embryos for adoption. Nightlight, which also does regular adoption, has been doing embryo adoption since 1997. Such an adoption differs from embryo donation to a fertility clinic in that genetic donors choose the parents of their unused embryos by way of letters, biographies, and photos—much like a birth mother chooses an adoptive family for her unborn child. The genetic parents sign release papers before the embryos are transferred. This adoption can be open or closed, depending on how much contact the parties want. Unlike traditional adoption, however, embryo adoptions allow the adoptive mother to experience pregnancy. Nightlight's program is called the Snowflakes Frozen Embryo Adoption Program, and through 2004, almost fifty adopted embryos had been born.

If you will have unused embryos, talk to your fertility doctor and ask what he or she suggests. Check the ever-changing laws in your state. Remember, not all frozen embryos will go on to become viable children, but it's best to have a plan. Have peace of mind. Be aware.

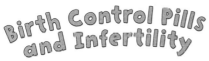

Birth Control Pills and Infertility

We know what the medical community says about birth control pills and fertility. We also know what women have told us. There are mixed messages everywhere, so you have to be aware of your body and how it reacts.

We think if you had irregular periods before you went on the Pill—like Julie—and you have irregular periods when you get off the Pill—like Julie—you need to go to a fertility clinic sooner rather than later. The Pill does a good job of masking irregular periods because it creates your periods hormonally.

Other birth control methods like Norplant, Depo-Provera, and Seasonale are long-term hormonal treatments. Norplant involves surgically inserting six flexible matchstick-size rods into your inner upper arm. These implants contain levonorgestrel, a progesterone-type drug, which is released slowly to prevent pregnancy for up to five years. Norplant suppresses ovulation.

Depo-Provera is an injectable progestin contraceptive given every three months that inhibits ovulation by suppressing the follicle-stimulating hormone (FSH) and luteinizing hormone (LH) levels, among other things.

Seasonale uses the same types of hormones as regular birth control pills (estrogen and progestin) for twelve weeks straight (rather than three) before a week of placebos that allow a woman to bleed. The result? Four periods each year rather than one every twenty-eight days.

Does all this sound normal and healthy to you? Long-term birth control may be convenient, but at what cost? We're not sure. We're not doctors. Doctors we spoke with feel that if you suppress ovulation with hormonal birth control for more than ten years, stop, and are not pregnant within six months to a year, something is wrong. We suggest you ask your doctor. Use your body as your guide.

It's Never Too Late

Midlife moms are the latest trend. According to the National Center for Health Statistics, the number of women over forty having children has more than doubled. That's us and probably the only thing about us right now that is trendy!

As forty-something moms with no nannies, we were both pretty bleary-eyed with round-the-clock feedings and babies that just normally got up early. We cannot imagine giving birth in our fifties, but some women can. According to the U.S. Center for Disease Control and Prevention, 263 children were born to women age fifty to fifty-four in 2002. In November 2004, Aleta St. James gave birth to twins in New York City. She turned fifty-seven two days later. St. James went through three years and $25,000 worth of in vitro fertilization to achieve this goal. She used donor eggs and donor sperm. She is a single mother. Wow. Bet she's exhausted—unless she has a bunch of help.

When is it too late to have a baby? Are you ever too old to start parenting? Is it politically correct to even ask this question? Who are we to challenge the reproductive decisions of another person? There are different schools of thought on this, but we have some doubts about the wisdom of the doctors who decided to help a fifty-seven-year-old single woman have twins. Sure, there's no assurance any of us will be around to parent our children to adulthood, no matter how young we are when we give birth or adopt them. Yes, age is a state of mind. Yes, it's easier if you have help.

But do the math. When a woman who gives birth at fifty-seven takes her children to kindergarten, she will be sixty-two years old. When they learn to drive at sixteen, she will be seventy-three. When they graduate from college, she will be seventy-nine. Most likely, this woman will not be a mother of the bride. She will not be a grandmother.

What about the kids? Will they worry about whether their parent will live to see them graduate from high school? college? elementary school? Will they wish they had one of those younger parents who run, jump, and play with them like those of their friends?

We're not playing favorites here. We have a problem with guys who father kids in their seventies for the same reasons. Is it fair to the kids? Most often, however, older men parent with younger wives, so at least someone is around to continue on after Dad heads to heaven. Whose going to be around for a single, fifty-seven-year-old mother of newborn twins should something happen?

We are not discouraging anyone. God knows, we did it ourselves. We love midlife motherhood—all of us late blooming mommies who beat Mother Nature and Father Time. We are just saying do the math. Be sure it is fair to the children and not just something you don't want to miss. Selflessness is part of being a parent. Then take your vitamins, quit smoking, and start exercising so you can be the best parent possible. And put a plan in place to take care of the kiddos in the event God calls you home sooner rather than later.

MAUREEN

When I got pregnant with Ava at age forty-one, my husband was fifty-one. Definitely late in the game for both of us. Our son, Quinn, was ten at the time.

I will never forget what Quinn said when we told him we were pregnant. He looked at my husband and said, "Dad, people with gray hair should not be having babies." Later, Quinn took me aside and said, "Are you sure Daddy isn't too old to be doing this?"

Will and I both got a laugh out of that, but our son wasn't kidding. He was coming from a place of good common sense, from the mouths of babes!

Going Solo

We support women taking charge of their fertilities. If you are pushing the envelope on motherhood and Mr. Right is nowhere in sight, by all means become a single mother. Just be sure you think it out first. It takes a village to raise a child, especially if you have no partner. On this there is no doubt. If you don't have someone else nearby to hold that child's hand while you grab a quick shower, well, you won't be taking many showers.

In the past, women had one another—their sisters, mothers, and female neighbors upstairs. There were other loving arms in which to place that child while Mom grabbed a moment of sanity. So if you plan to go through fertility treatment to become a single mom, put the village in place first, then have your baby.

Success Rates

Don't put off having a baby just because you think science will give you one when you want one. Ignore those who say it is never too late to have a child. Don't be so gullible as to assume that medical technology will rush in and save the day.

Let's be honest about success rates on fertility treatments. To begin with, there are no guarantees you will have a baby. Fertility treatment is less successful for women who are older than thirty-five. Assisted reproductive technologies like IVF don't compensate for the old age-related decreased fertility. It doesn't mean it won't happen; it just means that it may not happen as fast as you hoped or on the first try.

Henri Leridon, Ph.D., an epidemiologist with the French Institute of Health and Medical Research, researched this topic in a report in a 2004 issue of *Human Reproduction*. The study took into consideration a variety of details and determined the following.

Of women who try in vitro fertilization:

Thirty percent will give birth at age thirty.

Twenty-four percent will give birth at age thirty-five.

Seventeen percent will give birth at age forty.

What this says to us is that women need to have realistic expectations. IVF rates vary from country to country (with the U.S. having some of the highest success rates), clinic to clinic, and doctor to doctor. Do your research. Find doctors and clinics with the highest success rates.

Do what you need to do to up your personal chances of success—change your diet and exercise regimen, quit smoking, and so on. Taking good care of ourselves really doesn't change the biological clock. It comes back to priorities. If you want a baby and are over thirty-five, don't delay. Get aggressive sooner rather than later. If you don't get pregnant in an IVF cycle, ask what could be reviewed or changed to optimize a better chance of success the next time. Don't get suckered into the "just keep doing it; we'll get it right some time" game. Some clinics move to the next IVF without reevaluating the situation. As a result, couples may miss opportunities of fresh and more detailed looks at their problems and the reasons their IVF cycles are failing to result in babies.

Legal Questions

When you choose to use donor sperm and eggs, you need to be aware of the potential legal issues. What would happen if the sperm or the egg donor decides to assert parental rights? Unless you have covered all your legal bases (and we aren't lawyers, but we hire them), those donors will most likely be successful. In 2004, a Pennsylvania court ruled in favor of a woman hired by a single man to be a surrogate mother. The woman decided she wanted to assert her parental rights. The judge agreed.

You must think about these things ahead of time. What would happen to your family if your sperm and/or egg donor decides he or she wants to be part of your child's life? Don't assume the legal system will protect you. Even anonymous donors could litigate their ways through the courts should they want to find "their" babies.

What if you have no biological tie to your children? What if you are a single, older mother, like Aleta St. James, who used both a sperm and egg donor? What do you tell your children? How do they fill out their genealogical tree at school? In an odd way, they are almost like adopted children—adopted egg, and adopted sperm.

Do you tell your kids a donor was involved? What if the kids decide they want to find their "biological parents?" What if the egg and/or sperm donors don't want to be found? Currently, courts rarely respect anonymity in the face of such requests.

These are questions both couples and single would-be parents need to answer before going forward with any procedures.

JULIE

With my first pregnancy, Dr. Cohen suggested I do daily shots of heparin, a blood thinner. I have an antibody problem that causes clotting, and we hoped the heparin would prevent clots in the placenta as it formed. While the other drugs I was taking to support my pregnancy would be tapered off once the placenta kicked in and started doing its job, heparin would be my daily companion for the duration of the pregnancy.

Heparin shots use tiny short needles, but they hurt. Within a week, both my upper thighs were covered with black-and-blue-and-green bruises. It was awful. I cried every night when Robert shot me up. I was so stressed, my husband even commented that surely my attitude couldn't be good for the baby.

Unfortunately, I lost that baby at eight weeks. (Nobody blamed my stress over the heparin.) When I got pregnant the second time, I told Robert, "I can't do the heparin." He agreed.

We shared our decision with our OB/GYN, and asked Dr. Yarbrough what other options we had. Baby aspirin, he said, reminding us that heparin was better; heparin was what Dr. Cohen had recommended. Robert and I weighed the choices and did more research, knowing our decision might result in a placental clot that could harm or kill our unborn child. We took full responsibility for our choice and went with the baby aspirin. Dr. Yarbrough supported our choice, but let Dr. Cohen assume we were doing heparin. Why have two doctors worrying for nine months?

Make Informed Decisions

Having fertility treatments means you'll be making dozens of decisions—some of them heartrending. Some need to be made immediately, but most decisions can be made with some thought and consideration. Unless a situation is life-threatening to the mother, we suggest you take your time when you make these decisions.

Our friend Martha, who lives on Long Island, wants you to hear her story. "All my life, I dreamed of having kids. That's what I wanted."

When Martha was five and a half months pregnant with her first child, she went in for an amniocentesis. The results came back fine, but the sonogram didn't look right to the doctor. He determined that the baby's head was not fusing properly, and that he would not live beyond one day after birth. He recommended that Martha terminate the pregnancy. A medical professional herself, Martha immediately sent the films for a second opinion. She got the same diagnosis from the second doctor. Distraught, she and her husband decided to terminate the pregnancy, which was too far along for a D&C. Her labor was induced, so she could deliver the baby in a hospital. While the doctors told her it would "be all over in twenty-four hours," she labored for three days.

"I felt like my baby boy was fighting *not* to come out," says Martha. "It was awful."

When the baby was born, he was not only breathing, but there was also nothing wrong with him. His head was fine, just a small skin growth on the back of his head that could have been easily removed later. The doctors made a mistake. Martha's perfect son died in the palm of her hand.

It is impossible to fathom the depth of this tragedy. "If I had to do it again, I would take more sonograms, get more opinions," she says. "My advice to other women is take your time, and get your information." Martha did eventually give birth to a healthy daughter.

Do not make rash decisions in the heat of the moment. Wait. Take a deep breath. Think. Get a few more (at least three or as many as you need) opinions. If something doesn't feel right in your gut, go with your instinct—whether it is a treatment protocol, an adoption or surrogate situation, or a suggested termination of a pregnancy.

When Bad Things Keep Happening to Good People

Although our friend Martha with the misdiagnosed sonogram eventually did give birth to a healthy daughter, but her saga continues. Martha and her husband wanted more children. So soon after her daughter's birth, Martha got pregnant again, only to suffer a miscarriage at six weeks. She then got pregnant again and had another miscarriage at eight weeks. Finally, after a few months, she became pregnant with another little girl. When the amnio came back, the couple was told their baby had Turner's syndrome, a genetic disease in which there is a complete, or partial, absence of one of the two X chromosomes normally found in girls. One of the most common chromosomal abnormalities, Turner's syndrome occurs in approximately one out of every 2,500 live female births annually. Common characteristics of this syndrome include a short stature and no ovarian development, as well as the possibility of a webbed neck; turned out arms; cardiovascular, kidney, and thyroid problems; curvature of the spine; and hearing problems.

Martha opted to terminate this pregnancy as well. Again she delivered this baby in the hospital. After this Martha picked herself up from the depths of despair and got pregnant again, only to miscarry at eight weeks. On the seventh try, she got pregnant and didn't miscarry. The amnio can back fine. At six and a half months one evening she felt the baby boy kicking furiously. She thought it was odd and commented it to her mother on the phone. The next day she had a scheduled sonogram. Shockingly, the baby was dead. No reason given. Martha had to deliver him in the hospital—again—surrounded by all the same nurses and doctors from her previous deliveries. Pathology reports came back with no reason for the baby's death.

In total, Martha had seven pregnancies, three miscarriages, four deliveries, and only one living baby. After seeing various specialists about her experiences, Martha was told she was simply experiencing "bad luck." There was no other explanation. Our thoughts are that maybe some of the currently "investigational" and "not politically correct" tests were not done at the time. We'll never know.

Sometimes bad things simply happen to good people.

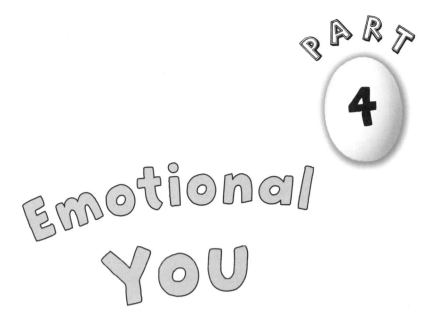

PART 4

Emotional YOU

Infertility is not only a physical burden. It's insanely emotional as well.

There are hormone injections that make you weep one moment and contemplate manslaughter the next. There's the giddiness of a positive pregnancy test followed by the gut-wrenching news of miscarriage. How do you deal with your best friend's baby shower, your brother's bumbling attempts to make you feel better, the melancholy of miscarriage, your nosy neighbor's inane comments all while deciding who you should kill first, your husband or your doctor.

You are so not alone. Neither of us ever thought trying to conceive would be such an emotionally draining experience—the highs, the lows, the thrills, the spills. We're emotionally exhausted just reliving it again while writing this book.

Julie

I never thought I would be that one-in-six statistic who would be infertile, or that one-in-five woman who loses her prized pregnancy to miscarriage. But I was, and nothing prepares you for that gut-punch to your psyche. The shock, the loss, the guilt, and the insanity can make you nuts.

Infertility's emotional low points were balanced by the births of my son and daughter, which were the highest of highs. My kids are still the high points of my life, even when they make me nuts. It is a privilege to parent them.

Maureen

Infertility challenged me in ways even I can't believe. I had to pull myself together after each heartache and despair and continue to move ahead. The pain of missed cycles, missed opportunities, and miscarriage never really goes away. It lives with me forever. The sorrow, while buried, is part of who I am now.

Infertility challenges your emotions. This emotional journey will change you as a person forever. The reality of this is humbling, yet you will triumph. Like us, you will find your family.

CHAPTER 11

Who to KILL ...
Your DOCTOR or
Your HUSBAND?

Julie

Here is what I have learned about fertility drug therapy.

Fertility drugs are expensive.

Clomid is a waste of time for me.

Progesterone suppositories are messy because they melt inside your vagina, then drizzle out.

Parlodel makes me so light-headed I have to pencil extra time into my schedule just to stand up.

Shots (any kind, but particularly the blood thinner heparin) can really hurt.

Traveling with natural progesterone suppositories means you have to pack a small cooler with frozen packs or baggies of ice because this drug has to be kept cool.

Also, it takes forever to explain all the vials of powdered HCG (human chorionic gonadotropin) and the big stash of syringes to an airline-security agent, and the people in line behind you *will* get irritated. At least the daily dose of baby aspirin is not suspicious, pain-free, and cheap. Did I mention that fertility drugs are expensive?

And I won't even go into the hormone-induced rages and weepiness that left my husband, Robert, backed against the kitchen sink, eyes wide, wondering what the heck happened to his happy-go-lucky wife.

If illicit drugs had all the cost, hassle, and just half the side effects of fertility drugs, I don't think we'd have as many addicts.

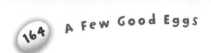

When my reproductive endocrinologist advised that I start taking Clomid, my first question was, "What are the side effects?" He told me I might have hormonal mood swings, some bloating, and general malaise. I had great reservations about it all—I don't like my body being invaded by a drug.

Within a month of taking Clomid, everything about me was swollen—my boobs, stomach, legs, and head. I turned into a big-breasted hell on wheels. Hormonal mood swings? Please. I was homicidal! I didn't just hate everybody. . . . I wanted to kill them. I just couldn't figure out who to kill first—my husband or my doctor.

On top of all this, I became hoarse. It was difficult to speak, and for me that is criminal! My ear, nose, and throat doctor sent cameras down my throat and found I had severe edema in my vocal cords. They were swollen, too.

When I asked if this could be a result of the Clomid, my doctor claimed no study had ever shown swelling in the vocal cords. I would have screamed, but no sound could come out. If my body could swell, why not my vocal chords? This horror went on for more than five months with no successful conception and, fortunately, no murder. I went off Clomid, and eventually my vocal cords relaxed—along with my weight, my personality, and my husband.

Ten Tips for Handling Hormone Havoc

1. Realize it's the drugs that are making you crazy.
2. Keep telling yourself weight gain is good.
3. Remember that fertility drugs may help you get pregnant—they are supposed to be your friend.
4. You're crying because of the drugs, not just because you're sad.
5. Consider telling people you deal with daily that you are on hormone therapy, so you don't end up friendless or fired due to crazy behavior.
6. Make friends with your new body.
7. Make friends with your new mind.
8. Enjoy and accept your insanity.
9. All of us want to kill someone at some point while fertility drugs are in our system. Don't act on it.
10. Accept that this, too, shall pass.

Infertility Is a Total Body Experience

Hormonal hazards are part of the infertility game—kind of like the sand traps on a golf course. But unlike those pesky sand traps, it's hard to find advice on getting through them. So let's talk about it.

Most fertility drugs prescribed are hormones or affect hormones that deal with your reproductive function, and that entails major mood swings, PMS, crying jags, and the surprise fertility treatment bonus—weight gain. This is weird science at its finest. Expect it to affect every part of your body, mind, and soul. These drugs can wreak havoc on your life, your husband's life, your boss's life, the dry cleaner's life—really, the life of just about everybody who gets in your way.

While you are on fertility drugs, you can kiss the old you good-bye and greet the new you—the new and insane you: the crazy lady who occasionally came calling in the past along with PMS but who now permanently resides in your every waking minute.

Our friend Wendy turned into her evil twin when her doctor put her on a double dose of Clomid. It was not pretty—but in hindsight, predictable.

"I was wacko," says Wendy, who was thirty-nine at the time. "I became an insane person, someone I didn't recognize. I used to scream at people on the street for no reason. It was like an out-of-body experience. I was glad when it was over. So was everyone who knew me."

Your Body as a Biochemistry Experiment

When you begin fertility treatments, you are going back to science class, and you are the experiment. Once your doctor has pinpointed your particular problem, he or she will most likely suggest a cocktail of fertility drugs to solve it. What your doctor is really doing with these drugs is trying to tweak the hormone production of your reproductive system. Some drugs stimulate hormone production, and others shut it down. Used in conjunction with one another, these drugs can actually let your doctor run the whole monthly show. At this point, you are not in control of the mother ship.

Drugs this powerful affect many parts of your body. The side effect of certain drugs like clomiphene citrate (Clomid or Serophene) or human menopausal gonadotropins (Pergonal or Repronex) may be an increase in the number of eggs released each month, raising the chance for multiple babies. Your doctor will give you a list of most of the other side effects—fatigue, nausea, dizziness, and so on. None of the literature we read, however, detailed that these drugs have the potential to make you nuts . . . and fat. By the way, side effects like blurry vision, severe headaches, abdominal pain, or painful legs are not good and should be reported to your doctor ASAP.

Your doctor needs to monitor you carefully to see how your reproductive system is handling these strong drugs. Depending on the drug cocktail you are ingesting, you may be in the doctor's office daily for blood work and/or sonograms and/or pelvic exams. While it's a pain to get out of work or travel to the crosstown clinic that often, monitoring is the only way to make sure you are being given the right medicine or amount of medicine to do the trick safely. By monitoring, your doctor will know to raise or lower the amount of medicine you're taking.

Occasionally, fertility drug therapies can lead to ovarian hyperstimulation syndrome, a rare but serious side effect. (According to the American Society of Reproductive Medicine, severe ovarian hyperstimulation syndrome occurs in less than 1 percent of all women undergoing assisted reproductive technology.) We've heard how awful this is—ten years ago, our friend Candy suffered from hyperstimulation and gained almost 90 pounds in three weeks. She was taking part in a medical study and was placed on large doses of fertility drugs. Fortunately, her doctors caught the problem, and she is fine now. This is why monitoring is crucial. Monitoring also ensures that you don't suffer fertility drug fiascos like overstimulated or ruptured ovaries, or maybe worse of all, conceiving six, seven, or even eight babies that end up handicapped, miscarried, or born horribly premature. More common, however, is the inconvenience and expense of frequent monitoring. On the bright side, consider this to be a great opportunity to learn to read an ultrasound of your ovaries and uterine lining. To minimize hassles, ask where the monitoring is done before you begin. Ideally, it should all take place in your doctor's office the way Julie's monitoring was handled. If you can't find a shop with one-stop monitoring, at least be sure you are not having the sonogram done in one building of the hospital complex, and your blood drawn at the other side in another building, like our friend Samantha.

A thirty-four-year-old West Coast furniture designer, Samantha had to drag herself between her doctor who was in one building, the ultrasound technician in another building, and the nurse who did blood work in yet another building.

"Not that I ever really dressed up for the clinic anyway," says Samantha, now the mother of four-year-old IVF twins. "But I remember specifically wearing running shoes so that I could make the trek without breaking a blister. One time, I wore a pedometer for the heck of it. To do that loop between offices was half a mile. One month, I put in about ten miles just getting checked out while on drugs."

By the way, a real fertility clinic is not closed on weekends. We've said this before, but it bears repeating—infertility is a 24/7 situation. We don't just ovulate Monday through Friday, 9:00 A.M. to 5:00 P.M. It's mandatory that you be monitored after-hours and on weekends. That is not asking too much.

The Fertility Pharmacy

Let's take a look at some of the most common fertility drugs your doctor might prescribe. Don't be surprised if your doctor advises you to take a combination of these. Also, the industry changes constantly, so no doubt there will be a bevy of new or investigational wonder drugs that will be available by the time this book is printed. Use the following as a guide to quiz your doctor on what he or she is prescribing, why, and what its effect may be on you.

Clomiphene citrate: Also known as Clomid or Serophene, clomiphene citrate is your fertility "gateway" drug—the first tool in the toolbox most doctors pick up. (For ease here, we'll just refer to it as Clomid.) Simply put, Clomid works to increase the amount of FSH released by your pituitary gland, and this may result in more than one egg being produced in a cycle. Because Clomid superstimulates ovulation, there is a chance that you might release multiple eggs each month, and this could result in multiple births.

If you are prescribed this drug, we would suggest questioning the doctor about his plans for doing a mid-cycle ovarian sonogram to determine whether Clomid is (1) working, (2) working too well by creating ovarian overstimulation, or (3) you are pregnant. Ovarian overstimulation results in your ovaries producing too many eggs, becoming enlarged, or becoming cystic—not good.

Clomid can also be given to men to stimulate FSH and LH as well as sperm production.

By the way, Clomid is very similar in structure to the drug diethylstilbestrol, more commonly known by its acronym DES, a synthetic estrogen prescribed during the 1950s and 1960s to help prevent miscarriages. If taken during pregnancy, Clomid can be associated with metaplastic changes of the reproductive tract similar to those seen in the offspring of women who took DES during pregnancy. Therefore, it is essential to avoid inadvertently taking Clomid if you are pregnant.

The side effects of Clomid include hot flashes, nausea, headaches, weight gain, mood swings, blurred vision, and abdominal pain if suffering from ovarian overstimulation.

Pergonal/Repronex: Pergonal and Repronex are for women who don't normally produce (enough) estrogen and who do not respond to Clomid. Unlike Clomid, which comes in pill form, Pergonal is delivered by a shot to the butt.

JULIE

Clomid is usually the first fertility drug prescribed, whether you need it or not. We say this because it seems Clomid is prescribed right off the bat by gynecologists before a patient is even seen by a fertility specialist. As in, "Oh, you think you might not be able to get pregnant. Hmm. Well, here, let's try some Clomid." Some doctors hand out Clomid to their patients like parents hand out candy to their children—to appease them.

Maureen and I both have several friends who casually (or in a panic!) mentioned their unproductive baby-making sex to their OB/GYNs and walked out minutes later with prescriptions for Clomid. The following month, they were pregnant. We also have friends, ourselves included, for whom Clomid didn't work because it didn't address our particular problems.

When I went in for an annual exam complaining of not getting pregnant after trying for three months, my (former) gyn doctor simply flipped open his prescription pad and wrote out a script for Clomid.

"Here," he said, glancing at his watch. "Take this for a couple months, and let's see what happens." There was no discussion about what he was giving, what it was supposed to do, or why he was doling it out.

I had been with this doctor for several years. It never crossed my mind to ask questions about side effects. It never crossed my mind he should have set up some kind of mid-month monitoring procedure. It never crossed my mind that he should have at least quizzed me about my periods, let alone done some infertility workup first. Nope, I just filled the prescription I didn't need, paid money I could have saved, and took the Clomid, which did nothing for my real problems of low progesterone or scarred uterus. What a waste.

Made from human menopausal gonadotropins (HMGs), this drug provides the LH and FSH necessary to stimulate ovulation. As a result, your ovaries go into overdrive, producing adequate hormone levels and may even expel multiple eggs in a given cycle. It can also be used on men to stimulate sperm production.

By the way, most gynecologists have no experience with these drugs and should refer you to a reproductive endocrinologist if they believe HMGs are the way to go. Your new proactive self should be asking about these drugs and demanding a referral to an RE if you are not pregnant after three Clomid cycles. And it goes without saying that you won't let a gynecologist prescribe these medicines for you, right?

Pergonal has all types of side effects, including weight gain, bloating, fatigue, mood swings, depression, hot flashes, and severe ovarian hyperstimulation syndrome.

Parlodel (bromocriptine): Parlodel is a pill that suppresses prolactin, a hormone produced by the pituitary gland that inhibits ovulation. Women produce prolactin when they are breast-feeding. Producing too much prolactin screws up your ovulation. If you take this drug, you will probably be advised to increase the amount of fluids you consume (except alcohol, which is a huge no-no) and take the medicine with food.

Side effects include headache, stuffy nose, nausea, fatigue, and dizziness. Dizziness and nausea are the most common.

Estradiol: This form of estrogen is used to stimulate the development of the endometrium (the lining of the uterus). Estrogen can be given in pill or injectable forms (estradiol), depending on your particular needs. Estradiol is the natural estrogen your body produces. In women who have too much of estrogen, either naturally or artificially, the endometrium can become too lush and possibly precancerous. This is why it is imperative to use estrogen only as directed by your doctor.

Side effects include dizziness, light-headedness, headache, upset stomach, bloating, or nausea. If you take the pill form, take it with food or right after a meal. If you take the shot form, bite a bullet—it could be painful.

Bravelle: While similar in effect to HMGs like Pergonal and Repronex, Bravelle is actually pure FSH. If your ovaries produce to much biological LH either on their own or stimulated by other drugs, Bravelle is often prescribed to try to get some balance. It is also prescribed to women who suffer ovarian hyperstimulation on other drugs. Other medications similar to Bravelle are Gonal F and Follistim—also pure FSH. By the way, these drugs are no more efficient, but some may be more expensive than the others, so ask your doctor if he or she prescribes one over the others.

Side effects of Bravelle include weight gain, bloating, fatigue, mood swings, depression, and hot flashes, just like Pergonal and Repronex.

Progesterone: It is a drug derivative of the hormone that helps create the lush uterine lining crucial to implantation and nourishment of a fertilized egg. It also works to keep the uterus relaxed when a woman is pregnant. Progesterone is prescribed in three forms: shot, pill, or vaginal suppository. It's also available in natural or synthetic form (we recommend only the natural as synthetic progestins have been associated with increased risk of birth defects and miscarriage).

Side effects are the same as if you were pregnant, which can be confusing: tender breasts, bloatedness, nausea, and slightly elevated body temperature.

Lupron (leuprolide acetate): Unlike the other fertility drugs that stimulate your hormones, a regiment of Lupron shuts them down, putting the ovaries to sleep—like menopause. Lupron actually suppresses the pituitary's ability to stimulate the ovaries. This injectable drug puts your doctor in charge of when the ovaries will start up again, so as to prevent ovulation from occurring before your eggs can be retrieved.

Some doctors use Lupron to coordinate your ovaries to the ovaries of an egg donor so you ovulate at the same time. It is also used for IVF treatment cycles, where research shows Lupron use increases IVF pregnancy rate. Lupron makes it easier for your doctor to schedule procedures with the precision needed. Antagon (Ganirelix) is another LH antagonist that has gained in popularity in IVF treatment cycles.

Side effects for Lupron are similar to menopause—hot flashes, vaginal dryness, depression, irritability, and increased body hair. Oh joy. Well, think of it as practice for the real thing.

Where's the Drugstore?

Having a drug prescription is not enough. You have to find a pharmacy to fill it. If you live in a big city, no problem. But if you don't, frustration can occur. Don't start any medicines unless you have the full dosage. Few things are worse than taking that last Pergonal shot or progesterone suppository because the hometown pharmacy promises they'll have the rest in tomorrow and then doesn't. Without taking the medicine on time, you will waste not only the drugs you've ingested and the money you've spent, but also another month trying to get pregnant. Do not let this happen to you.

Be sure you have everything you need in hand before you start the process. Ask your doctor to recommend a pharmacy. The REs know who can and can't provide the goods in a timely fashion. Some of these drugs have to be compounded on site, so you want someone who knows what they are doing. Because Julie lived in a small-town suburb of Dallas at the time of her treatment, she always had her prescriptions filled in the hospital pharmacy where her clinic was located. It was quicker, easier, and more efficient to use the big-city pharmacy than trying to find someone in her own town.

Hormonal Hazards

Losing your mind, gaining weight, weirding out—it's just fertility drugs doing their job. You're not insane, just out of balance. You're not alone. Every other woman sitting in the clinic's waiting room is experiencing (or about to experience) the same thing. This was comforting for us to discover; we weren't the only ones feeling like soft, pudgy, dough girls who somehow had to entice their husbands to the bedroom while wanting to strangle them for not bringing home the dry cleaning we forgot to tell them to pick up. The best way to describe the drug-induced hormonal mood swings that make murder manageable? PMS to the max.

Our friend Darcie didn't handle the hormonal havoc very well. "Part of the reason I was so quick to move forward to IVF was that I didn't want to stay in the 'body as biochemistry experiment' any longer," says this forty-something mom of fraternal twins. "The various drugs I was on changed me; I gained a lot of weight, became lethargic, very depressed, dealt with a lot of drug-induced ovulation pain. I felt like a miserable, fat cow, and I could not enjoy any aspect of life in that state.

"It's too easy, I think, when you're in the thick of things, to think that the mood changes are because of the emotional stress of the situation—with me, it was clearly drug-induced. Taking breaks on the treatments really helped me to realize that, yes, just facing the fact of infertility is depressing, but I could function well in life; I was happy and enjoyed life when I wasn't on the drugs, despite my sadness about not getting pregnant. When I went back on the drugs, my mood plummeted."

Since we know drug therapy to get you pregnant may make you nuts in the short term, and so you don't go through a fiasco like Darcie, ask these questions before filling your prescription.

Questions to Ask Before Ingesting Any Medicine (Bring a notepad. Write the answers down. Refer back.)

1. What are you prescribing for me . . . in English, please? And what exactly does it do?
2. Why do I need this particular drug?
3. What do we hope will be accomplished during this drug therapy?
4. What side effects should I be aware of? Looking for? Calling immediately about?
5. How is this drug therapy going to affect the rest of my body? (Will I gain weight or get hormonal?)
6. Is there anything I should/shouldn't do while on this drug?
7. How safe is this drug . . . really?
8. What are alternatives to this drug?
9. How do you monitor me while I am on this drug?
10. Is your clinic open on weekends to monitor me?

MAUREEN

One evening, while on Clomid, I went to the movies with my husband and son. I am a fairly patient person, but this evening, I felt the sharp edge of Clomid-induced agitation. Still, I hoped the light comedy we came to see would ease my hormonal mind. I settled in with popcorn and my men.

Once the movie started, I noticed a group of young girls in the front rows. They kept getting up from their seats, running in and out of the theater noisily and disturbing everyone. I missed whole scenes of the movie because of them. In and out they went many times, making a racket.

Their timing could not have been worse. Here I was, trying so hard to have a baby, and these kids were out of control—clearly because their parents didn't give a damn about disciplining them. Their parents had just dropped them off at the theater and left. All of these thoughts and emotions started to fester inside of me. I could feel them rising like lava in a smoldering volcano.

I started to tap my feet; Will tried to soothe me—no go. My eyes were so blurry with rage, I couldn't see the screen. I shouted at them a few times as they raced out of the theater. Suddenly, the most important scene in the movie came up, the one where the actor was explaining why he was commitment phobic. Again the girls jumped up with a raucous indifference and exited the theater. I missed the most important line in the movie!

That was it. My internal Clomid-fueled volcano blew up. I jumped up and ran after them screaming. Will and Quinn were stunned. The rest of the theater, probably relieved. This raving hormonal crazy woman was fixing the problem. I was at a new level of aggression—one my own family had never seen, let alone a theater of strangers. When I got to the theater door, the girls were trying to come back in. I opened the door and told them they were not allowed back into the theater.

They were stunned. One teenager said, "You can't yell at us!" which enraged me even more.

"Someone has to do it," I screamed back, slamming the door in their nasty little faces. I stood by the door of the theater and held it closed with all my might to prevent their reentering the theater—Me against five thirteen-year-olds. They didn't go easily. They screamed, kicked, and pushed the door, but I stood firm. I remember my adrenaline pumping—Clomid courage! There was no way even a stampede of bulls was going to get through those doors. This is what fertility drugs can do to you.

When the movie was over (I missed the rest of it because I was standing guard), I opened the doors. The girls were gone, thank God. I proceeded directly to management, followed by a still stunned Will and Quinn, complained, and ended up with free tickets to that movie theater.

I still have those tickets. Why? Because we have a baby now, and we have no time to go to the movies.

When Weight Gain Is Good

Weight gain is another surprise fertility treatment bonus. We know this will upset some people, but the hormone therapy necessary to help you conceive will most likely also make you fat. But wait—in this instance, a few extra pounds are actually a good thing. Very thin women can have problems menstruating, and if you aren't menstruating, you aren't getting pregnant. If a woman is too thin, she can lose her period altogether. Women with more cushion, however, boast the fat stores that can push a pregnancy along.

Julie gained twelve pounds within two weeks of hormone therapy. Maureen gained ten. Our friend Peggy gained twenty. Weight gain is pretty unavoidable when you are on fertility drugs. Our fertility doctors all thought we looked great, tons better, more fertile. We just thought we looked tons larger, like supersized, weepier versions of the old us. We tried to feel sexy and rounder in our new, pumped-up-on-hormones, potentially fertile bodies. Wow, we were round in all the right sexy places: boobs, butt, tummy, and thighs. Of course, then we had to look in the magazines and remind ourselves that all those skinny actresses were not the norm.

Being skinny and boney just doesn't cut it in the fertility game. Enjoy and embrace your roundness. Dress it up, show it off, eat, drink (preferably not alcohol), and have babies. You can go on a diet later. As Maureen likes to say, "This is a life thing, not a food thing." Suck it up (or in) and try to enjoy the more womanly you. Fortunately, hormone-induced body fat tends to get back under control as soon as you quit the drugs. Well, think of it as opportunity to buy a whole new wardrobe. Besides, gaining all that weight is good practice for when you actually do get pregnant.

By the way, if gaining weight is too much of a frightening thought, perhaps you should reconsider having a baby. Gaining the necessary weight is the first selfless move in the motherhood journey. All of us know selflessness is an essential quality for good parenting later.

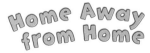

Home Away from Home

When you are doing fertility drugs, you run your existence by a calendar. You have to take your shots and/or pills at certain times every day or on certain days of the month. You will have to be monitored by your doctor certain days of the month. You will have to have sex on certain days of the month. And you will have to do all of this clandestinely, taking an hour or two in the morning to visit the doctor or leaving parties early in the evening to get home for those shots. Unless, of course, you have a really understanding boss or you've told all your friends what you are doing.

Our friend Deb is an East Coast schoolteacher who went through three years of fertility treatment before giving birth at thirty-six to her son and two years later to her daughter (unaided! after she'd given up hope!). She kept her treatments secret, which was quite the juggle.

"I wished so much had been more out in the open," she says now. "I mean, it all seemed like such a secret 'illness' or somehow something that could not be talked about. For example, I had to tell my principal I would be late for school every day for several days a month, and I didn't tell her why, just that it was a health problem. I'm not sure why I didn't tell her; I guess I just didn't feel comfortable enough—and I didn't want to be asked if it was working, I guess. Luckily I was team teaching, otherwise I can't imagine how I could have done it."

For Deb, the logistics of scheduling the doctor appointments was extremely disruptive. Her job situation was not flexible. "I don't know how people who travel for work manage it all," she says.

The mid-month monitoring can be a pain. This has to be done at the clinic and usually involves drawing more blood and/or sonograms. Driving an hour to the fertility clinic while under the influence of very expensive fertility drugs, well, talk about road rage. A short-tempered, exhausted, fat woman with a touch of depression and maybe a headache, all drug-induced, on purpose, driving in traffic en route to the fertility clinic—we'd get out of your way, too.

So how to handle the stress of practically living at the doctor's office—other than remembering you are not dealing with a sane you? Check out books on tape from the library or buy a satellite radio for the car trip. Use the time to catch up on phone calls. Read all those magazines in the doctor's office (we particularly like doctors with copies of *People*). Keep repeating the mantra "this too shall pass." The silver lining? Once you go off the drugs, you will revert back to the person everyone knew and loved—and hopefully have a baby.

The manic moodiness is a living nightmare. If you don't have a sense of humor it will make you nuts. The best thing to do? Dance with the chaos. Accept the weight gain. Laugh at the insanity. Don't kill your husband. Spare your doctor. Remember, it will all come to an end when you go off these drugs. It is just a short stop during the game of trying to create life.

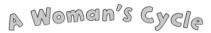
A Woman's Cycle

"I want my wife back." This is the plaintive call of the hormone-haggard husband. Infertility has the ability to weave itself into the very fabric of your soul.

Don't let it define who you are. If you are desperate and at the breaking point, take a break.

Cinda, thirty-nine at the time, did not react well to fertility drugs. She gained a lot of weight, suffered debilitatingly painful mid-cycle cramps, and sweated through hot flashes. Worst of all, she got very, very depressed.

"My RE put me through the paces, cookie-cutter style, like everyone else," says our pal, who eventually gave birth to IVF twins at age forty-one. "Try this, try that, very specific steps. I was on Parlodel, Clomid, then the injectables, then IUI plus injectables. My side effects from Clomid were terrible. And along with the emotional letdown of successive failed attempts, I had arms that looked like a drug addict's from all the blood they had to draw every other day.

"I just felt I could not live my life like this for very long. It was too physically, mentally, and emotionally taxing. When I'd take a month off from treatment, suddenly my mood, energy, everything, returned to normal. My husband would say, 'Welcome back.' I became the person I had always been again."

Amen to that. There's no place like home.

CHAPTER 12
A Pregnant Pause:
MISCARRIAGE

Maureen

I was the first of my friends to have a miscarriage. Most of my pals were in their late thirties, early forties. I learned that single career women are not the best post-miscarriage shoulders to cry on. All of them said the wrong things very lovingly. They sent flowers. They had good intentions but no experience.

My family wasn't much better. My mother told me it was for the best, "and besides, you don't really need another baby, Maureen." No help there. My sister one-upped my miscarriage with her own story—how her (now ex-) husband told her she was ruining his Super Bowl party by having a miscarriage. It wasn't about me and making me feel better, it was about her and her miscarriage. She was trying to help, and her intentions were good, but it didn't comfort me. Nothing could. My father cried. I never heard from my brothers.

There is no emotional indulgence in my family. In a way, it's good because it shortened the grieving time for me. I learned to handle it myself. Sometimes grieving alone can make you go insane, and at other times it can strengthen your overall character. My mother kept telling me these miscarriages would "build character," but by the third miscarriage, I didn't want any more character. I had enough, and I cried. I wanted my babies. I still miss them.

My best friend, Dee Dee, who had no children at the time, sent me a short, comforting paperback book on grieving over a miscarriage. She didn't know what to say (you'll find few who do). Receiving this book during that sad and lonely time was more helpful than she will ever know.

Julie

Here's how it has gone for me: Can't get pregnant. Infertility treatments. Still can't get pregnant. Prepare to adopt. Get pregnant. Miscarry. Get pregnant. Have a son. Get pregnant with twins. Lose one immediately. Miscarry the other midterm. Get pregnant. Have a daughter. Get pregnant. Lose another baby.

The fear of maybe miscarrying yet again prevented Robert and me from trying to get pregnant anymore. Miscarriage is emotionally draining, and we came to a point where we just couldn't go through it anymore. You are excited and pregnant one day, minus a baby and depressed the next. And when you do get pregnant and carry a child for nine months, you worry endlessly every day until that baby is placed in your arms. When the thought of being pregnant again scared me, I knew I had lost my warrior spirit—the mentality necessary to fight for any more children.

My multiple miscarriages did have a silver lining of sorts. They helped us figure out some of my fertility issues. In turn, that information helped me carry my subsequent healthy pregnancies to term.

Honestly, however, I'd rather have all those lost babies than all the knowledge garnered from the ordeal. But I know I'm one of the lucky ones. I ended up with two healthy babies. And four I'll meet up with in heaven someday.

This was on one of the cards I received from a friend after a miscarriage. It still speaks to me.

"In one of the stars I shall be living. In one of them I shall be laughing. And so it will be as if all the stars were laughing when you look at the sky at night."

—The Little Prince by Antoine de Saint-Exupery

Ten Things No One Tells You About Miscarriage

1. You probably know several women who've suffered a miscarriage. They just haven't told you.
2. Nothing can prepare you for the loss you will feel.
3. When you miscarry further along in a pregnancy, your body may act like you delivered the baby and produce milk.
4. Miscarriage hurts both emotionally and physically.
5. Miscarriage knows no socioeconomic boundaries.

6. Most women don't talk about their miscarriages.

7. You can't expect your friends, family, and/or husband to understand your grief.

8. You will bleed a lot after a miscarriage.

9. You will feel alone.

10. You will feel guilty, but you *should not*.

The Melancholy of Miscarriage

Miscarriages happen. A lot. To everyone. It's just that women don't talk about it very much. And until recently, you never heard a celeb or famous person admitting to miscarriage misery.

But one out of every five pregnancies ends in a miscarriage. Sometimes you miscarry without even knowing it. Before we had those pee-on-a-stick pregnancy tests, many women who had what they thought were just late periods were actually miscarrying.

These early detection pregnancy tests have their plus sides. They also catch pregnancies that aren't viable. We have friends who took the test, got the "I'm pregnant" double lines, and by the time they got to the doctor a few days later, were no longer pregnant.

While unsettling and surprising when it happens to you, miscarriage is actually pretty common. According to statistics provided by the American College of Obsetrics and Gynecology, one in five pregnancies ends in miscarriage. That translates to 20 percent of all pregnancies. Most of these miscarriages happen in the first three months.

Thanks to high-tech equipment, sonograms, and blood work, doctors can tell if a woman has lost a baby before she notices any symptoms. A woman strolls into the office, beaming because two weeks ago she found out she's pregnant only to discover she's lost her baby, needs a D&C, and they can do it tomorrow. Whoa!

There is something heartrending about losing a child you only knew through black-and-white sonogram shots. You grieve not for what was, but for what could have been. You cannot intellectualize miscarriage.

There are also the physical realities of miscarriage, which nobody bothers to tell you about! Having a miscarriage when you are further along in your pregnancy than just a few weeks puts your body through the same rigors of childbirth—such as labor—except you don't walk out of the hospital with a baby. In addition to their loss, women who miscarry also have to deal with the hormonal shake-ups of new mothers. You may experience night sweats; your milk may come in, making your boobs hard as rocks with no child to relieve the pressure. We have this from a good source—our own bodies.

What Did I Do Wrong? Probably Nothing.

When you have a miscarriage, the first thing you worry about is what you did wrong. Let's eliminate some guilt. You did not miscarry because of any of the following reasons:

- You rode the exercise bike too long.
- You drank a glass of wine at dinner last night.
- You sat or stood too close to the TV, the computer screen, or the microwave oven.
- God is mad at you.
- You had raunchy sex with your partner.
- You had an abortion at one time in your life.

You need to know for your own psyche that you probably did nothing wrong at all. We'll look at some of the real reasons for miscarriage in a minute.

Early Miscarriage

Don't let anyone tell you that miscarriage at six, seven, or eight weeks isn't tough. You might not be very far along in your pregnancy, but you are pregnant. It's easy to become attached early to something you have been wanting for a long, long time.

If you ask around, you will discover a lot of early miscarriages, even among your friends and family members who went on to have problem-free pregnancies. Julie never knew her own mother had suffered a miscarriage until she had one of her own, and they finally got to talking about it.

Gail, a twenty-eight-year-old administrative assistant, had been trying to conceive for a year when they finally sought help. The doctor put her on Clomid, and she became pregnant on the first cycle.

"We were elated," she says. "Then I miscarried when I was six weeks along. It was devastating. It really took me several months to accept that my baby was gone. I piled on the guilt for not pushing for progesterone and more tests. I cried myself to sleep for weeks."

Gail and her husband tried to get pregnant again for a few years, but with no success. "The hardest thing for me?" she says. "Watching my friends have babies. I couldn't bring myself to go to baby showers. I was a bitter woman. I wonder if I should give up on kids altogether—and I'm still young!"

Midterm Miscarriage

Midterm miscarriage means losing your baby in the second trimester, which is even more devastating. These pregnancies often fail because the uterine envi-

MAUREEN

It was Quinn's first day of kindergarten; my husband and I brought him to his classroom with tears in our eyes. I was twelve weeks pregnant and one of three expectant mothers in the classroom. Everyone knew we were having a baby—even Quinn. I was also thrilled to know as I kissed my son good-bye that I had another life growing inside of me.

I drove to the doctor for my twelve-week appointment, where I spent one hour with the nurse practitioner going through all the details of my delivery, due date (which happened to be my mother's birthday), and so on. Finally, I jumped on the table, so she could check the heartbeat. I see it in slow motion now—the heartbeat monitor being laid on my belly and no sound coming through. In that one moment, everything changed. A sonogram showed what we couldn't hear—a small black sac with a dead fetus my body had not yet expelled. My body, like my mind, wouldn't let go.

"I'm so sorry," she said. "Your baby is gone."

My choices? Schedule a D&C to remove it or wait to miscarry, which could take up to three months. I drove back to school to pick up Quinn in a daze. When I got there I hugged him, a smile pasted on my face. My husband was there, too. When we got in the car, my husband asked excitedly about the appointment. I replied simply, "Oh, it was fine."

I wanted to spare my son any unnecessary heartache, but children are more perceptive than we give them credit. Quinn looked up from his booster seat in the back and said, "That baby is gone, isn't it Mama?"

Stunned and teary, I answered yes. Will's jaw dropped. It was a quiet trip home.

The next day I had a D&C, my doctor sucking my baby out of me while I lay there. The horror still lives with me to this day. Unfortunately there are things in life that are out of our control. This was one of them. I just had to accept that, and try to move on.

ronment in which the baby is growing can no longer support the pregnancy. In some cases, there are problems with the baby itself. But you've had much more time to be pregnant and excited.

The hardest part, in our opinion, is that all of us hold our breaths until that magic first three months is past, then breathe a sigh of relief. Most pregnancies that survive that critical stage will make it the next six months, but not all of them. Again, we speak from experience.

When you miscarry at this time, different doctors do different things. Some doctors will make you deliver the baby you are losing as if it were a normal pregnancy. You will go through labor even though the baby will die or is already dead. Other doctors will put to you to sleep and perform a D&E (dilation and evacuation) to ease the mental anguish you will experience. Still others will do neither and send you to an abortion clinic. Most women never ask the tough questions about midterm miscarriage. Be sure you do. Before it happens, ask your doctor what his office prescribes for mid- to late-term miscarriage. You need to know your options, and you might not like the answers you hear.

JULIE

While all miscarriages are tragic, they are particularly so to women who had to fight extra hard to get pregnant. It's crushing to finally become pregnant only to lose your precious baby-to-be while still breathless from pregnancy's thrill.

Miscarriage also takes your words away—along with the words of everyone else. Friends and family have trouble expressing their sorrow or sharing the grief, unless they've been through it, too. When my best friend miscarried years ago, I said all the wrong things. I was still single, not yet bitten by baby hunger. She was married with one daughter. She called me, crying, and said she had just lost a baby. I said something stupid like, "Well, you're lucky you already have a baby," and "It's God's way; something was probably wrong."

What was wrong was everything I said to my friend. I know now I was no help—emotionally out-to-lunch. She should have removed me from her Good Buddy Rolodex, but thankfully she didn't.

When I lost my first baby at eight weeks, after almost two years of trying to conceive, the wrong things I said to my friend came back to me from the inane mouths of others. Suddenly I realized my blunder. Just like I probably didn't comfort her, these friends (who didn't get it) didn't comfort me.

Recurrent Miscarriage

Recurrent miscarriage—suffering three or more miscarriages in a row—is really being put through the ringer. Multiple miscarriages happen to only about 4 percent of women and more than half of those go on to have a baby, but it is no fun along the way. Ask Maureen, who's had her share of baby loss. Or listen to the wise words of our friend Colleen, a fifty-year-old writer who lives in Long Island. She had her daughter at thirty-five and her son at thirty-nine. Along the way, Colleen suffered through fifteen miscarriages. Fifteen! Imagine.

"It took me two years to have my daughter, which I now know was a lucky break, and three years to have my son," she says. "Like a lot of Baby Boomers, I assumed I had plenty of time to have a baby. The world of science, according to my optimistic reading of news articles, promised me years of fertility. My adolescence had lasted through my twenties, and at thirty I was ready to settle down. I married the love of my life and stopped using birth control two years later.

"For the first time, after always getting what I wanted when I wanted it, I didn't," said Colleen. "I felt young, but my eggs knew better. Over the next eight years, I had two beautiful children and fifteen miscarriages, most of them ending ephemeral pregnancies detected with the little urine-testing wands I bought at the pharmacy. Pregnant one day, but not pregnant a week or so later.

"Surviving miscarriage is done only with the help of a supportive spouse and the words of other women who have been through the same experience," Colleen adds. "My mantra was to thank God my body was efficient and able to toss out the bad eggs—think of the alternative. After my daughter, Amy, was born, I began to think the child I was meant to have would be the child who could survive this very tough weeding-out process. My son, Jack, is indeed a warrior child."

In our opinion, not being able to carry a baby to term is a fertility issue just as much as not being able to get pregnant. Fortunately, doctors can figure out what's wrong and fix the problem in about half of the women who have recurrent miscarriage.

Here are the most prevalent reasons for recurrent miscarriages.

- Hit-or-miss chromosomal errors.
- Chromosomal boo-boos passed on to the embryo from Mom, Dad, or both.
- Hormonal abnormalities, including low progesterone.

JULIE

I don't dwell on my past miscarriages, but I remember every one. The first one was at eight weeks, another at seven weeks. But the hardest one was losing our son at seventeen weeks—a healthy little fellow we had come to know as we watched him grow during weekly sonograms at Dr. Yarbrough's office.

It had been a problem pregnancy from the beginning, complete with a vanishing twin, sporadic bleeding, clotting, the works. But naively, I thought once I passed the "magic" three-month period, I was home free. That's what all the pregnancy books told me.

So when Robert and I went to the amnio at sixteen weeks, we were in high spirits. We were past four months. We were safe! I had just bought a slew of maternity clothes in celebration.

But we weren't safe. The sonogram showed a healthy baby, a boy, but very little amniotic fluid. It was seeping out, leaving our son high and dry. The doctor told us he was sorry, but there was no reason to do an amnio. Our baby was healthy, but his environment was not. He left the room with the suggestion we go immediately back to our OB/GYN to discuss this.

I was shaking as I peeled off the hospital gown and pulled my clothes back on. Robert was stunned. We drove in silence across the street to Dr. Yarbrough's office. What was happening?

That's when our doctor told us he had been concerned about the fluid, but hadn't wanted to worry us until he got a second opinion via the amnio specialist. He was sorry. The nurse cried. I cried. Robert was stoic. Our choices now? Pray for a miracle, but expect that I would go into labor and then more choices. I could chose to miscarry (deliver the fetus) at home (and then what? bring it in the next day in a baggie?), or I could come to the hospital when I felt contractions. Those aren't really choices.

A few days later, the unwanted contractions arrived. Cursing my body for its betrayal, I went to the hospital and had them sedate me for the whole thing. When I woke up, I wasn't pregnant anymore.

I sent Robert home and sat in bed staring out the window. My brother stopped by, but he didn't know what to say, so I sent him home, too. It began to rain. Heavy sheets of water pounded the parking lot pavement below; lightning sliced the sky above. Heaven and earth visualized my sorrow. I spent the deep night writing a letter to my lost child, chronicling my feelings onto the pages of a reporter's notebook that I later locked in a drawer with his sonograms.

The next day, Robert and two-year-old Graham came to pick me up. Dr. Yarbrough was in my room, sitting in a chair after finishing his rounds. My son jumped into my lap, and I cried—tears for the other women who have lost babies like me through miscarriage, but who didn't already have someone small to snuggle in their arms and help heal the hurt.

At home, we found a beautiful bouquet from our friends Betty and Barbara. Their card said simply, "Heaven weeps, too."

Those three words summed up the whole event most eloquently.

Now, whenever I drive past Presbyterian Hospital in Dallas, I think about the ashes of this baby, our almost-boy, sprinkled in the memorial garden they maintain for angel children like him. It may be a fleeting thought, a glance, if I'm on the way to the pediatrician with the kids, and the radio is blaring, and someone is demanding my attention, or a momentary prayer if I am in the car alone. I call him R. J.; initials that stand for two names we had considered for a boy.

- Infections.
- An abnormally shaped or scarred uterus that doesn't allow the baby enough room to grow.
- Antiphospholipid antibody syndrome (APLS), an autoimmune disorder.
- Constricted uterine arteries, which cause poor blood flow to the uterus and cut off the oxygen and nutrients to the growing baby.
- A weak cervix that tends to dilate before the baby is ready to be born.

Ten Miscarriage Misconceptions

1. Miscarriage always means there was something wrong with the fetus.
2. Miscarriage always means there is something wrong with you.
3. Miscarriage can't happen after the first three months.
4. Miscarriage won't happen to me!
5. My doctor's explanation of my miscarriage must be true. (We can't blame everything on old eggs!)
6. Miscarriages can't happen twice.
7. The miscarriage was caused by something you did.
8. A miscarriage is no big deal.

9. A miscarriage is God's way of telling you something.
10. Miscarriage means you are a bad person and an unfit mother-to-be.

Miscarriage Causes

Most women who miscarry hear the proverbial "bad luck" as the reason. We're here to tell you most miscarriages happen for a reason that has nothing to do with luck. More than half of all miscarriages are due to a random chromosomal blunder that doesn't happen the next time you get pregnant.

How do you know which type of miscarriage you had? This is tricky, since most doctors won't refer you to a specialist, much less check out the cause of a miscarriage, until you've suffered through two or three miscarriages in a row.

JULIE

The physical realities of miscarriage were almost more shocking to me than the emotional drain. I had *expected* to be depressed and miserable!

Some women lose their baby before they even know they are pregnant—for them, it's just a heavier period when they're a few days late. But if you are a few weeks along, as I was with my first pregnancy, and miscarry, you will go into the hospital for a D&C. Some doctors suggest you let your body spontaneously abort, but your body might not expel everything, and you don't need to worry about infection on top of everything else.

A D&C is an outpatient procedure. By the afternoon, I was home in my own bed watching chick flicks and crying my eyes out.

My next miscarriage, at seventeen weeks, was even more emotional. I knew this baby. I had felt him move, just a butterfly flutter, but movement nonetheless. Physically, however, it was much harder. A second trimester miscarriage throws your body into some of the same rigors of childbirth. You will actually go into labor to expel the fetus, unless you choose to go into the hospital before that occurs. It doesn't stop there. Women, like me, who miscarry later in a pregnancy also have to deal with the hormonal shake-ups of new mothers. They might experience night sweats and mood swings—I had both. Their milk might come in. Mine did. These things are bearable if you have a baby to share them with. Without a baby, they suck.

The physical aspects of miscarriage were something for which I was not prepared. Even if I had known what was coming, I would never have been able to process it all—until I went through it myself.

MAUREEN

After my second miscarriage, I chose to have the fetal matter tested. I wanted to know if it really was old eggs or if something else was wrong.

When I finally had the energy to get up from the table and get myself dressed following my D&C, the nurse asked if I would do them a favor. Could I bring the sample from my pregnancy next door to the hospital for them? In a post-anesthesia fog, I said yes.

It wasn't until I was alone in the elevator going up to the lab that I realized I was holding my baby in the brown paper lunch bag. I wanted to keep that bag. I didn't want to give away a bit of my baby. When I handed the bag to the lab tech, a piece of me died inside. It still baffles me that a nurse would give me that task in the first place.

Unfortunately, their testing showed nothing. They claimed there was not enough tissue present to make a determination. I found myself wondering if my doctor did this intentionally. Perhaps her "old egg" theory wasn't right, this miscarriage could have been prevented, and she didn't want to tell me.

It wasn't until years later when I found out I had low progesterone that I realized my miscarriages had occurred because of my hormone levels, not simply "old eggs." With the addition of a simple progesterone suppository in the beginning of my pregnancies, I'd probably have two more children today.

Most doctors just assume miscarriages happen because of arbitrary chromosomal abnormalities. But it's never good to assume, especially when there are definite symptoms you can look for to determine if your miscarriage is the result of something else. If you can identify the cause, then you might be able to treat it and save your next pregnancy.

Because we are not doctors, you should talk to your own doctor. But based on what we've read and experienced, here are some likely scenarios.

- If you showed no symptoms, only to be told during a sonogram that a heartbeat had never developed or that the heart had stopped beating some time before, most likely, your miscarriage was due to chromosomal misalignment—particularly if you are over thirty-five years old.
- If you experience cramps and bleeding while the baby's heart is still beating, then look for problems in the uterine environment or placenta as the cause of miscarriage.

- If your miscarriage is particularly painless, ask your doctor to check you for possible cervical incompetence.
- If you continue to have miscarriages, ask your doctor to send the fetal tissue for chromosomal testing. (That's one of the reasons women who miscarry at home are given the onerous task of collecting "samples" to bring to the doctor.) If the results come back normal, it is likely that your body is the culprit—not misaligned chromosomes.

Here's a rundown of some of the most common causes of miscarriage.

Chromosomal Defects

Creating a viable pregnancy is much more complicated than just sperm and egg getting together and BOOM!—baby in the making. We'll leave the specifics to the real medical professionals, but here's our take on the basic procedure: your twenty-three-chromosome egg must merge correctly with his twenty-three-chromosome sperm to create one embryo with twenty-three *perfectly matched* pairs of chromosomes. A minor error in this merger can result in extreme genetic boo-boos that embryos can't survive. The result is a miscarriage of some type. If these errors occur early, you might not even know you were pregnant. If they occur later in process, the result could be a blighted ovum (where the embryo doesn't develop, so all you see is the gestational sac) or even a fetus with no heartbeat.

The chance of chromosomal abnormalities increase as you get older. It's those old eggs again. When you are twenty-five, less than 20 percent of your eggs might be chromosomally abnormal. When you hit forty, however, there is probability that as many as 45 percent of them may be abnormal—and up to 75 percent, if you are older than forty. This translates to an increased risk of miscarriage and greater chance of babies with Down syndrome in older women—more reasons not to wait too long to be a mommy.

Chronic Illness

Having a chronic health condition such as uncontrolled diabetes; thyroid problems; or heart, kidney, and liver disease can cause miscarriage. If you suffer from a chronic illness, your doctor should treat you as the high-risk pregnancy you already are. If not, find a doctor who will monitor you closely.

Infections

Some infections can play a role in miscarriage. Toxoplasmosis (from cat litter or eating undercooked beef like rare hamburgers or steak tartare), listeria (from processed meats), malaria (from mosquitoes), chlamydia (a sexually transmitted disease), and mycoplasma (bacterial infection) carry a risk to the fetus. Ditto for German measles, mumps, herpes, parvovirus (also known as fifth disease), and hepatitis A and B.

Fevers

A high fever early in pregnancy can trigger miscarriage. It seems that a core body temperature of 102 degrees or more can be toxic to a tiny embryo, particularly if it occurs before six weeks.

If you get a fever, don't blow it off. Call your doctor immediately and treat the fever right away with acetaminophen, which is safe for pregnant women to take. You might even consider a cool bath or shower while waiting for the fever-buster to kick in.

Of course, it goes without saying that you should stay out of the hot tub. But we'll say it anyway. Stay out of them. There are studies that suggest sitting in a hot tub or whirlpool may increase the risk of miscarriage, especially early in pregnancy. The higher the temperature, the higher the possibility.

You could be pregnant in those early weeks and not even know it. So, better safe than sorry. If you are trying to get pregnant, and there is even the teeniest possibility you might be, stay out of hot tubs and fight any fever that comes your way.

Hormonal Problems

Creating a baby depends on an intricate balancing act starring our hormones. A simple ovulation is an Olympic endeavor. For approximately 15 percent of women who have multiple miscarriages, the hormones involved in their monthly cycles are to blame. There may be too little progesterone produced in the back half of the menstrual cycle, resulting in that "luteal phase defect," which hinders implantation of a fertilized egg and undermines a pregnancy from the start.

For an accurate diagnosis, your doctor can do a blood test and a biopsy of the uterine lining near the end of your menstrual cycle. For treatment, your doctor may suggest ensuring the adequacy of your cycle by taking three to four days of progesterone, beginning after ovulation. If you get pregnant, you may be given progesterone pills and/or suppositories until you reach ten to twelve weeks. (This is what Julie had to do with all her pregnancies.)

Immune System Malfunctions (Antibody Problems)

With immune system malfunctions, your body produces antibodies that essentially attack your own growing baby. The main symptom is recurrent miscarriage and antibody problems that can be diagnosed with blood tests.

Julie had an antibody problem called antiphospholipid antibody syndrome (APLS). Women with APLS produce antibodies that cause their blood to clot in the tiny blood vessels of the placenta—deadly for a developing fetus. Left untreated, these clots can cut off oxygen and nutrients to the embryo, mess with the amniotic fluid, and result in miscarriage.

Fortunately, APLS can be counterbalanced by blood thinners given after ovulation or once you are pregnant. For some, baby aspirin and/or heparin shots will do the trick. For others, like Julie, HCG shots (human chorionic gonadotrophin, a special hormone your placenta manufactures when you're pregnant) are necessary in addition to facilitate growth of the placenta across the surface of the uterus.

Our friend Betsy, a forty-two-year-old Boston paralegal, also had a clotting problem. She got pregnant at thirty-eight and had a miscarriage at six weeks.

"I was so surprised that I had gotten pregnant in the first place because we had just started trying," she says. "My doctor told me that 20 percent of pregnancies miscarry, and she didn't think mine had implanted properly in the first place, so I really wasn't all that upset. The doctor chalked it up to statistics and bad luck. She didn't test the embryo to see if there was any other cause for the miscarriage."

After a second miscarriage at ten weeks, Betsy's doctor referred her to a fertility specialist, who discovered the APLS after a battery of testing. Off she went to a hematologist who specialized in these disorders and diagnosed her with antithrombin deficiency, which also caused clotting. She was told to start aspirin and heparin as soon as she became pregnant, which she did. The next year, when she was forty, she gave birth to a healthy baby girl. At forty-two, Betsy had her second child, a son.

Natural Killer Cells

Natural killer cells are yet another way your body can sabotage your pregnancy. While rare, they are worth discussion. Some women produce an overabundance of these white "killer" blood cells that secrete a protein called TH1 cytokines. These, in turn, may cause clots to form in the placenta or create proteins that kill the growing embryo. Blood tests can determine if this is your problem. If so, some doctors will use immune serum (gamma globulin) to stop damage from the natural killer cells or in rare instances, use the father's white blood cells to immunize you. Of course, when someone else's blood is injected into you, there is always a risk of HIV, so be sure your partner is tested prior to any transfer of his white blood cells.

Uterine Problems

Here's the kicker with a defective uterus—you probably won't know you have one until you miscarry. Unless you have had infertility workups and sonograms, you can't "see" uterine problems.

So what could be wrong? Let's take a look.

- Fibroids can grow inside the uterus, taking up space and the blood supply the baby needs. Our girlfriend Kim was put on bed rest because the fibroid in her uterus was almost as big as her growing baby. She was one of the lucky ones. She went on seven-month bed rest and, rather than miscarrying, delivered a healthy girl only slightly premature by way of C-section.
- A wall of tissue called a septum dividing the uterus. Septums keep an egg from implanting properly.
- Uterine scarring (yet another of Julie's multiple miscarriage reasons!), which prevents blood flow and the building of a lush lining for the embryo.
- While not technically the uterus, an incompetent cervix fits into this category. This defines a cervix too weak to hold the baby's weight as it grows. This plagued our friend Celeste, who actually had a stitch (called a cerclage) placed in her cervix to keep it closed as long as possible before the birth of her daughter at thirty-nine weeks.
- Abnormal blood flow to the uterus can also cause miscarriage. This occurs when one or both uterine arteries are constricted, preventing oxygen and nutrients from reaching your baby. If you have had previous infections or uterine surgery, diabetes or high blood pressure, or are over thirty-five, you are at higher risk for this occurrence. Ditto if you had a prior premature pregnancy. Treatment for abnormal uterine blood flow revolves around correcting the lining of the uterus (a procedure called ploughing) and sometimes the use of vaginal Viagra (yep, the guy get-it-up drug) before ovulation, as it allows greater blood flow.

To determine whether you have any of these problems, your doctor will examine you, take an X-ray of your uterus, check your cervix, place saline in your uterus while observing the sonogram (saline infusion sonogram), or do a hysteroscopy by looking in the uterus with a hysteroscope (like a lighted telescope). The saline infusion sonogram should only be done by someone who has expertise in this field. The resulting films should be reviewed by a fertility expert as well. The hysteroscopy is actually the superior method to evaluate the uterine lining.

Once diagnosed, uterine defects can often be corrected.

The Rest

There are also other baby losses not diagnosed as a regular miscarriage—ectopic pregnancy in which the fertilized egg attaches itself outside the uterus; blighted ovum, in which the embryo doesn't develop, even though the gestational sac does; and molar pregnancies, in which a pregnancy becomes a benign tumor in the first trimester.

However, just as there are those of us diagnosed with unexplained infertility, there are those diagnosed with unexplained miscarriage. They are the ones, like our friend Martha in chapter 10, who get the bad luck diagnosis.

We would also be remiss if we didn't mention that sometimes your miscarriage affects your doctor, too, although he or she may not let on. This doesn't surprise us. The relationship between patient and doctor becomes very intimate because infertile couples see their physicians so often. As a result, doctors can become very involved with their patients' cases.

"You go through medicine, hormone treatments, and surgeries with these people," says Dr. Yarbrough, Julie's OB/GYN. "It's a roller coaster of high, low, high, low. A patient finally gets pregnant and then something happens. It's hard. All pregnancies are important, but it's so much harder when a woman has been doing infertility treatment.

"It's the hardest thing I had to do, bringing the worst news possible to people who are pregnant," he continues. "They come in happy and hopeful, and then *boom*, we have to be the carrier of bad news. This is a small office. We know our patients. We become more involved emotionally, so it's tough. I've had women with their fifth pregnancy—after four miscarriages—miscarry again. We try not to cry in front of the patients, but it does put a damper on your whole day."

We can imagine.

MAUREEN

Recently, I got into a conversation with a salesclerk in the Sak's Fifth Avenue children's department. She was in her late sixties and expressed surprise at the ten-year age difference in my children. When I told her I'd had several miscarriages in between Quinn and Ava, I opened the floodgates. She began telling me about her miscarriages. Clearly this information had been heavy on her heart for years. In her generation, there was no outlet to talk about miscarriage. She had tears in her eyes as she shared that she still thinks of those babies and how old they would be today. We talked about miscarriage like two men who had fought in the same war.

Before we parted company, she told me that she had never spoken of these miscarriages to anyone in the forty years since they had occurred. Finally talking about them, she said, brought her great relief. The simple act of communicating with another woman who had suffered the same hardship helped lift some of her sadness.

How Can I Prevent a Miscarriage?

Before we give you a laundry list of bad habits to break, here's the truth: You may have no bad habits and still have a miscarriage. You may do everything exactly right and still have a miscarriage. But that doesn't mean that you shouldn't at least do the following:

1. Don't do recreational drugs—marijuana, cocaine, and all the rest of them are toxic to your unborn baby.
2. Don't smoke—a no-brainer.
3. Don't go nuts on caffeine. A cup of coffee or tea or a Coke won't hurt you, but don't drain the pot daily or slug back a six pack of cola.
4. Avoid diet soda. We are not fans of fake sugar and chemicals in these beverages.
5. Back off the soft cheeses and processed or undercooked meats such as hotdogs, which can carry the listeria bacteria.
6. Don't habitually drink alcohol. An occasional glass of wine may be fine, but why take the chance?
7. Stay out of hot tubs.

8. Watch your weight, both up and down.
9. Don't overexercise. Running three to five miles every day can certainly mess with your ovulation and increase your chance of miscarriage, even if you've "always done it!"

If It's Not My Fault, Why Do I Feel So Guilty?

Along with disbelief and sorrow, guilt forms the triple crown of miscarriage emotions. Why do we feel guilt over something we probably had no control over? A psychologist could probably answer that better than us, but here's what we know—almost every woman suffers undeserved guilt pangs after a miscarriage. With the betrayal of your body, you feel helpless. It is something that you should be able to rely on, and you can't. Your own body has hurt your unborn child, and there is a sense of anger toward your own physical self. It is a conflict of your spirit and your physical being.

JULIE

Journalizing is cathartic for me, so I did it with each of my miscarriages. I jotted my pain into my journals, taped sonogram pictures there, tucked in the cards, and then locked them away. Once I poured my soul onto the paper, I felt better. By writing my miscarriages out, I honored my lost children. If the stories were on paper, they were off my mind.

I didn't realize how important this exercise was until I couldn't find one of my notepads. I panicked and tore around the house, upending things in search of it. My husband, who processes his grief differently, didn't understand.

"What's the big deal?" he asked as I rooted through the bedside table, shaking and almost in tears.

The big deal, I realized, was fear. I was afraid if I didn't find that notebook, I would lose it all—the memories, the feelings, the fact I had been pregnant at all. I needed to know where the only vestiges of my lost children were. Fortunately I found the notebook, and all was well in the world again.

MAUREEN

When I lost my babies, I went to Grace Cathedral in San Francisco, where I lived at the time and where my son went to school. I lit a candle after each miscarriage, setting their spirits free in this beautiful cathedral. Quinn would often remark to me how he could see them flying around the cathedral during school's morning chapel. He told me these babies were girls, who looked like angels and were happy. He told me they wanted him to share that with me. When I think of them, I feel sure they are indeed safe and happy inside Grace Cathedral, which makes it more bearable.

Coping with Depression: It's Okay to Grieve

Depression usually follows hot on the heels of guilt, which, as we've established, happens right after the miscarriage.

Betsy, the Boston paralegal, didn't grieve her first miscarriage. "I had gotten pregnant almost immediately and miscarried very early on . . . at like six weeks. I just assumed it was a fluke, that I'd get pregnant again immediately, and everything would be okay."

But her second miscarriage at ten weeks was another story. "There was an eight month gap between the two miscarriages. I was devastated, hysterical for days. Even shopping didn't make me feel better. Frankly I was upset about it until they figured out what the problem was.

"I don't think I was grieving a lost child per se," she says. "Just my inability to have the thing I wanted more than anything else. My husband was pretty upset, but for the most part he's a very analytical/nonemotional type. So he just kept saying 'We'll figure out what happened, and we'll fix it.' He didn't mope around or obsess the way I did."

Since Betsy didn't tell anyone until way after the fact, she and her husband had to grieve alone. Here's her advice now. "Having had a miscarriage, here's what I would tell another woman to prepare her for this situation: Don't panic (which will be hard), and try to be very scientific as opposed to emotional about it."

Here's what we say. Suffering a miscarriage is tough. If you don't give yourself time to mourn, you will have a harder time dealing with it later. A wise doctor (or girlfriend) will try to point out something positive from the whole experience—like the fact you were able to achieve a pregnancy. Being able to get pregnant is half the battle.

To help you mourn, here are some things that helped other women through the grieving process.

- "I planted a rosebush in memory of my baby."
- "I held a funeral for her."
- "I wrote a letter to him."
- "I named him. Right after I miscarried I knew I wanted the name Benjamin. I promised myself I would never forget my first baby. Because from the moment of conception, they are unique—there's no replacing that."
- "Due dates and the like are very difficult, but I always light a candle and pray for him in heaven."

Ten Tips for Surviving a Miscarriage

1. Allow yourself time to grieve.
2. Keep a journal.

JULIE

My girlfriend Meg, who had never had a miscarriage to my knowledge, was one of my friends who "got it," when she found out I had lost a baby. She sent me a CD of the Dixie Chicks with a note that said, "Get in the car with Robert, play 'Cowboy Take Me Away,' and go for a drive."

So we did. It was great to open the windows, blast the music, and belt out the song into the wind. Just getting out of the house in a mindless way was good. Singing to songs that are upbeat and have nothing to do with loss was good. Having a friend care about me enough to come up with a creative way to share my grief was really good.

I still keep that Dixie Chicks CD in my car, and "Cowboy Take Me Away" is our family's favorite tune. There was a period of time where I came to define distance by how many times "Cowboy Take Me Away" can play—from our house to the preschool is exactly one rotation of the song; to the grocery store, two song's worth; to the mall, too many times to count.

But even today when I listen to it, I think of my good friend Meg, who understood how to make me look forward again with a simple song.

3. Honor your lost child in some way—plant a flowering bush or tree.

4. Write your lost child a letter, pour out your feelings, then tuck the letter away.

5. Don't go it alone. Talk about the miscarriage with your partner, your parent, or a friend.

6. Give yourself a break. It is not your fault. You are not a bad person. Let go of the guilt.

7. Yell, curse, pound your fist on the table, go for a run, curl up in your bed and sleep . . . then start living again.

8. You are not the only person to whom this has happened. Find others who understand.

9. Take care of yourself—go to a spa, get a manicure or facial, buy yourself something special.

10. Realize that these feelings will pass, but never be forgotten—and that's okay.

Will It Happen Again?

Honestly? Maybe yes, maybe no. The biggest problem in infertility is that there is so much that is not yet understood. Miscarriage is like that, too.

There is also confusion among the medical community—one doctor saying baby aspirin is great for those like Julie who have antiphospholipid antibody syndrome. Other doctors say no, we need more information on APLS before handing out blood thinners. Ditto for whether a woman should be given progesterone to help stabilize a pregnancy. Julie's doctor said yes; Maureen's said no. For something medical to become commonplace it seems as if you have to have multiple studies and guidelines in place first. These conflicting messages can make you crazy and confused. Which way do you turn? Who do you believe? That's why women have to talk to one another—we learned as much from talking with girlfriends and acquaintances as we did from our doctors.

Miscarriage is traumatizing. After you suffer from one (or more), you will never be able to enjoy pregnancy believing you are home free—not until they put that baby into your arms. Then you understand just what a miracle normal really is.

THE HUSBANDS

When it comes to miscarriage from a guy's perspective, it sort of depends on how much work went into the conceiving. Miscarriages affect men more who are involved in fertility treatments. It's not just our opinion; here's what a couple of guys who've been through it told us—our husbands.

Robert: Sure, all miscarriages are painful, but most guys don't realize the whole importance of that lost pregnancy. When you are involved in fertility treatments, you understand the preciousness of that lost baby, and you pray like hell it doesn't happen again because you are forced to a level of compassion that is just not there for most men.

That compassion takes so much effort, when in reality you want to say, "Okay, we can't have kids, here's some money, let's go adopt" . . . or something like that. You don't want your wife to keep going through the miscarriage ringer.

Will: This is a tough one, as having had the experience versus not having had the experience is night and day. Having now been through it, I would tell another man that if your wife has a miscarriage, seek out anyone else who has had the experience themselves and arrange some kind of confab. The idea would be to get counsel on the potential elements involved—a support group. Family and close friends are the best, given the personal aspect. That emotional support is important. In addition to supporting himself through the miscarriage, he also needs to be empathetic to his spouse. That is pretty paramount.

CHAPTER 13
Who Do You Tell? (Or, When People You Love Say STUPID Things)

Julie

Not talking about my infertility soon became exhausting. About that time, I had the first big breakthrough—at my friend Grace's kitchen table. Out of the blue, Grace started talking about her infertility problems.

What? Grace was having problems, too?

Neither of us had realized the other was having trouble conceiving, although we saw each other regularly. With her secret out, I spilled my story. It felt good to talk with another woman. Here was someone who could actually relate. Here was someone who knew what Clomid was and how much heparin shots hurt (no matter what the doctor tells you), who couldn't get her hormone-induced body fat back under control, who was seeing a side of medical science she never anticipated she would need. We compared stories and treatments, and I got the name of her reproductive endocrinologist.

It was so liberating to finally have a girlfriend to talk with about this whole process. It was pivotal for me. I changed doctors and changed my mentality. I started talking to friends and colleagues. What an eye-opener! The (lack of) response I got when I brought up infertility in general, mine in particular, blew me away. People didn't want or know how to talk about it. I'd found a topic that made them as uncomfortable as their pregnancy questions made me. They changed the subject or piled on the pity, or worst of all, plied me with their pregnancy tales. Few seemed to get it. It made me nuts. Wish I'd known Maureen back then!

Maureen

When I got pregnant with my son, I did what everyone naturally wants to do. I told everyone—every friend, every family member, my dry cleaner, my deli guy, my hairdresser—with no consideration whatsoever that anything could go wrong. I was blessed, and everything went as planned.

When I got pregnant again six years later, I did the same thing, but I lost the baby at twelve weeks. I had told several friends and acquaintances, then had to update people as I ran into them. I didn't see one woman until a few years after the miscarriage. I ran into her on the street, and the first thing she said was "Where's the baby?" It was so awkward. If I hadn't told her I was pregnant in the first place, I wouldn't have had to relive the miscarriage with her. I wouldn't have had to deal with that. Explaining everything to people was in some ways more painful than dealing with the miscarriage itself.

After suffering through that first miscarriage, I decided to deal with my fertility issues and future pregnancies by myself. Pregnant again, two years later, I changed tactics. I told only my best friend, my mother, and my husband. Then, twelve weeks later, I miscarried again. That I had told only a few people made a big difference in my recovery. The same happened with my third miscarriage.

When I got pregnant again one year later, I just assumed the worst and told only Julie, my friend Dee Dee, and my husband. I was convinced I would lose this baby, too, and just waited for it to happen again. When I hit twelve weeks, I worried more and still told no one else. When the amnio brought back great results at sixteen weeks, I was still afraid to spread the news. If I could have hidden my pregnancy until the day I gave birth, I would have been happy. I realized that people constantly asking me about everything made me feel worse. I decided it was no one's business what I was doing to get pregnant and if I got pregnant at all. So I just told everyone except for those closest to me that we'd quit trying. Then, when Ava happened, it was a miracle—a surprise. They didn't need to know details.

At six months, I finally relented and announced I was pregnant. Everyone was shocked, although a few admitted they thought I was looking a little rounder. I also asked my girlfriends to hold off on giving me any baby gifts. I didn't want them in my home for fear something would still go wrong, and I would have to face little booties, cute outfits, car seats, and strollers. I did not breathe a sigh of relief until I saw the sparkle of my newborn daughter's eyes.

My advice? Keep it to yourself and those closest to you. You will want people to be there for you in a loving way if things go wrong—because sadly, sometimes they do.

Ten Snappy Answers to "When Are You Going to Have a Baby?"

1. When we get to it, I promise you'll be the first to know.
2. When we are rich and famous.
3. Why do you want to know?
4. I've already had several miscarriages. (This usually shuts them up)
5. Why are you so nosy? (Said with a smile, this comes off playful, although serious works well, too.)
6. I'm so glad you brought that up! I'm having fertility issues. What do you want to talk about first—my uterine lining or John's sperm count? (Don't be surprised if they spit out their coffee at this one.)
7. When we win the lottery. (They'll never guess it's the baby lottery!)
8. We're trying, and we're having a hard time of it. Do you have any other friends with fertility problems?
9. We've decided not to have kids; thanks for asking. (When it happens, they'll be surprised.)
10. We're in a quandary—puppy or baby. Which do you think would be better?

How many times has this happened to you? You're out with family or friends (it doesn't seem to matter), and someone you either (1) know really well or (2) hardly know at all says for all to hear: "Now, honey, tell me why aren't you pregnant yet?" or "No kids yet? Why not?" or "When are you going to start a family? You're not getting any younger, you know!" Then, everyone in the group (or room) quiets down and turns expectantly in your direction.

We always hated those moments, which seem to increase at each passing birthday. In our roaring twenties, when we were specifically trying hard not to get pregnant, we'd laugh it off with some smug comment about being too busy having too much fun, then regale them with the latest job-related escapade.

Babies? At *my* age? Boring!

When we were in our mid-thirties, however, and up to our elbows in baby lust and fertility issues, those same questions began to grate on our hormone-frazzled nerves. Usually, we'd laugh off their rudeness or make some offhand comment. What we wanted to do was shout, "Shut up! It's not for the lack of trying!" But, of course, as we tell our kids today, that would not be appropriate behavior.

These questions and comments cut to the heart when you are fighting infertility because infertility is one of the most personal physical challenges a couple can face. It's emotional. It's draining. It sucks. Besides, who wants to start a conversation you can't finish without bursting into tears?

At the same time, you *do* want with talk about it to someone! However, deciding *who* to tell *what* to is one of the tougher first steps you'll take.

The Big Secret

When a woman finds out she's got fertility issues, she doesn't tell anyone—even the people who love her most. If pregnancy rates as a badge of honor, infertility ranks as a big, black mark against our womanhood. We feel sad, guilty, and confused, so we keep quiet.

"My wife and I differ a little on that one," says Terence, who has been struggling with infertility for more than two years. "She feels ashamed, and she's told only one friend and her parents. She'd be happier if fewer people knew. My wife doesn't even want her brother to know. I'm different—I find support and strength by telling others. I've told my family and a few of my friends. We haven't told our pastor yet but may at some point. Everyone is different."

Because we don't talk about infertility the way we candidly discuss other diseases, nobody knows how to react to us. Until very recently, no one in the celeb spotlight—Hollywood or otherwise—would admit to infertility, either. If everyone else seems to be having babies and the infertile people are clammed up somewhere in a corner, where's the point of reference? With all this silence, one wouldn't think infertility was as widespread as it is.

"We try to shrug off the insensitive remarks—I can't tell you how many times people have told us to 'relax' or that maybe we should 'take a vacation,'" adds Terence. "I know that I would have said the same things a few years ago. I don't blame people for not understanding our problem. But infertility is a more common problem than most people know."

Listen to what happened to our friend Krista, a thirty-five-year-old marketing director from New Jersey. After finding out she had fertility issues, Krista hit the first bookstore she drove by in search of info. Not seeing what she wanted, she asked the woman at the counter for help. After explaining to our pal that she was in a Christian bookstore, the bookseller then asked Krista why she wanted a book on infertility. Without going into detail, Krista told the woman she was having trouble getting pregnant. While she didn't have a book for Krista, the woman did have some advice.

"Honey," she said, meaning well, we're sure, "That's easy. Just grab your husband and jump in the back of a Chevy like all those sixteen-year-olds do. They sure don't have any problem getting pregnant."

Well, okay, then.

These types of remarks do not solely come from those we don't know well. Our non–pregnancy challenged girlfriends who were generally compassionate women turned into boors on this topic. Few seemed to realize how comments like, "Hmm, I've just never had a problem with that." could shut us down. And who wants to continue a conversation with a woman who, at the mention of your infertility, simply sighs, shakes her head, and tells you she has no clue how she keeps getting pregnant. One actually laughed and said her husband could "just look at her," and she was on the nine-month roller coaster. One friend made her husband get a vasectomy after bearing two kids because his sperm was "so powerful." Another told Julie she'd "get over all this baby insanity" if she and Robert just spent a weekend alone with her three kids.

Those of us who desperately want children don't want to hear our pals preach about their problem-free pregnancies and wild family lives. We're sure these gal pals never meant to make us feel bad. We're sure your friends don't either. They just don't get it.

How About My Husband?

Soon after they started exploring treatments, Julie quit talking about her infertility to everyone except her husband. This was not good, for a few reasons.

1. After the initial shock of the infertility diagnosis, women want to talk.
2. After the initial shock of the infertility diagnosis, men don't know what to say.
3. He's going through it, too.
4. He's doesn't want to talk about it as much as you.

Women are communicators by nature. We love to talk, and we want details—all the details. Men are wired differently. Husbands never bring home enough details about what's going on. A guy can spend half a day playing golf with a buddy who is going through a nasty divorce or whose wife just gave birth to triplets, and when we ask how the buddy is, he says, "I don't know. We never talked about it."

Rare is the man—even the most compassionate, loving man—who will want to spend every waking minute thinking and talking about infertility. Rare is the woman going through it who won't. So consider giving your partner's ear a break occasionally.

Breaking the News. Should You or Shouldn't You?

There are two schools of thought on this. Let's discuss.

The Keep-it-to-Yourself Philosophy

The following are some valid reasons for keeping quiet about your infertility and treatment:

1. You don't want the hassle of explaining everything to the uninformed.
2. You don't want everyone to know your business.
3. You don't want to hear totally unhelpful comments such as
   "It will happen if it's God's will . . ." or
   "You have so much to be thankful for already," or
   "Maybe you aren't supposed to have a baby at your age."
4. You don't want people worrying about you or pitying you.
5. You married a guy who has the girlfriend's gift of gab and will talk about this topic in-depth any time you feel the urge.
6. You don't want the pressure of people asking, "How's it going?"

The Sharing and Caring Philosophy for Finding the Right Confidante

There are also several valid reasons to share the news. While we each feel differently about who and how many people to tell, we do agree that you should tell someone what you're up to, even if it's just one soul. The question is who do you tell and how much do you reveal?

Here's our rule of thumb: If you don't send them a Christmas card, don't bother sharing the most intimate details of your baby quest. However, if the opportunity presents itself and the mood grabs you, feel free to talk about your treatments with acquaintances. Ask them if they know anyone else going through fertility treatments. We have met many women struggling with infertility just by opening our mouths when the opportunity proved attractive. However, you don't have to overwhelm the uninformed or uninterested with every teensy detail of your baby quest.

Sadly, infertility is considered a taboo topic by a lot of women and most men, particularly when it's *their* infertility. Our friend Melinda wanted to organize an infertility support group through her church. Before she launched her group, she quizzed women via Internet fertility chat rooms on how they would like to see a support group run. She was astounded when many said they didn't really want face-to-face contact with other women about this subject—even other women who were going through the same thing! While they were desperate for the friendship and information, they were just too embarrassed about sharing publicly. Isn't that interesting? Here we are, the gender known for chatting about everything for hours on end, and the one thing that we all want to talk about—babies and how to get them—shuts us up? By the way, Melinda started her group anyway—although with a core group of five women, it hasn't turned out to be the roaring success she'd hoped for.

MAUREEN

When I finally admitted I had fertility issues, the first thing I did was call a girlfriend who had been going through infertility as well. She hadn't gotten pregnant yet, either, so I thought she would be helpful. I soon discovered the more I questioned her, the more she didn't seem to want to answer me! It felt as if she wanted to put this behind her. This is the problem with infertility. Most people don't want to talk about it or admit their own problems, and it can make it difficult to get the information you need. Here I was lost in this maze of "what comes next?" and "is this normal?" and "what does that mean?" and I couldn't find anyone—other than Julie—who could give me the real story.

If we keep our infertility a state secret, we can't help one another or get the nurturing we need to go through it all. Besides, if you start talking about your infertility to those in the know, you will find help for other things you might need to know later—like how to find a birth mother or a surrogate, or how other couples made it through high-risk pregnancies.

There's no need, however, to bare your soul to everyone in the office, all the neighbors, or the guy who fixes your car. While most of your friends will want to know the challenges you are facing, not everyone wants to know every detail about your hysteroscopy, progesterone levels, or husband's sperm motility. Some things are best left said only to your best friends.

We're not so foolish as to think everyone can run right out and start chatting up infertility. There are a lot of us who are incredibly modest, private people who hate to divulge any personal information. But infertility secrets are not helpful to anyone. Look, if people can go on reality TV or spill their guts to *People* magazine, it's worth a try to open up to our closest friends.

So, when does your infertility become someone else's business? When a conversation leads to a natural opening and you feel ready to share your stories.

Filling in the Family

You may want to start with family. If your parents are desperate to become grandparents, this can be tough. Unless your mom and dad went through infertility themselves or happen to be OB/GYNs, they will probably not relate to what you are experiencing. Such things were kept hush-hush in their generation, and they really may not know anyone who's been where you are. But that doesn't mean they won't be interested in your condition and concerned about your health and emotional state. No matter how old you are, you are still their baby.

Even the most loving parent with the best intentions will say something that sounds heartless, like "When am I going to be a grandparent?" Try not to be too caustic in return with a retort like "I don't know, when are you?" particularly if you haven't yet told your parents about your infertility.

The grandparent question is often partnered with a sigh or chuckle, depending on how guilty the commentator wants you to feel. No doubt about it, this is a selfish question. It is all about them and rarely about you or your condition. They simply want some reassurance that in living your action-packed life, you have not forgotten their desires—wallets stuffed with grandbaby pictures and someone small they can spoil rotten, fill up with sugar, and send home to you.

Mary, a thirty-four-year-old teacher, told her parents she wanted children as much as they wanted grandchildren. She then moved on to discuss what was going on in her life that made having kids on cue such a challenge. The result—Mary's parents are less cavalier in their comments, and Mary has found an ally and a sympathetic ear in her mom.

The good thing about moms is that they've been through pregnancy and can talk the body parts. Even if saying "uterus" makes them blush, they at least know where the organ is. Fathers, however, have a harder time talking reproduction. The trick to parental ease is to speak in their language. You obviously know your parents better than we do, so each case is different, but there are some generalities we can make here.

With mothers, conversations about feelings, hopes, and dreams can combine with the procedures you are going through. These conversations seem to just flow. Fathers, however, seem to like a more scientific, technical dialogue. Don't go too deep into it. Try to give him the gist without using too many words, like penis, sperm count, or vagina. For some reason, Dads seem to cringe when their darling daughters talk that way. In his eyes, you are still seven years old. And remember, that generation of men were rarely allowed into the inner sanctum of the OB/GYN office or the delivery room. This is new territory for most of them.

The other men in your family (brothers, male in-laws, and so on) will most likely fall into the category of people who are intrigued but embarrassed by infertility in general and your infertility in particular. These guys want to empathize with you, but they really don't want or know how to talk about infertility as they do cars, sports, or fishing. For the most part, they want a simple explanation and some reassurance that nothing you are doing to your body will hurt or kill you. In these situations, keep it simple, answer their questions, and watch their expressions. No need to embarrass all the men in your life. Your husband doesn't have a choice.

Sisters seem to fall into the "best girlfriend" category. Our friend Sheree put off telling her parents and friends about her infertility until she and her husband did their first in vitro fertilization. However, she wasn't alone. Sheree had chosen to tell her sister everything in the beginning. She is very close to her sister, who also happens to be a doctor. So, while friends and the rest of the family were surprised, Sheree had gotten her sister's support (and free medical advice) from the get-go.

"I didn't tell the rest of the family right away because I didn't think I could handle their expectations," says Sheree. "I didn't want them putting too much subconscious pressure on me, and I didn't want to feel as if I were failing them, so I just told my sister."

Telling Friends and Acquaintances

The great thing about those closest to you is that regular conversations usually provide plenty of opportunities in which to broach this subject. Show us a child-free woman who has hit thirty years old and has never been asked, "When are you going to have kids?" and we'll take odds she's either a liar or a nun. Some women hear it even sooner, but it is the rare woman who never hears that infamous question at least once. When friends ask, consider it carte blanche to answer honestly if you want.

So what to say and when? We base that on a couple of apt clichés: "honesty is the best policy" and "timing is everything."

Trite, yes, but true when it comes to infertility.

If you're going to talk, you have to tell the truth. If you're like us, either you can't lie or you're so bad at it that you always get caught. After a while, we get our stories so convoluted that we can't remember the truth from the lie. So we stick with the truth—or say nothing.

JULIE

Once I got that first conversation out of the way, it wasn't as bad as I thought it would be, which empowered me to have the next conversation and the next.

Because my best buddies hadn't had problems conceiving or carrying their babies to term, infertility was foreign to them. Once they got up to speed, however, I got a lot of encouragement, magazine clippings, and phone calls about websites or TV specials.

Of course, most sitcoms and TV dramas are more fiction than fact when it comes to fertility. For example, there was that episode from the final season of HBO's *Sex and The City*—the one in which Charlotte tells an unattached Carrie that at age thirty-nine, there's still time to decide whether she wants to have children. Those of us in the know will tell you frankly that Charlotte was giving her pal some bad advice. Thirty-nine may be too late. But trying to educate friends who advise you based on sitcoms might be too time-consuming. Thank them for their interest, then sift through the information and disregard the rest.

It's best to have met with your fertility doctor at least once or twice when you start talking to others about your infertility. This way, you will be out of the disbelief and denial stages. You'll also be better able to answer any questions. Most people you talk with will have questions, so be prepared to educate them, particularly if they haven't been through the process themselves.

The hardest conversations about your infertility will be the first ones. If you don't talk about it, infertility almost doesn't seem real. And if you're like us, you don't want anyone to pity you. Pity seems to be a corollary to infertility. But infertility is a reality, and pity doesn't get you pregnant.

But once you spit the words out the first few times, you will find that the conversation flows.

How to Handle the Ignorant and the Inane

Be prepared. Some of the most well-intentioned people say the most stupid things. These well-meaning people usually don't know what to say to you, so they say the first thing that comes to mind. Or they might truly believe their inane comments like, "If you just relax, you'll get pregnant, like so-and-so did." Poor souls. They are so wrong.

We can promise you that at some point during your infertility, your dearest pal or closest family member will unwittingly say something insensitive to you. Almost every one of our best, dearest, most loved friends made a comment at one point or another that we found inappropriate, inane, or inexcusable. However, we have forgiven them all their social blunders, and we still speak to them. You will, too

One girlfriend suggested that perhaps Julie and Robert were doing something wrong, as if infertility weren't a medical condition, but a sexual disorder or related to some specific bedroom position. A friend of Maureen's, who shall remain nameless, advised that it was "just God's way." Another friend, being philosophical, mused that maybe it was nature's way of saying we shouldn't be parents.

To help out, here are a few things not to say to anyone experiencing infertility.

1. Just don't think about it, and it will happen!
2. Maybe you're trying too hard.
3. But I bet it's fun trying! (Sure, it's a real blast!)

JULIE

And now for my favorite—the comment that continually pissed me off: "When are you going to quit working so much and start a family?"

This remark never failed to annoy me because it assumed my priorities were screwed up. It assumed I was selfish, and, as a woman, I couldn't be proud of my job or the advancements I had made. Wow. Let's just negate everything else I've ever done in one sweeping comment. I don't think I was lacking as a person. But that one question summed me up as a failure, despite all I had accomplished. It never failed to me make me feel bad, especially when my husband and I were working diligently after-hours to create the family they were asking about.

People don't realize how time-consuming working through infertility can be. With the slew of doctor visits, shots, sonograms, procedures, and pre-planned sex, infertility is like having another job—a job for which you don't get paid! So when people ask you when you are going to slow down the work pace and start making babies, I suggest you tell them the truth. You are currently working two jobs—a career during the day that earns you money and an after-hours occupation trying to get pregnant that spends it.

4. Just start to adopt—then you'll get pregnant! That happened to my friend.

5. You're really lucky—you can do anything you want. We never get to go out anymore.

6. Don't worry, you're still young.

7. Why do you want kids anyway?

8. Did you ever think about adopting? (No, it never crossed my mind. What's adoption?)

9. Pregnancy is easy for me. I'll be your surrogate. (Followed by a self-deprecating giggle.)

10. Anything new on the baby front?

11. Are you keeping your legs up after sex?

12. Are you getting drunk before sex?

13. Is your husband wearing loose underwear?

14. Are you taking your temperature?

15. Are you using an ovulation predictor test?

16. Are you doing it doggy style? That worked for us!

17. Are you doing it in public? That worked for us!

MAUREEN

I heard a few zingers, too. In addition to "What's the matter with you?" and "How are you affording this?" I also got "What the heck are you thinking?"

We already had our little boy, Quinn, so when it got out we were trying to get pregnant, some family and friends actually told us to quit while we were ahead. We heard "Why take a chance on another child when your son is so wonderful?" and "Feel grateful for what you have," and "It sure would be hard to top that great boy!"

Needless to say, those comments didn't make me feel any better. In fact, they scared the pants off me. I started second-guessing myself, so I shut up. When my mother would come over to watch Quinn while I went to the fertility clinic, I'd just tell her I was going to the store. Everyone has an opinion, but some opinions are not helpful. Be ready for those.

18. You should have more sex.
19. It's probably for the best.
20. Don't worry, you'll get pregnant soon.
21. You probably need a vacation.
22. I get pregnant when I look at my husband.
23. Give it time.

Listen, these comments aren't meant to be mean, even if they hurt like hell. Words are pretty powerful because they hang around in your mind long after the conversation is completed. We have found the easiest way to handle these comments *is to simply not respond in kind*. Bite your tongue. We know . . . it's hard, particularly when you really want to say something sarcastic. But don't. You'll only feel better for a minute, and you may shut a door you'll want to walk through later.

WHAT TO SAY TO A FRIEND EXPERIENCING INFERTILITY

"I don't want to keep asking about the baby stuff. Just know that whenever you want to talk I'm here."

This is the perfect thing to say. We plan on putting this on a bookmark to hand out to friends and family, but feel free to jot it down and hand it out yourself.

The best thing to do is tell your pals their comments don't help because you are having trouble getting pregnant. Let them know you appreciate their concern (if you do), and that you're glad they haven't had any problems because you wouldn't want them to go through what you are dealing with. Often people say inappropriate things because they don't know what else to say, and they are grasping for something they think is helpful.

Your job is to educate them if you choose, not make them feel better about your infertility at your expense. When people you love say stupid things, don't waste energy getting mad at them. Use their comments as an opportunity to educate them about infertility—or just let it go.

Look, you can't be infertile *and* be thin-skinned. No time for it. There are better things to do with your energy. Yes, it's a bummer that after all those years of trying *not* to get pregnant, you suddenly can't get pregnant quite as easily as you thought. Infertility isn't personal, so don't let the uninformed make you feel as if it is. Also remember that your infertility isn't really anyone's business—unless you make it so. But being rude isn't really the best choice. The world is full of boorish people. No need to give the infertile a bad rep.

You Can Always Adopt!

Another comment every infertile couple eventually hears is, "You can always adopt."

This is usually a clumsy attempt to downplay your infertility and make you feel better. Your friend is probably trying to show you that things can't be all bad if you've got options. Unfortunately, it also assumes if you can't have your own biological child, you will most certainly go the "next best" route and adopt.

This comment does not elevate adoption to the level it deserves, and it leaves no room for the other choices you have should fertility treatments fail—such as surrogacy or not having children. But before you bark back with a biting response, realize the person making the comment is most likely trying to help, not drive you crazy. Tell them adoption is an option you are considering, if that's the case, then drop it.

Our friend Susan, a thirty-nine-year-old journalist, was plenty aware that she could adopt, but she wasn't there yet. "Well-meaning people say things like, 'Oh, well, you can always adopt,'" she says. "But I want the whole experience—including pregnancy and childbirth—not just a child. Comments about adoption can make you feel guilty. But anyone experiencing infertility problems should decide for themselves what it is they want."

And in some cases, however, adoption might not be right for your family. Remember Julie's pal Grace? She was interested in the adoption option as soon as she found out she was battling secondary infertility. But her husband wasn't so sure adoption would work for him. So how do you answer the adoption comment in situations like that?

Well, you can take the easy way out and simply say, "You're right. We can." or "That's an option." and leave it at that. Or you can tell them how you really feel. You want the whole experience, and you are not ready to think past that at this point. Or you've carefully thought through adoption, and as a couple have decided it is not for you at this time, but you'll keep them posted as you go forward.

Any News?!

Once you tell people you are fertility-challenged, you've invited them to your party. Particularly if you are vocal about your cycles or the procedures you are doing, someone will eventually ask if there's any news. This is not a trick question. What they really want to know is if you have any good news—like you're pregnant and just forgot to tell them.

This is one of the harder parts about sharing the details of your infertility with a lot of people, as Maureen learned. In addition to handling your own disappointment over failed procedures, you have to handle their disappointment as well. This can be emotionally draining, so we suggest you only tell those closest to you about the actual timing of your fertility procedures. It's also best to establish some ground rules to avoid hurt (yours) and embarrassment (theirs). Tell everyone in the know that you will call them with any results as soon as you can (or want to). Ask them to please not call you. You will have to remind them that infertility is one of those rare times when no news is really not good news at all.

If the "Any news?" question comes from a random source—someone acquainted with your infertility, but not intimately so—keep your response short and sweet. Tell them things are status quo, and you'll let them know the minute you have some good news. Then change the subject if it is too painful for you or if the loss is too recent.

You can try Maureen's trick. Simply tell everyone that you have stopped trying. That way, when you do become pregnant, they will just be happy and surprised. Not everyone has to know *all* the details. When she got pregnant with Ava, everyone just assumed it was IVF. She ran into a friend's mother who had experienced infertility decades ago who marveled at modern medicine today and how doctors could just get anyone pregnant these days. She assumed Maureen had done IVF because she was over forty and pregnant. It was hard to convince her otherwise. So why bother?

Womb Envy

The emotional upheaval, which we call womb envy, is something all of us go through, something we don't really talk about. This is the feeling we get in the pits of our stomachs (or maybe our hearts) when we see a new mother with her infant, a child in the park playing on the swings, or a coworker's pregnant belly. Why them and not us?

"No one really talks about the powerful hate/jealousy you feel for other people who are able to get pregnant/be pregnant/have babies," says Ellen, our East Coast pal who went through several years of infertility before having her two babies. "But I felt it. It is an ugly feeling and not to be expressed in polite company, but for me it was very, very real. I avoided places with kids at all costs. I couldn't go to church on Mother's Day, and other church holidays were excruciating."

Ellen adds, "The emotional part of infertility is totally unbelievable. I felt like a totally different person while I was in the middle of all of that. I was trying to find solace in church, but I couldn't stand to sit in a service behind a baby, which was a little tricky."

To survive, Ellen depended on her RESOLVE support group and her therapist. "My family was not very helpful—it's an area that is extremely touchy for me. I mean, my family didn't know what to make of me, and I couldn't handle it very well with them. I just felt constantly on the brink of breaking down—I remember a holiday, Christmas or Thanksgiving one year, when my sister-in-law had a baby, and I couldn't even stand to be in the room with him."

Ellen's case is not unique. While you are going through treatments trying to get pregnant, someone you know *will* get pregnant. While in the midst of our own infertility, Julie's friend Caren got pregnant twice, as did Maureen's good friend Rena. When these girlfriends tell you their good news, it is your job to be gracious. If they know you are working through infertility, then they probably had some misgivings about sharing their news with you for fear of upsetting you. The truth is that hearing that others are pregnant while you are still trying will probably upset you. We felt like we were being cheated—again—while someone else got to hold up the brass ring. There's no way to sugarcoat it—it sucks. The best way to respond to this type of news is to simply congratulate the friend or couple and move on—physically, if you need to. Leave the room and compose yourself, then return.

Being gracious doesn't mean you have to torture yourself. If the glowing mother-to-be is an office mate or casual friend, don't feel obligated to attend baby showers or sit in on all the gossip fests on how well the pregnancy is going. It's okay to excuse yourself. If someone says something about your lack of participation, be honest. Let them know you wish the mom-to-be the best, but frankly it's hard to be around others who are pregnant when you are having so much trouble. Don't be the wet blanket on her happiness, however. If you can't be congenial or don't feel up to the festivities, remove yourself. Do not have a public pity party. That's not fair, either.

It's harder when the expectant mother is your best friend. "My wife's best friend called on a Saturday afternoon to tell us that she is pregnant with her second baby," says our guy friend Dennis, a forty-six-year-old dentist. "My wife went through such a range of emotions that weekend. On one hand, she was happy for her, but [on the other] it reminded her that she hasn't been able to produce one baby when her friend had gotten pregnant twice. We cried a lot that weekend and supported each other."

Those emotions are normal and expected. It's difficult to see others get what we want. But when a good girlfriend is pregnant, things shift a little. It is your job to show up and be happy for her. You can mourn privately, but don't take it public. There's also the cosmic culture that believes being happy for others' good fortune with help yours show up as well. Besides, a best friend being pregnant means there will soon be a baby around to hold.

We know it sounds a little like character building here. It is. Sometimes you have to be happy for someone else's success when you can't find your own and hope the universe will balance it all out in the end. This can be tricky because our culture has become so self-absorbed. We are more selfish and wallow in self-pity more than in the past. But you have to accept that when it comes to babies and fertility, you don't have all the power or control. If you did, you'd be fabulously wealthy, gorgeous, famous, and pregnant! Okay, lecture over. Back to class.

Guy Talk

Let's talk about husbands. We have noticed that guys don't seem to mind discussing infertility as it directly affects their wives. Robert could discuss clinical

MAUREEN

When my girlfriend got pregnant after I had suffered three miscarriages and six missed inseminations, I was thrilled for her. Really.

I decided early on that my inability to get pregnant should not affect my joy for her pregnancy. My friend was actually more worried about how her pregnancy was going to make me feel!

I decided it was important to grin and bear it because, you know, not everything is about me—something that is really hard for those of us facing fertility issues to accept. I had to separate my issues from her pregnancy so that I could enjoy it and experience it with her.

My reward was the joy in Rena's face during her pregnancy and getting to hold that little baby after his birth.

procedures with the greatest of ease because they involved another human's body—Julie's.

But when men are physically involved in the whole inability-to-produce-a-baby process, things shift. What guy wants his sperm count or undescended testicles brought out as cocktail party conversation?

So with whom do you share your husband's infertility secrets? Your best bet is to talk with him about it before getting on the horn to the whole world.

Some guys don't mind if their family knows what's up with their plumbing. Others can't bear the thought of having their mother know. Still others can talk to strangers about things like sperm penetrating power and semen analysis but clam up around friends and family. We've seen more than one man melt into the furniture when his wife started nonchalantly discussing his manhood in a group setting.

Your partner is the most important person on your infertility team, so don't upset him by sharing too much too soon with too many people. Your best bet is to start off talking with him. Find out his comfort zone and then make a pact to stay within it. Touch base often. The further along you are in treatment, the more men are willing to talk about the whole process. They need time to buy into it, to get over the whole guilt thing you are going through, too. We have no scientific proof of this, but it probably goes back to the prehistoric cave man and his ego.

Talking It Out with Someone Who Relates

It's best to find other people who are going through the same thing as you. Friends and family members who don't have an infertility problem simply can't understand the pressure of what you are going through, even if they mean well. Someone who has kids and had no problem getting them cannot possibly understand how you feel, no matter how hard they try. Couples who are child-free by choice cannot relate. As we have told many "well-wishers," it's one thing to actively choose not to have children—and quite another to have that choice taken away. That's why it is very important to find a few infertile friends.

Grace was Julie's touchstone during her years of infertility leading up to her son's birth. She could relate. She was there, too, sharing insight on procedures and crying over miscarriages. Through her, Julie found others. They may not become your closest friends, but they will be the ones who get it.

Someone fighting infertility will never tell you "Just relax, and you'll get pregnant."

They will say, "This is hard," "You can go on," and "It's okay to cry." They will be the ones who give you the scoop on the newest procedures, herbal options, and the best reproductive endocrinologists. To find a support group, call the local chapter of RESOLVE, ask your doctor, or check out your local hospital.

Communicating Incognito

Not everyone feels comfortable in face-to-face infertility conversations, even with their friends. That's why the Internet can be so great—it allows you to "chat" with others who are in the same situation, while maintaining anonymity. Besides, it's easy to use. You don't have to be a great computer whiz to zip along the information highway. Use a search engine like Yahoo.com or Google.com to help you find appropriate websites.

While we have posted some questions and left some responses, we are mostly Internet voyeurs. Our friend Terence and his wife, who have been trying to conceive for more than two years, love the Internet and use it as a tool. They join chat rooms and post questions on various website bulletin boards.

"The best advice I could give couples who are facing infertility is to find an online support group," says Terence. "It helps so much to talk to others with the same problem. My wife and I have found a lot of support and information on those boards."

CHAPTER 14

MONEY
Mind Games

Maureen

I was lucky that my insurance covered most of our treatments, but injectable fertility drugs were not covered. I was ambivalent about doing injectables anyway, so we chose to opt out of that and saved a great deal of money and aggravation. IVF wasn't even in our budget—too cost-prohibitive, which made me angry because it's as if only those people who are well off financially can afford these procedures. It's not as if we don't have a good income, which made it even stranger when we realized IVF would be an unreasonable financial burden on us.

I was unwilling to ruin our financial future with unsuccessful IVFs, especially since we already had Quinn. We decided to just put that money aside for his college.

Julie

Robert and I decided from the start we would pay for one year of infertility treatment. One year of balls-to-the-walls, go-for-it therapy. Boy, did we spend a lot of money that year.

Everyone assumes infertile couples already know how costly treatment is, but even though I consider myself a smart consumer, the numbers we wrote on the checks to doctors stunned me. Sticker shock continued when I went to the drugstore to pick up my prescriptions. I still wonder if one Clomid pill was really worth seven bucks.

Neither my RE or subsequent high-risk OB/GYN were on any insurance plans. At each visit, I was expected to pay for services rendered (they took cash, check, or credit cards) and was provided with a duplicate copy of my bill and receipt to file with my insurance company on my own. I would never choose a medical professional solely because they are covered by my insurance. I don't like some insurance clerk in Omaha dictating my medical processes, so I don't begrudge a doctor for feeling the same way. Besides, out-of-network physicians on my plan were covered once I reached the deductible—not too hard to do with infertility treatments.

On the positive side, we reached our sky-high insurance deductible rather quickly, allowing my husband to get one of those fancy, full-blown physicals he'd always wanted at the Cooper Clinic in Dallas—fully funded by insurance!

Ten Financial Facts You Need to Know

1. Infertility is an expensive condition to battle.
2. Your insurance company probably will not cover all of your treatment.
3. Insurance companies often consider infertility treatments to be investigational and therefore don't cover them.
4. While your insurance may not cover infertility, they may cover the diseases that cause it.
5. Some doctors will let insurance coverage dictate your treatment plan.
6. There are creative ways of financing infertility treatments.
7. Some clinics offer a reimbursement program if treatments like IVF are not successful.
8. You need a budget and a financial plan if you are undergoing infertility treatment.
9. Infertility treatments are a financial gamble because money doesn't guarantee success.
10. Nothing in life is free.

The Money Game

Here's a tidbit no one bothers to share up-front—infertility is expensive. It is not only time-consuming and emotionally and physically demanding, but also requires an open wallet.

If you're rich, congrats. Money is no object. You'll have fewer problems. You can skip this chapter and move to the next. For the rest of us, fertility costs a lot, which can be devastating if you are not careful. Infertility is on par with weddings and funerals because your emotions get so wrapped up in the process you forget the price. It's easy to forget the ramifications and spend without thinking. You're trying to have a baby; damn the cost! But left unchecked, you may find yourself shelling out money faster than a baby goes through diapers.

The only way to avoid a monetary meltdown midway through is to decide ahead of time how much you are willing to spend. Establish your financial limit from the very beginning, then stay within that framework. Budget baby making, just as you would groceries and vacations. The most successful couples—as in those who end up staying together—take charge of all aspects of their fertility, including the financial one. Sadly, we know a few couples who got divorced over the financial strains infertility put upon them. Occasionally, the husband was a jerk, too, but that's besides the point.

Dollars and Sense

Sometimes it all boils down to making sense out of the dollars. To put it into perspective, we've costed out a few fertility treatments (without insurance coverage considered) to give you an idea of what you might be possibly spending. All costs are averages, of course, and subject to change at the whim of the industry and your doctor. Interestingly, the cost of various procedures can vary greatly depending on where you live. In our limited study, it seems to be the bigger the city, the higher the price.

Fertility drugs: These meds are not cheap and make up the major cost of each treatment cycle. Expect to pay between $50 (for one cycle of Clomid, excluding doctor visits) to as much as $2,500 to $4,000 (for one cycle of gonadotropin injections, including doctor's visits) per cycle, depending on your treatment plan and the drugs involved. Some cycles will demand several drugs.

We suggest checking different pharmacies around town to get the best prices on drugs. It's interesting how much costs can vary for the same darn thing. We suppose if you live near the border, you could get your drugs in Canada or Mexico—at least until the bureaucrats in Washington shut down the over-the-border prescription pipeline.

Also, make sure you buy what your doctor ordered. For example, if your doctor orders progesterone, make sure it is natural progesterone. There is an increased risk of birth defects associated with synthetic progesterone.

Artificial insemination (AI): The cost for having the doctor inject sperm into a woman's uterus through a catheter is $250 to $750.

Sperm wash: Washing sperm is a multiple step procedure that removes as many weak or unhealthy sperm as possible so that the resulting concentration boasts the strongest swimmers. The average cost is $150.

Ovulation induction with artificial insemination (AI): The average cost of ovulation induction is $1,600 for office visits, injection training, baseline FSH test, and estrogen and ultrasound monitoring throughout the cycle. This price excludes fertility drugs.

In vitro fertilization (IVF): The average cost of removing eggs from a woman's ovaries, mixing them with her partner's sperm, and implanting the resulting embryos into her uterus is about $9,000, although fees for this procedure range from $7,000 to $15,000, depending on the doctor, clinic, and hospital. This cost estimate includes office visits, baseline tests, estrogen and ultrasound monitoring, hospital retrieval costs and embryo freezing, in-lab fertilization expenses, hospital transfer costs, and physician services. The price excludes fertility drugs.

Intracytoplasmic sperm injection (ICSI) combined with IVF: The cost of injecting a single sperm into a single egg and having the embryo that results implanted into a woman's uterus is $10,000 to $17,000, depending on the doctor, clinic, and hospital. ICSI combined with IVF adds an additional $1,000 to $1,500 to cost of IVF.

Gamete intrafallopian transfer (GIFT): This procedure mixes the harvested eggs and sperm in a lab. The resulting mix is injected into a woman's Fallopian tubes with the hopes fertilization will occur naturally there. This costs the same as IVF—$7,000 to $15,000, depending on the doctor, clinic, and hospital.

Zygote intrafallopian transfer (ZIFT): Again, the harvested eggs and sperm are mixed together in the lab. The difference is that the doctor ensures that the eggs are fertilized before putting them into a woman's Fallopian tubes. Same cost estimates as IVF—$7,000 to $15,000 depending on doctor, clinic, and hospital.

Donor eggs: The cost is $10,000 to $50,000 and includes compensation to the egg donor as well as the egg retrieval and subsequent IVF. The donor's eggs and egg retrieval are never covered by your insurance.

Surrogates: The cost is $15,000 to $60,000, with the money going to the attorneys and agencies, as well as toward the surrogate's medical expenses. This is never covered by insurance.

Hysteroscopy: This uterine surgery can range from $350 to $600.

Laparoscopy: Average costs are $3,000 to $10,000 for a doctor to perform this surgery.

In addition to these specific procedures, there are constant tests, blood work, office visits, and sonograms. There is also anesthesia to pay for. Okay, you get the idea. It's involved, and it's expensive.

How Much Is Too Much?

Now that you have ballpark figures on what some fertility procedures will set you back, it's time to determine your limit. How much money you budget for fertility treatments is a personal decision. Money is an integral part of the whole big baby-making picture, so spend some time thinking and talking about it. Here are a few questions to get the ball rolling.

How much time will you devote to trying to have a biological child?

How much money will you budget to trying to have a biological child?

Do you want to have money left for adoption, donor eggs, or surrogacy should treatment fail?

How will you pay for all this?

Will one parent quit his or her job to stay home with the child after he or she is born? How will that affect your family's insurance coverage or your ability to pay off your fertility debt?

When it comes to family finances, all things are relative. If you're both hot-shot lawyers, you might not sweat losing six figures to infertility in your quest for kids, like our Texas pals who spent more than $150,000 to conceive their two IVF tots. Dual career couples with no kids have more disposable coin than their married-with-kids cohorts—which is why the budget may change for those experiencing secondary infertility. It's tougher to pay for Pergonal and preschool at the same time.

Sometimes you have to get creative. We have several friends who are still paying off the loans they took out to create their kids. One pal calls the monthly payment to a line of credit her "Melanie mortgage" in honor of the precious IVF daughter the money helped them create.

Remember, however, that when you charge your fertility—whether on plastic or with a line of credit—you also pay for the failures. Lucinda, who lives near Maureen, has had numerous fertility failures that she and her husband financed on a credit card. It tortures her to pay that bill—a monthly reminder when she pays the minimums that she is still childless. When Maureen had her first miscarriage, she was billed for many months for the D&C her insurance was supposed to cover. It haunted her each month when it showed up on the bill, until it was finally straightened out.

We compare investing in your fertility with gambling—or investing in the stock market. There are no guarantees. Spending more money on infertility may give you more chances at conception, but there is still no assurance you will have a biological child. Money can't always buy everything. Even for the wealthy, spending $200,000 on several unsuccessful IVFs, the way one of our West Coast girlfriends did, has to be a bit of a hit.

Know Your Limit

Starting the process with a clear picture of your reality makes budgeting easier. Before you write even one check to a fertility doctor or pharmacist, sit down with your partner and discuss how far you are willing to go *emotionally* with this process. Emotions impact financial decisions. Once you dive into treatment, it's easy to fall into the trap of thinking, "I shouldn't take a month off from infertility treatment for any reason. . . . I just know that this next month will be the one!"

But it is equally important periodically to reassess your treatment plan, finances, and parenting goals. Continuity in treatment is important, but sometimes a break can provide needed rest and renewal for the next steps—as well as a chance to regroup financially.

"For me, after three years of tests and surgeries and pills and shots, I finally had to stop," says our friend Susan, who recently adopted a little boy from the Ukraine. "I was emotionally bankrupt, and Roger and I had exhausted our bank account. It was hard, but we reached a point where we needed to set all of it aside and just start living a normal life again."

Create a Financial Plan

When you have a plan, you are in control. Start by determining how much time, energy, and money you want to invest in trying to conceive a biological child. Decide how far you are willing to go with surgeries and procedures. When you figure out where you draw the line, develop your backup baby plan, so that when the time comes you will be ready to consider options like adoption, foster parenting, or surrogacy.

Having a defined game plan helps you pull yourself out of the whole situation when it gets to be too much. But few of us think to sit down and have the discussion early on. We didn't. In fact, Laura is our only pal who really tried to reach an early agreement with her spouse on the conception cash flow.

"I would advise every couple to have a 'what are your limits conversation' right at the start," says forty-two-year-old Laura, married to Evan for seven years, and finally pregnant with IVF twins.

After much cajoling on Laura's part, Evan finally admitted that it was paramount to him to have his own biological child and that he was willing to spend up to $100,000 to achieve that goal. "Once the decision was made, we knew what we had to do," says Laura. "We didn't have the money, per se, but we knew where our comfort level in spending was." The couple put a second mortgage on their house, borrowed the rest from their parents, and began intensive fertility treatments.

"Evan wanted a baby so friggin' bad, I was willing to do a donor egg if we had to, but I really didn't want to shell out $70,000 for a surrogate," adds Laura, who ended up getting pregnant with her own eggs on their third IVF. "I saw *that* as money we could use to adopt and start a college fund."

The point of Laura and Evan's story is this: The time to talk turkey is right now—before you are in too deep. No sense in being both emotionally and financially bankrupt at the end of this ordeal.

Here are a few questions to help you and your partner get a clear picture on the limit of your fertility finances.

1. Do you understand how much money this will cost?
2. Do you understand that we may spend all this money and still not have a baby?
3. How will we pay for this?
4. How far into debt are we willing to go to finance this?
5. Does our insurance cover any of this?

6. Where will the money come from to pay for treatments that are not covered by insurance?

The Baby Budget

Now that you know your limits, let's talk about your insurance companies limits. How much you pay depends on your problems, your treatment plan, and how much your insurance company is willing to cover.

Insurance is a crap shoot. Some companies have good coverage and some don't. We were lucky. Maureen had great insurance, and Julie good insurance coupled with doctors willing to go to bat with her when the insurance company balked over an expenditure. We still spent more money than we ever expected, but at least some of it was covered.

Insurance coverage of infertility is nothing if not confusing. Some insurance companies cover nothing fertility related—other than pregnancy itself. Others cover some procedures but no medications or IVF. Still others cover almost everything once you reach your deductible and stay in the plan. In still other cases, insurance may not cover infertility treatment, per se, but will cover treating some infertility-inducing medical conditions.

"There is so much you don't think about before you go through infertility," says our buddy Ellen, a schoolteacher who endured three years of treatment. "I never thought to check out my insurance so closely before. And then trying to dissect it all! Our coverage handled most of the cost of the drugs, which was very helpful. It also covered all the tests I had up until we went out of the HMO to the specialist for the IVF consultation. They would not have covered IVF if we had gone that far. Thank goodness I got pregnant before we had to figure out how to fund that!"

Fortunately, many clinics have a staff member who specializes in dealing with the insurance companies and will help you. Others will file your insurance for you once you meet your deductible.

Here are three ways you can take charge of your fertility finances.

1. Understand your insurance coverage: Look at all the plans available to your family through both spouses' jobs. Determine which plan offers the best coverage and go with that one. To get the full info, read the benefits booklet (we know, they are tedious) and talk with someone in the company's human resources office.

2. Understand your fertility issues. Make your doctor explain your specific fertility issues to you carefully. Take notes and understand everything he or she is saying so that you can explain it to your insurance company. This in-depth knowledge about your issues will help you when you deal directly with the insurance company.

3. Be persistent. Just because an insurance company says no the first time, doesn't mean the answer is really no. They may need more details, or you may need to speak to a supervisor. Ask questions. Demand answers. Be prepared to fight for your fertility coverage.

Reading the Policy

Each insurance policy is different, and things change constantly in this industry (usually not for the best of the patient, but that's another congressional-based story). To ensure you understand your benefits regarding infertility testing and treatment, you need to understand your policy, which can be more confusing to read than a computer manual. Check out your insurance handbook, call your insurance company's customer service department, or stop by the human resources department of your company to get the full scoop on what is and isn't covered. Before you start shopping for better insurance, check to see if you can upgrade your (or your spouse's) existing policy. There may be other possibilities available. Of course, you may have to pay the difference in the premiums, but it may be worth it.

But just because your insurance doesn't cover something doesn't mean you should bypass it. Why do fifteen IUIs because your insurance pays for it when you really need IVF—which isn't covered? Does that make sense? No. This shouldn't even make sense to the insurance company. We can't figure out why they would want to pay for a less expensive procedure that has been determined won't work for you, when they could pay (or partially pay) for a procedure that will. Maybe you can explain it to them and perhaps they will change their minds. It's worth a shot.

Our friend Lee was inspired by a woman in her RESOLVE support group who had expressed the same feelings, then decided to get out the big guns, so to speak, and go straight to IVF, with success. "After nine months on various drugs, I decided to take her route and go more immediately to IVF," says this mother of twins.

In putting all her eggs into one IVF basket, Lee went against the advice of two very respected reproductive endocrinologists. "One RE I loved. He treated me as an equal, and even though I went against his advice, he acknowledged that I did so having sound knowledge and information about the issues, the chances, and my health."

Lee acknowledges that she was able to go this more rapid route because she and her husband, Bennet, had the financial resources to pay for IVF without becoming impoverished. "When I was going through this in the nineties, other less successful, less expedient procedures were covered by insurance, while IVF was not, which incentivized doctors and patients alike to continue month after month trying what insurance would cover," says Lee, whose kids recently started kindergarten. "I really believe that insurance companies might save themselves money if they just covered IVF—so that fewer people would choose to spend all this time waffling around in the never-never land of laparoscopies, inseminations, and everything else. If paying for IVF is a huge financial burden, couples are not going to move toward it so quickly, and as a result, may spend more months, even years, doing fertility treatments that are less likely to result in success."

We couldn't say it better ourselves.

Time to Move On?

Some of our friends actually changed jobs to get better insurance coverage. Really.

Our friend Jimmy is a practical guy. A thirty-three-year-old insurance agent married to a thirty-nine-year-old computer analyst, he believes in proactive planning. Infertility has been ruling their lives since they married and began trying to conceive two years ago. Their old insurance covered only some of the procedures but did not cover medications nor IVF.

"My wife is a researcher," Jimmy says of Gail. "When we first started thinking we may have an infertility problem, she was on the Internet and in the library gathering information. Every medication or procedure she's had, she researched first. She researched insurance coverage as well and actually just changed jobs specifically for better insurance benefits for infertility."

The duo is waiting for the grace period to end on the insurance before resuming fertility treatments. Then, their plan is move straight to IVF. "Gail's new insurance will cover three egg retrievals for IVF," says Jimmy. "If we surpass that limit and we're given hope from the docs that further attempts would succeed, we'd find the money to continue."

Our friend Sam is also making a job change for his future family. "The most surprising thing for me is how many couples have infertility problems," says Sam, a forty-year-old executive married to Tammy, a thirty-five-year-old administrative assistant. "I was really shocked. I was also surprised to learn how little most insurance plans cover."

Under Sam's insurance coverage, the couple has been able to do a basic fertility workup, three IUIs and an HSG for Tammy. "It also covered a laparoscopy for her, where the doc found Stage II endometriosis," says Sam. "But, now for us to go further, we need different insurance. The docs have suggested we try injectables, which may cost as much a $1,000 per month. We're most likely going to skip ahead and go right to IVF if we can find a job with insurance that covers it."

Sam has an application in at a company that employs some friends. "We found out about their insurance when they were successful with IVF," he says. "They told us their insurance covered the procedure, so I applied there."

Our suggestion is to ask to review the specific insurance plan of any prospective employer. If they can't make that available, at least try to get the plan name and the insurance company. You can then check the insurance company's website for more details. Also, it might be wise to mix up your questions about infertility coverage with questions about other coverage issues so as not to raise a red flag with the insurance company or the prospective employer. Who wants to hire someone who might be pregnant within a year or two?

Skip the State?

If you would consider changing jobs for infertility coverage, you might also consider changing states. Here's why. Our friend Deb, felt her insurance was adequate, although it didn't cover the three artificial inseminations and the one IVF she eventually had.

"My insurance covered most of the other stuff at 80 or 90 percent," she says. "Our prescription plan covered the drugs; I had a $5 co-payment, which was great because one of my prescriptions was $1,200 for one cycle."

But lack of insurance coverage limited the couple to one IVF. "It was all we had money for," she says. "There's a lot involved with IVF—several somewhat painful tests to undergo, shots to get the maximum number of eggs, retrieving them, all the lab work, inserting the embryos, then the waiting, which is the worst. Then, our procedure didn't work—the embryos didn't attach. This made it like a very expensive experiment . . . that failed."

Had Deb, who lives in Utah, relocated to Arkansas prior to IVF, however, her insurance would have covered the procedure. It's true. Some states have regulations mandating fertility coverage and actually require insurance companies by law to cover in vitro fertilization. Arkansas, for example, requires that IVF be covered up to $15,000 in most cases, unless either partner has had a surgical procedure specifically to prevent pregnancy. State laws change frequently, but when we went looking, we found fifteen states with either mandates to offer coverage or mandates to actually cover some aspects of infertility, including IVF.

A "mandate to offer" is a law requiring insurance companies to make available health policy that covers some aspects of infertility treatment. Employers, however, are not required to pay for the infertility treatment coverage. States we found with some type of mandate to offer are California, Texas, and Connecticut.

A "mandate to cover" is a law requiring insurance companies to provide coverage of infertility treatment as a benefit included in every health care policy, with infertility treatment coverage included in the policy premium. Some states have several conditions that must be met or limit the number of IVF cycles. Others mandate coverage but exclude IVF. States we found with mandates to cover include Arkansas, Hawaii, New York, New Jersey, Maryland, Massachusetts, Ohio, Montana, Illinois, Louisiana, Rhode Island, and West Virginia.

Two organizations that keep tabs on the latest state legislation are RESOLVE and the American Society of Reproductive Medicine. Both have great websites. Check out RESOLVE's at www.resolve.org and the American Society of Reproductive Medicine website at www.asrm.com.

Buy the Best

Having said that infertility is expensive and is not completely covered by all insurance policies, we are now going to sound contradictory by telling you to get the best medical advice and treatment you can afford. Like Julie's husband likes to say, it doesn't cost any more to go first class, you just can't go as far. So find the best doctor and clinic in your area and hotfoot it over there.

Insurance companies, however, may hamper your quest. The best doctor in your city, for example, may not be on your plan. Some physicians are not on any insurance plans because they don't want the insurance companies dictating their treatment protocol. The expectation is that most insurance policies don't cover the testing and treatment performed at their clinics, so why bother with the hassle of dealing with them? These clinics will supply you with a duplicate form to file with your insurance company. Most are also happy to assist you in getting information on your policy or providing extra information for your insurance claim.

But don't write off a doctor just because your insurance doesn't cover him or her. Before choosing another doctor, calculate the costs and consider paying the difference your insurance doesn't cover when you go out of plan.

Final Fiscal Thoughts

We don't recommend that you finance your baby quest by taking out a second mortgage, stripping your retirement account, or piling on credit card debt. But we aren't your mothers, either. We know you'll do what you feel you have to do. Some friends borrowed from family members or pinched pennies until they turned into needed dollars. Others maxed out credit cards or took out loans, which removes any chance of keeping your infertility secret. Still others spent wildly and had to file bankruptcy. It's really your choice.

Some fertility clinics offer special financing packages, as do some creative doctors. Some doctors or hospitals might offer a reduced rate for those interested in participating in clinical trials or trying new procedures. It doesn't hurt to ask.

Some clinics also offer a refund policy for IVF. Often, a refund plan returns a stated percentage of in-cycle expenses if the patient meets certain criteria. For some, it may be "if a pregnancy sustained through the first trimester (twelve weeks) does not result in a baby." Other criteria may state that "all frozen embryos resulting from the initial egg retrieval must be transferred in order to qualify for refund." Some programs apply only to couples for whom IVF is medically indicated. Others cover egg donation but not in situations requiring a gestational surrogate. Any clinic offering such refund programs will outline in detail the eligible expenses and the procedures necessary to recoup any dollars.

There are even grants around for those who need some assistance financing their infertility. Our friend Christa participated in one in New York that was based on yearly income.

"You had to pay a percentage of the $12,000 according to what the chart said you could afford," she says. "There were guidelines for participation—in this case, you had to be under thirty-eight years old and had to have done IVF fewer than three times. Technically I had done it twice before with my first doctor, so I was only eligible to use the grant one time. I'm not sure how medications figured in, since my insurance did cover them, but I guess they figure that into the scale. I wound up paying less than $2,000 for my IVF that time because our income from 2003 was very low."

Christa found out about the grant program from a nurse her sister knew. "I did all the paperwork through the participating physician's office, through the coordinator who worked with the Department of Health. Guess they are the ones who financed the grant. The coordinator asked me the questions, then mailed me the paperwork. I had to give her copies of my W-2 forms from the year before, and she came back to me eventually with a percentage that I would be responsible for. I paid my $2,000, and the rest of the doctor's fee was covered by the grant."

No matter how you pay for your treatment, consider it practice for when Junior arrives. Once you have children, you might as well open your wallet and leave it on the kitchen counter with a sign that reads, "Take Me." Diapers, food, cute outfits, and college tuition ain't cheap, either! Luckily, most toys will probably be supplied by overindulgent grandparents and friends.

CHAPTER 15

SELF-care IS SELF-preservation

Julie

The first thing my reproductive endocrinologist suggested (demanded?) was that I quit all my exercising, other than walking. That may sound easy to you, but exercise is my outlet, my stress-buster, my me-time . . . , and our couple time. Robert and I met at a health club, and working out together is part of who we are as a couple, part of the glue. Suddenly no more running, no more biking, no more weights, and no more rowing machine relegated us to what . . . walking the dogs?

Walking the dogs it was.

It was awfully hard at first to slow down to a stroll, but eventually walking the dogs became our nightly routine. We'd leave our house, walk downtown to the Square, and make multiple loops while we looked in shop windows and debriefed each other about our respective days. It became our new couple time. The dogs loved it. And, eventually, I slowed down enough to love it, too.

I had to stop running, stop biking, and start walking to find my quiet center, to give my body a chance to round out and soften for a baby, to give my mind a break, to finally relax enough to see the big picture of my life. Why was I running everywhere when walking could get me there, too . . . eventually? I'm not going to tell you I really enjoyed watching my hips and upper arms lose their gym-trim tone. I hated it. But in the grand scheme of things, is that really so bad?

Maureen

When I got pregnant with my son I was a lean, mean machine. But I wasn't meant to be.

When I was studying dance, I remember my ballet teacher coming up to me one day and telling me I could be an incredible dancer if I would just lose those last ten pounds. Ballerinas just don't have my round hips and ever-present tummy. I remember thinking when that teacher made this potentially life-altering comment that although I might not be built to be a dancer, I was sure built to have babies. My friend Eric used to tell me the reason my legs were short was so that when I spit those future kids out they wouldn't have far to fall! Still, I exercised like a fiend for my dancing instructor. But I was convinced that, having paid on the dance front with not being the right body type, I would reap my rewards on the birthing front—wrong. They had to use a vacuum to suck Quinn out of me — and even that didn't work. Finally, after twenty-six hours of labor and five hours of pushing, the doctor basically sliced me to the rear, stuck a hand up, and pulled him out . . . kind of like a cow. Apparently all the exercise I did was no help at all.

But I continued exercising. Along with the everyday strain of life, I was constantly spinning. If it wasn't on a bicycle, then it was in my head. When I suffered infertility, it didn't dawn on me to slow down. It never occurred to me that my life was affecting my hormones. I thought I was superwoman, and I wasn't. Eventually, I realized my body was crying out to me, and I hadn't been listening. I stopped immediately and changed my life. I began to get my rest, breathe, and take in the world around me. I rounded out my body and my life. I may carry a few extra pounds around with me now, but when I look into my children's eyes, I am proud of each and every ounce.

Ten Reasons Why You Need to Keep Your Sanity

1. You are the mother ship; everything really revolves around you.
2. You can't depend on your husband to remain sane.
3. You don't have time or energy to expend on going wacko.
4. The fertility drugs will keep you nuts enough.
5. A calm environment within your body makes it more hospitable to conception.
6. You deserve it.

7. Life is too short.
8. You need to make rational decisions.
9. Insanity requires too much energy—energy you need to save for the baby you want.
10. Calmness breeds introspection, which can help you deal with the insanity of infertility.

Surviving Life in Thirty-day Cycles

Infertile women hate the word "relax," but putting the process into perspective is critical to your sanity. When you are involved in fertility treatments and know the inner workings of your reproductive system like never before, you finally understand the importance of each day of the month. Day one? Better start that Premarin. Where's the Parlodel? What about the baby aspirin? Honey, I need you to give me this shot! What day is today? Honey, I need you to give me this shot! Oh, there's that good cervical mucus! Honey, I need you to give me this shot! Felt a twinge—must be ovulating! Honey, we need to have sex now! Honey, we need to have sex again. Now! Okay, where's that progesterone? Am I pregnant? I don't feel pregnant . . . or maybe I do? I don't want to think about it. Honey, do you think we're pregnant? I'm going to buy a pregnancy test just in case. Am I pregnant? I don't feel pregnant . . . or maybe I do? I don't want to think about it. Oh . . . Honey, I got my period. Shit.

In addition to all this homework, you may be driving daily to the clinic for monitoring, bloodletting, and sonogram scanning and to the pharmacy to ensure you have all the drugs you need to get through the month. You will also have to find time to actually go to your real job (if they haven't fired you yet for absenteeism or falling asleep in your cubicle), clean your house, and go grocery shopping. Oh yeah, and have a romantic date with your partner to keep the love alive while you try to conceive a couple of kids to add to the mix!

Infertility is daunting. It's overwhelming. But this we know: You can do this. You can survive this.

Baby Madness

Infertility creates stress? That's a no-brainer. Research shows undergoing infertility treatment can produce a level of stress similar to dealing with serious illnesses such as cancer and heart disease. The roller coaster begins each month with the hope that you will become pregnant and ends with disappointment if you don't. Along the way, there are prescriptions to take, sex to schedule, doctor visits to juggle, and checks to write. Who wouldn't be stressed? Unfortunately, obsessing about infertility will not help you get pregnant, which is too bad, because obsessing about our infertility is what we all do so well. And now we're telling you to stop.

Here's why you have to focus on taking care of you—stress can mess up our bodies. Too much stress can tinker with hormone levels, cause irregular ovulation, screw up your periods, and decrease sperm production in a guy. It can also cause your Fallopian tubes and uterus to spasm—not good.

Stress can mess up your sleep patterns, increase your heart rate and blood pressure, and lower your immune system's defenses. Stress and age affect your progesterone levels. (Maureen is our test study.) We deduce this from our own experiences and those of our friends.

MAUREEN

I think stress caused my infertility. Not only because a doctor told me stress can alter progesterone production, but also because, in retrospect, I was stressed out. Stress is part of my generation. We're the women who were told we could have it all, so we are out there fighting for equality in the workforce and trying to balance career with having a family. Stress is part of my life.

At the time I was trying to get pregnant, I was also orchestrating a cross-country move for my family. Add to that the biological clock ready to ring its alarm for that second baby. We moved back to New York in July 2001. Two months later September 11 changed the world as we knew it—right in our new backyard.

The additional stress definitely affected my body. I began to have tremors in my arms and hands, blurry vision, and extreme fatigue. A neurologist diagnosed me with "dead arm syndrome" and put me in intensive physical therapy for six months to remove the adrenaline trapped in my muscles that was beginning to affect my entire system. While this was going on, I went through a battery of tests to determine what had caused my miscarriages.

Stress doesn't have to be visible to amass inside of you, change your chemistry, and affect your hormones. In a cosmic sense, perhaps it's God's way of keeping a baby safe by not giving it life inside the body of a stressed-out woman. Perhaps this is to prevent new life from being brought into a toxic environment.

JULIE

Like Maureen, I have a stress story. Stay with me, there is a fertility point at the end.

In order to prepare for the family reunion we offered to host in June 2004, Robert and I decided to finish some renovations on our house. We tore out walls, moved a bathroom, and totally redid the kitchen. We started in January. In February, we decided to also renovate a rental house at the back of our property into a guest house—and have it done in time for the reunion. Then in March, we decided to landscape, too.

Soon, we were down one bathroom and entering the construction zone that used to be our kitchen through a wall of plastic. All our food staples were stacked in the dining room, the coffeemaker sat in the master bathroom, and the refrigerator had been moved to the back porch. To get milk, you had to go out the front door, down the driveway, and onto the back porch. Simply preparing breakfast was an aerobic exercise. It stayed like this right up to the first of June.

As if this weren't enough, I helped start a private kindergarten at my son's school, began potty training our daughter, planned a four-day bash for sixty family members, and worked on this book, which sold to the publisher in May.

One week before my family reunion, I went to the doctor covered head-to-toe in a splotchy rash. Not only did I have strep throat, but also mononucleosis and parvovirus B-19, more commonly known to moms as fifth disease—a childhood rash disease that can manifest itself in adults for several months complete with recurring rash and arthritis-like joint pain. I was falling apart, knocked out by a bunch of kid's diseases. I was exhausted, splotchy, and achy for most of the summer—all stress-induced.

More interesting, however, was the havoc this was all wreaking on my menstrual cycle. Beginning in April, those regular every-twenty-ninth-day-of-the-month cycles that had come with the birth of Amanda disappeared. One month, my period would show up on day forty-two—and last seven days. The next month I would have cramping like clockwork on the twenty-ninth (two weeks from my last period!), but wouldn't bleed for four more weeks and then bleed lightly for three days. Four weeks later, I would get my period and bleed for eight days. This went on for seven months.

Talk about inconvenient. I never knew when I was going to get my period. For a while, I thought I'd hit perimenopause at age forty-four. Then I thought maybe I was pregnant, so every month I'd buy a pregnancy test just in case, wasting a total of $52. I finally quit diagnosing myself and went to my gyn doctor. Dr. Hunt told me that given the stress in my life, coupled with my body being so sick (also an immune system reaction to the stress), it was no surprise to him my periods were irregular. He said to try to take it easy for a few months and come back and see him if things didn't get back to normal.

I worked to remove the stress from my life over the summer. Surprise! By mid-fall, my periods were back to normal. So I have firsthand knowledge about the physical power of stressful situations. Here's my analysis: Stress messes up hormones, messes with ovulation, and messes with your mind. Stress can alter your monthly cycle.

If your period is screwed up and you don't know when the heck you're ovulating, you tell me how you expect to get pregnant.

It's a vicious circle. As we know from personal experience, if you can't conceive on cue, it's easy to feel depressed, angry, and anxious. The spontaneity disappears from sex—as well as most of the fun!—which adds even more stress. Stress leads to infertility, which can lead to stress, which messes up fertility, which messes up your mind. It's a variation on the old chicken and egg quandary again. Which came first—stress or infertility?

A 2001 study by the Magee-Women's Research Institute found increased levels of the stress hormone cortisol in reproductive-age women who had amenorrhea (stopped menstruating). Called "functional hypothalamic amenorrhea" (FHA), this condition features erratic or totally absent periods and affects about 5 percent of women in their childbearing years.

Basically, this is stress screwing up your periods because researchers determined that FHA is not caused by any defect in the women's reproductive parts. Women with this condition were often perfectionists, tried to get too much done in one day, or made poor nutritional or lifestyle choices. Gee, what woman doesn't that sound like? When women were treated with stress-relieving behavior therapy and nutritional counseling, most got their periods back to normal. Want to hear something funny? Most of the women in the study didn't even realize they were under stress! Just like most of us!

The emotional upheaval of infertility can also impact your ability to conceive. Some men will suffer impotence when they discover they have a low sperm count. Some women won't want to have sex because they feel like failures. Others are exhausted by the time and energy consumed by fighting for their fertility. So is stress the cause or the effect?

Me First

Let's focus on that stupid word "relax" for a minute. Here's why we hated it so much when we were in the throes of our infertility—because we kept hearing it from everyone in the wrong context. Like "If you'd just relax, you'd get pregnant." Well, there is some truth to the fact that you need to relax—for your sanity's sake, as well as your fertility's. The big dilemma is how to overcome the guilt of taking time to simply breathe.

We have some ideas.

We're pretty much a Me Society. Baby-making is pretty much a selfless act or should be. So it seems at odds for us to remind you to remember yourself. But it's too easy to lose yourself in infertility, the process, and the outcome. It's easy to get wrapped up in it all. You have to keep the process in perspective to keep your sanity. You are important because your body will house your baby. Without you, there will be no baby. You have to learn to nurture yourself first, so you will have the ability to nurture another life.

If you don't, if you allow yourself to be consumed by the quest to conceive, you will end up like a car with no gasoline—empty. Eventually all the parts will freeze up, and the engine will no longer work.

Nourish Your Spirit

The miracle of our children's births reminds us daily of the existence of a higher power. You need to support your spiritual side to survive the challenges of infertility, so search out that solace, whether you are a religious or nonreligious person.

How to do this: Take some time to reflect on who you are and what you really want in your life. Clear the cob webs from your brain and get in touch with your soul. Meditate. Pray. Sit quietly. Start out with just five minutes a day—five minutes to allow yourself a chance to breathe. Shake the tension from your shoulders. Drop your head. Listen to your heart. Increase it to ten to fifteen minutes, and you will find that the intensity and pressure of infertility will begin to lift. Becoming philosophical about things we cannot control is one way to deal with them. At some point it is out of our hands, out of the doctor's hands, and in the hands of a higher power, something that is bigger than all of us.

Really Relax

What if we told you learning to relax might help you to conceive? Would you take a break then?

Well, there is scientific evidence that stress causes infertility. A relaxed, peaceful body is more apt to function "normally," normalize your periods; normalize egg production, fertilization and implantation; and increase your desire to actually make love to your partner.

How to do this: Give yourself a break. Slow down. Walk when you want to run. Don't just hear the music of life, really listen to it. Smell the air—really suck it in deeply into your lungs and blow it out hard. It will definitely help your state of mind—a more relaxed body, a more relaxed mind . . . a sense of balance.

Lie Down

Your body does its best work at night when you are asleep. This is the time for your mind to reflect onto itself, and your body to repair all the daily damage it incurred while moving you around the planet. If you don't go to bed, however, none of this can happen.

How to do this: Get some sleep. Go to bed earlier. Can't do it? Used to working until midnight on all those projects? Stop it. If you have to wean yourself slowly, then start by going to bed thirty minutes earlier, then increase it to another thirty minutes. The goal? By the end of thirty days, have your butt in bed by 9:00 P.M., lights out by 9:30 P.M., 10:00 P.M. at the max. You'll be surprised at how much better you start to feel. After your body catches up on the

MAUREEN

When I got pregnant, my friend Greg, who is very centered and spiritual, kept telling me, "Go lie down and rest." He wanted me to rest my body, mind, and spirit and reduce my stress.

I didn't listen to him, kept going, and kept losing my babies to miscarriage. After six inseminations and no success, my doctor gave up on me. I cried and mourned my loss.

Then, one day, it dawned on me. Maybe Greg was right. Maybe all that had happened to me was a sign to slow down, so I did. I bought a very expensive down comforter, put it on my bed, took the weight of the world off my shoulders, and snuggled under that comforter as often as I could. Within six months, my life was different. I quit mourning. I moved on. We made an offer on a house and took a romantic weekend trip, during which I got pregnant with Ava.

I had my nest, I had some sanity, and I had my health back. My progesterone levels throughout that pregnancy were perfect. There is no science that can support all of this, but that down comforter was the best investment I ever made.

sleep it was lacking, you will actually find yourself beginning to wake up earlier and earlier, giving you plenty of time to do some stretching, walk the dog, drink your decaf, or make love to your husband without having to rush!

Get Your Priorities Straight

The most important priority in your life right now is fixing your fertility. Everything else is secondary, except your relationship with your partner!

How to do this: Schedule everything. Write it down in your date book, Palm Pilot, or BlackBerry. Write down when you have to be at the clinic, when you have to have sex, when you need to go to the dentist, when you want to have coffee with your best friend, and when you must be at that business or civic function. Schedule some "Me" time in, too. Time to buy those holiday gifts. Whatever you have to do in your life, write it down. Then stick to your schedule. Don't cross out one thing for another. Once you write it down, you can forget about it until you flip to that page. You have suddenly prioritized your life. You can look and see what you think is important—and ditch the stuff that ain't. By the way, you are scheduling your priorities here—with baby making and all that entails at the top of the list—not simply prioritizing your current schedule. You are going to drop the stuff that doesn't matter and replace those with time to nourish your spirit, relax, lie down, and remember yourself. Sounds impossible? Try it. Put the priorities in place first, then schedule the rest of your life around it. Presto—a balanced week, a balanced life. And time to get it all done!

Get Negative Out of Your Life

We are borrowing an idea from a brilliant woman for whom Julie used to write speeches. Jinger Heath, former head of Dallas-based BeautiControl Cosmetics, realized one day that being surrounded by negativity had a way of encroaching into her own personal life. She shared the message of getting negative out of your life with the thousands of consultants who sold her company's products. Julie helped Jinger write that speech. Its message of "get negative out of your life" has been Julie's mantra ever since. We believe this philosophy of getting the negative vibe out of your life will help your fertility.

How to do this: To keep the positive attitude necessary for surviving infertility, get everything negative out of your life. Turn off the television news if it upsets you. Bypass the front page of the daily paper. Don't read about every murder or watch those reality shows on which people air their dirty laundry. Why waste time on that crap? You've got better things to do.

Most important, get all the negative people out of your life. These are the constant complainers, whiners, and wailers who want to bring you down to their depths. You've got enough to worry about. Don't take on their burdens, too—even if they have been your best friends for years. You don't have time or energy to waste on all their negativity now—not while you are trying to keep yourself sane.

After you have your family, you may find you don't miss all the trauma and drama and decide to keep negativity out of your life forever. We did.

Overcoming Fertility Fatigue

If you don't take some me time, you will get hit with fertility fatigue. Since you probably won't take any time for yourself—no matter what we say—you will be run over with this exhaustion at some point.

Fertility fatigue happens when you just can't mentally go on anymore. You not only can't, but also really don't want to, either. Well, who wouldn't be exhausted? Look at everything you are doing. You're like that vaudeville guy—the one-man band who played like seven or eight instruments at one time while dancing a jig and wiggling his eyebrows. No one can keep that up forever. Even his act was only five minutes long.

You have to give yourself a break here. A break as in cutting yourself some slack. You can't do it all and do it all well. It's time to prioritize, plan your work, then work your plan. It's time to learn to say "no" and be okay with it. It's time to regain your sanity.

Here are some suggestions from the trenches.

Ten Tips for Keeping Your Sanity

1. Call an infertile friend: Nobody knows what you're going through like someone who's going through it, too. Put their number on speed dial and use it often.

2. Go for a walk: Grab the dog or just your sneakers and head out the door. All that stuff your mom said about fresh air being good for you was right. There's nothing like striding through the neighborhood or a nearby park and drinking in nature to clear one's head.

3. Get a hobby: Obsessing about infertility is not a hobby—although it probably counts as a second job. If you don't have a hobby, get one—learn to paint, try photography, start needlepoint or sewing, build model airplanes. Read a book, watch an old movie, knit a scarf (for yourself or your husband, not the baby you long for). There are a zillion fun things to do, and trust us, you need some fun.

4. Get a life: Remember who you were to help define who you are. Then do something fun the old you would have enjoyed. You're still in there somewhere, you know. Take the time to find you again.

5. Go on a date: Date nights remind you that you're a couple, not just parents-in-waiting. Schedule time together, even if you opt to stay in and rent a movie. Put your date nights on the calendar for every week, and promise not to break them.

6. Surf the Internet: Surfing the latest infertility advances can empower you. Joining an online chat group can comfort. Of course, we also have friends who also tout online shopping as a great distraction.

7. Take a trip: Sometimes simply changing the scenery adjusts an attitude. While a well-deserved vacation to a tropical paradise would be the most fabulous, a weekend getaway in your own town or a mindless trip to the mall also works well.

8. Just say no: You are not superwoman. You cannot do it all. You shouldn't even want to because overcommitment will suck the emotional life right out of you. So quit saying "Yes," as in "Yes, I'll chair that committee," or "Yes, I can pick up your sister at the airport," or "Yes, I can organize that going away party at the office." It's okay to say no when you're asked to do something you really don't want or have time to do. Guess what? It will still get done, just by someone else. Saying no is very liberating. Try it.

9. Write it out: You don't have to be a professional writer or even a good speller to wield the power of the pen. Jotting down your thoughts in a journal is a great way to clear your head and heart. If someone upsets you, write them a letter about how you feel, then tear it up.

10. Cook up some comfort food and eat it: Sure, macaroni and cheese or a hot loaf of fresh bread may not be the best thing for your hips, but what else soothes a weary mind like our favorite foods? Besides, if you're taking fertility drugs, you're already fat. If you don't want to eat that whole batch of chocolate chip cookies, pack them up for the neighbors, or take them with you to the fertility clinic. But for a little while, rejoice in how wonderful the house smells.

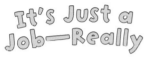

It's Just a Job—Really

All of us make choices every day about how we live our lives, how much work and responsibility we take on at the office, what extras we volunteer to do, where and when we eat and sleep, how many tasks—physical and emotional— we take on. When it comes to becoming and being a mother, everything else really is just a job. If fixing your fertility and creating a family is your goal, make it your priority, which may mean giving up some of the goodies—like that big promotion, redoing the kitchen first before getting pregnant, or that great, trim figure you've worked years to attain.

This is not always easy. Our girlfriend Suzanne was undergoing infertility treatments while finishing her Ph.D. dissertation. In that regard, she was lucky because her time was her own, and she had flexibility to go to doctor's appointments without having to sneak out past glaring coworkers. But she was also putting her career on hold.

"My decisions about jobs were directly affected by whether I'd be pregnant or not," the now mother of two says. "Like, if I don't get pregnant in the next year, this one high-pressured, tenure track job would be fabulous. But if I do get pregnant and have a baby in the next year, I don't want this job. And maybe I don't want to take this exciting high-pressured job anyway if I want to lower my stress levels to optimize the chances of getting pregnant. So here I was, putting myself on the academic job market, but having a hard time making career decisions because I didn't know what my (fertility) situation would be from month to month.

"It also was tough because I was faced with a choice: Do I accept an ideal career position that (because of location and time demands) would mean not pursuing a specific course toward pregnancy? Or do I decline the offer so as to

MAUREEN

When Quinn was three, I went back to work. I had been home with him since his birth and was haunted by that nagging feeling that I wasn't getting anywhere in my life. While I was thrilled to be a mother, I didn't want to be defined by that alone. I wanted more because I was raised to be a career woman. When I was home with Quinn, I secretly felt as if I were failing.

So I started my literary agency. We didn't have the money to hire a babysitter, so Quinn played on the floor while I hid in closets and made phone calls where I hoped no one would hear my child in the background. I worked around the clock for a year with little sleep and no computer or fax machine. Then one morning, my son changed my life (yet again). I was in my bathrobe and slippers with my telephone headset on, cutting up Quinn's waffles, and frantically trying to close a deal. He sat at the counter just staring at me, then suddenly shouted.

"Mama!!!!!!!!"

I shushed him with my finger to my mouth.

"Mama!!!!" Very insistent kid.

I shushed him again, not wanting my client to hear his little voice in the background.

"Mama," he yelled emphatically. "I have something to say to you!!!"

Stunned (because this was so out of character for him), I put my hand over the microphone of my headset and said "What is it, Quinn?"

He looked up at me with his sparkling, blue, innocent eyes and gave it to me straight.

"Mama," he said, "It's just work." Then he smiled at me and went back to eating his waffles.

In that moment, my life changed. His simple statement had such power behind it—and made such sense. I understood what he was saying to me, and I realized I really needed to get my priorities straight and be proud of my choice to be a mother.

Quinn was right. It's just work.

Today I have a healthy toddler and preteen running around my agency, creating all sorts of noises in the background. If anyone has a problem with that, I tell them, "It's just work," and I hang up, smiling.

undergo the surgeries and procedures that may be necessary—not knowing, in the end, whether the sacrifice would even pay off?"

Suzanne stopped fertility treatments for awhile, so she could accept a fabulous, high-intensity, interim job. Another year, she ended up declining a job she really wanted because it became clear that the job circumstances wouldn't let her pursue fertility treatments to the extent she felt might be necessary for success.

"I hated being so in limbo," says Suzanne (who really speaks for many of us!). "I felt like we were indefinitely postponing big life decisions and treading water endlessly, waiting for a resolution on infertility, so we could get on with our lives. Then, it dawned on me. Becoming pregnant was the priority, which meant putting everything else on the back burner temporarily. As it turned out, I wouldn't have the kids I have today if I had done otherwise."

I Need Help!

Infertility has the ability to define everything about you—how you feel about yourself, how you treat others, and how you view your life in general. The trick

JULIE

Back in the eighties, Bruce Willis and Cybill Shepherd starred in a TV series called *Moonlighting*. I have never forgotten a line Bruce's character told the relationship-phobic Cybill character during some boyfriend bungle—it went something like "A good job doesn't love you in the morning."

Boy, is that right. A job is a job.

A job . . . a career . . . whatever . . . will use you up and spit you out without even saying thank you. And if you think you cannot be replaced, you are wrong. Everyone is replaceable—even if you run the show. I am a freelance writer, and I like to think no one else can quite do the job I can. As a result, it took me a long time to learn that it was okay to say no to an assignment—particularly if it infringed on my family and their needs. Using that simple word removed a lot of stress from my life.

I work when my kids are in school. When they come home, I shut up shop. Robert and I try not to work on the weekends and never on vacations if possible. Sometimes I say no to assignments that I really want. Maybe the magazine or news-paper or corporate client will call me back. I always hope they do. But sometimes, they don't. Someone else gets the next assignment. The magazine, newspaper, or the corporation goes on without me.

I am not irreplaceable to a company. Neither are you. Your company will go on without you. But your family won't. Every husband needs a wife who is there. Every family needs a mom who is there. Those people care whether you show up or not.

I worked too hard to build my family—those people who love me in the morn-ing. Here, I am irreplaceable—exhausted, but irreplaceable. Now, that's a good job.

is dealing with this in the healthiest manner possible. For some of us, that means going to a spa, getting a massage, grabbing a decaf hazelnut latte with our best friend, or walking the dog across town and back. For others, it means calling a professional.

At some point, you may feel the need to seek out a psychiatrist, psychologist, or counselor who specializes in people like you—people facing infertility. Your partner can't do all your counseling! He may even need or want to go with you himself. Guys have issues, too. And there's only so much your pals want to hear.

How do you know if you need a few minutes on the couch? If you are depressed or anxious or if your infertility is so overwhelming it's taking over your life and sucking all the joy out of it, you need to call someone. If you have guilt or the blues so bad you cannot shake them or feel totally worthless because of your infertility, you need to seek help. Ditto if you have lost total interest in things that used to excite you; if your relationships with your partner, family, and/or friends are suffering; if you can't sleep, can't eat, or can't stop eating, or if you find yourself abusing alcohol or drugs (not fertility!) as an escape.

It's also good to get another perspective if you and your partner don't know what to do next—if you have unexplained infertility, for example, and are confused as to what you want or should do, or if you are considering donor eggs or sperm or a surrogate, or stopping the whole deal and living child-free, then a visit with a counselor can clear up any concerns.

Ask your doctor to suggest counselors experienced in dealing with infertility. Check with your place of worship. Consider contacting an infertility support group like RESOLVE for recommendations on individual and couple counseling to help you figure things out.

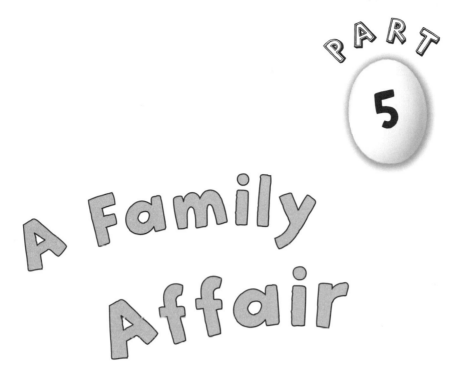

A Family Affair

PART 5

Infertile couples learn pretty quickly that it could take a committee to help them conceive. With all these people in the room, it's easy to lose track of each other and the goal for which you are going through all of this insanity—a family.

Infertility, with its associated guilt, gut-wrenching, and (believe it or not) occasional giggles, can pull a couple apart or stick them together like Velcro. Understanding what the other person is going through, communicating, and maintaining a sense of humor can help you survive.

Maureen

Walking into infertility is like entering a maze. You think you know where you are, but suddenly you're not there anymore. The changes are constant, and just when you think you've got it figured out, you're lost again.

Making a baby, something you always thought would be romantic and exciting, becomes bad theater. Your reproductive life suddenly becomes center stage—and you are the star! Bright lights spotlight you while procedures are going on . . . not exactly the candlelight that you always expected. You begin to see your husband as nothing but one giant sperm. You almost expect the medical staff treating you to break out in a musical kick line, singing, "One . . . sperm and egg sensation. . . . This is all it really takes!"

I told my RE that I was going to turn the entire experience into a Broadway musical and call it *IN-Fertility*. I had my husband, doctor, nurses, and technicians as my cast members. I had them dancing and singing in my mind during my most difficult situations. I envisioned the sperm meeting the egg by IVF with a song "In the Dish." My husband providing his semen sample to the tune of a song "In the Cup." It was a running joke throughout my treatment, and it was so corny that it added some lightness and laughter to a difficult situation. All of us got a kick out of this idea.

I'm sure a therapist would have a field day with how I dealt with all of this, but the most important thing is to find what works for you and use it. It sure beats the other option—sitting in a dark room, weeping.

Julie

Robert and I survived infertility intact and as a couple. It didn't break us, financially, physically, or emotionally. It made us laugh. It made us cry. It made us appreciate even more fully what it is to parent our two kids. We are lucky.

Some couples break up over or during infertility treatments. We've seen it happen in our own close circle of friends. With one couple, the husband went grudgingly into treatment, while his wife was almost manic to have another child. He was happy with their life and content with their only son, who was twelve. Infertility consumed my girlfriend's time and a large portion of the family budget. She missed a lot of time with her son in an effort to have a baby. She missed out on the fun of decorating the huge home her husband bought her in an effort to appease her. She hired a decorator instead. She rarely swam in the pool he installed for her. She focused entirely on adding to her family to the detriment of the family she had.

More than $100,000 later in failed drug therapies, IUIs, and three IVFs, she still was not pregnant—and she was furious. She took out anger on her husband. He felt guilty because he couldn't provide the one thing in life she apparently wanted—a baby. So he began spending more time away from home. Eventually, he found another woman who was happy with what he could provide. Today, she lives in that big fancy house and swims in that pool while my girlfriend lives alone. Her son turned eighteen and moved out on his own three weeks before her divorce became final.

Yep, after surviving infertility, Robert and I can survive anything.

CHAPTER 16

Hypodermic MOMENTS

Maureen

After failing our many inseminations, my doctor suggested we try injectable drugs. Will and I went to class, where we joined several other couples and one brave single woman. They gave us purple kits with syringes, Band-Aids, small cold packs, and assorted other things. The nurse in charge told us about the shots and how to administer them.

The entire experience was odd to me. Although I grew up with a diabetic sister who takes shots daily, I wasn't thrilled with the idea of having my husband shoot me up. When she showed us how to mix the powders and make the drug cocktail, my mind started to race. We're supposed to mix these? We have no experience! How many mistakes have been made by couples like us? I was frightened by the idea of strange drugs being injected into me and especially of the thought of mixing them wrong. It was intimidating to say the least. Then the nurse pulled out an orange and tried to demonstrate how you insert the needle, lift the skin, and shoot.

I looked around the room and saw a lot of queasy faces—men and women both. Everyone looked confused, scared, and in shock—me and Will included. We left the class with me knowing we would not do the needles. I chose to close that door. I'd reached our limit. I have great admiration and respect for couples who take this route, but even now I can't eat an orange without thinking of *injectables*.

Julie

"Shots! What do you mean, my husband has to give me shots?"

This was a shocker to the newly infertile me. Accepting that I had a problem conceiving was much easier than digesting the thought of Robert coming at me with a syringe.

"Shots?" asked my husband. "No problem."

If I close my eyes, I can still see the nurse's face when Robert told her he knew all about giving shots. Lana was standing in Dr. Cohen's office with a syringe in one hand and an orange in the other. I was already sitting down, silently freaking out as Robert calmly explained to us that he grew up giving shots—to horses.

This would be true. At one time, Robert's family had thirty horses—he and his dad went through a period where they went to the horse auction every weekend, buying a few horses this week, selling some the next week . . . it's a long story. They did all the doctoring on their animals. During the equine encephalitis epidemic in the seventies, Robert helped inoculate 1,500 horses in a weekend.

"I've stitched horses up with a leather awl," Robert told me later when I asked for his credentials. "I've had my arm all the way up the ass of horse checking for twist (short for twisted gut, when a horse's intestine twists)."

When you are up to your shoulder in a horse's ass, well, you are a cowboy.

He never practiced on the orange. I cannot count the number of times during our infertility treatment and subsequent pregnancies that he slapped me on the butt a few times before jabbing me with the needle. He was right. He was good. The slapping hurt more than the needle.

"Giving you shots was fun," he told me when I asked him about it as I wrote this chapter. "It's the only time I ever got to slap you on the ass and not get retribution for it."

Thank God I never had twist.

Ten Surprising Things About Infertility

1. Someone other than a doctor or nurse may have to give you shots.
2. You may have to give yourself shots.
3. You will be told when you can and should have sex. You will obey these orders, even if you have a headache.
4. Sex by the calendar loses its thrill pretty fast.

5. You will feel like an egg donor. Your partner will feel like a sperm donor.

6. This will be okay with you.

7. You will be able to say words like penis, vagina, scrotum, and cervical mucus without blushing. Yes, you will.

8. You will discover infertility's comical side and wonder why Jay Leno and David Letterman haven't.

9. You and your partner will find interesting ways to get freshly caught semen to its destination.

10. You will wonder why you are paying so much money to suffer such indignity.

The Indignity of Infertility

Here's the $10,000 (and probably more) question: How far in embarrassment are you willing to go to create a baby? Infertility is nothing if not embarrassing. Everybody in the clinic knows your business; you don't even know their names. You are a science experiment of your own making. One minute you are counting eggs, the next minute you're counting sperm. Your self-esteem is shot, your modesty is gone, and you're fat. You are being shot up by your partner, having sex on command, and walking around with body fluids in unmarked paper sacks. All because you want to. Oh, and you are paying a lot of money for this privilege.

Oh well, nobody ever once said infertility was fun. Funny, yes. Fun, no.

Sex on a Schedule

Get out the Daytimer. It's time to pencil in a little romance, on specific days, specific times, with specific positions. It really sucks, no pun intended, when sex becomes a chore. As one of our husbands said, "You know it's bad when the guy isn't even looking forward to getting laid again."

During infertility, your relationship with your husband changes. Anyone who tells you differently is lying. Julie's husband would refer to baby-making sex as stud farm duty. "Am I on duty tonight?" he'd ask when Julie would suggest an amorous adventure.

But you have to have sex to procreate. When too much sex becomes, well, too much—and it will—you have to get creative. Or just accept that sex is going to be a job for awhile and put up with the mundane aspect of it all. Frankly, jazzing things up is more fun. Not all sex has to have a purpose, although it's easy to get caught up in that cycle. Sex can be just for fun. Remember back when it was fun? Before the thermometers, the shots, and the frantic phone calls—"I'm ovulating. Get home now!"

When Gwen, who lives in San Francisco, was told she was ovulating and ripe for the taking, she immediately called her husband, Sandy, who was on a business trip in New York. He was in a meeting at the time with eight other men and was pulled from the meeting for the phone call. She told him to get on a plane and get home ASAP for some nooky.

Sandy returned to the meeting and announced to the other men, "Gentlemen, that was the phone call we are all waiting for. My wife wants me to get home right now to have some sex!"

The minute the meeting ended, Sandy snapped his briefcase shut and caught the next flight out of town.

We remember things like this. So does our friend Alma, who revved up sex when she started fooling around with how she and her husband fooled around. Alma, a thirty-nine-year-old West Coast designer, had been trying to conceive for two years. Sex was draining until they moved on to intrauterine inseminations (IUI), where the washed sperm is inserted directly into the uterus by a doctor. The result? A little more spontaneity returned to their lovemaking.

"Now that we've been doing IUIs, some of the stress of having to 'do it now' is gone, which has been great," she says. "When we have sex now, it's because we want to, not just because we're on a mission. When my husband has to make his deposit prior to the IUI, we abstain from sex for a few days. I use this opportunity to talk dirty and tease him sexually, knowing he has to wait. I don't know, maybe this helps our sperm count."

Let your hair down. Have sex in different rooms. Dress up in sexy lingerie. Play games. This is easier to do with primary infertility. If you have secondary infertility and a child or two already at home, the sex thing becomes even more complicated. You have to make sure scheduled sexual rendezvous don't conflict with your kid's schedule. Is he asleep yet? Is she awake already? Hurry up, he's going to walk in any minute. If you have to wait for a child to fall asleep before jumping your husband, you may very well be asleep yourself when sex time finally rolls around.

And how do you explain Daddy giving Mommy a shot in the hiney to a sleepy preschooler who walks into your room in search of a glass of water? This was Maureen's dilemma. She could just imagine the conversation. "My dad gives Mom a shot every night, and she says 'Ouch' really loud." Not exactly what you want the preschool kids hearing during show and tell—or the neighbors or your own parents. We suggest those experiencing secondary infertility send the kids to Grandma's before venturing out of the bedroom for sex.

Getting Needled by Your Partner

Even if you kind of knew fertility treatments involve shots, you never really expect your husband will really have to give you yours. Frankly, we never could understand why trained professionals would turn over a bunch of powerful fertility medicine and a stash of syringes to rank amateurs and expect us to do a good job. But this is how it works.

Many fertility drugs need to be injected. Since you don't live at the clinic—though you may feel as if you do—you will have to find some way to get this done at home. Usually your partner or a really good friend learns how to give you these shots. If you live close to the clinic, you might be able to work a deal in which they give you the shot, but this is really inconvenient. And in cases where there is no other choice, you may have to learn to give them to yourself.

You will need to learn how to mix the drugs. Most come in powdered form and have to be mixed with a special solution prior to injection. For those not interested in playing Mad Scientist, some clinics simplify the process for patients with a prefilled, pre-mixed cartridge of medicine that works in a pen-shaped self-injector. This device contains not only the medicine (with a convenient, easy-to-use dial-a-dose feature), but also a teeny needle. Just dial up the amount of drug you need and plunge the pen into your flesh. Done. No mixing. No mess. Pain factor, unfortunately, still exists.

Don't fear. Most offices let couples practice plunging the needle into an orange under supervision before attempting these shots at home. Usually a nurse will help you. Sometimes the doctor's office might show or lend you a video on proper shot technique. Nobody should ever leave the clinic without understanding how to administer a shot correctly, so keep asking questions until you understand it.

Our friend Lynne dragged her husband along to the injectables class necessary for their treatment protocol. "I told Leo, 'we are in this together,'" she says. "It was very, very important to my husband to have a biological child of his own. I felt bad I was having trouble giving him that child, but I also felt like if this is so important to you, and I am willing to do all this stuff to my body because

I love you, you are going to be the one who gives me the shots. I felt as if Leo needed some responsibilities, too.

"I told him, 'Honey, I need you to help me. . . . I don't feel comfortable giving myself these shots.' But my thought was, 'I'll be damned if I'm going to do this myself.'"

Like most of us, Lynne balked at the idea of two regular Joes heading home with their drugs, needles, and a red jug with a yellow "hazardous waste" label. "I couldn't believe they would trust us laypeople to do this," says Lynne. "The glass bottles, the powder, the needles, and syringes. I just kept thinking God will protect me. I had blind faith.

"To be on the safe side, I always mixed it up myself," she adds. "And tapped out all those air bubbles."

Playing Doctor . . . or Whatever Works

Sometimes you've gotta do what you've gotta do to get through the shots, the sperm donations, the poking and prodding, and the incessant anxiety that is infertility. Consider it comic relief or fodder for future family jokes. Why can't you have some fun with infertility?

To get through the whole shots scenario each night, Tom and Mary (not their real names) started playing doctor, literally. Tom would mix up the drug, load the syringe, and inject Mary—all the while mimicking their fertility doctor . . . accent and all.

"One night, Tom came out of the bathroom brandishing the syringe and wearing a surgeon's mask," says Mary. "I have no idea where he got it, but it just cracked me up. Another time, he gave me a lollipop for being a good patient because our doctor kept a glass jar of suckers on his desk. It seems silly to talk about now, but really it helped me relax for those stupid shots."

Stand on My Head? And Other Things You Never Dreamed You'd Do.

Can certain sexual positions increase or decrease your chances of conception? Which positions are best if you want to get pregnant? How does the couple down the street with four kids do "it"?

This would be water-cooler conversation in the fertility clinic waiting room—if we weren't too embarrassed to talk to one another. But inquiring minds want to know, so here goes. As far as we can tell, there haven't been many studies on this. Our take is any position that allows for deep penetration, which puts the sperm closer to the cervix and its eventual destination, is good. The "bad" positions would be any in which the sperm has to fight gravity to get to the egg. This would include sex with the woman sitting on her partner's lap, sex standing up, or sex with the guy lying down and the woman bouncing around on top. You have our permission to pass on those until you are pregnant.

The best bets? The sexperts we consulted consider the good, old-fashioned man-on-top, face-to-face missionary position to be the best for baby making. Toss a pillow under your hips so your bottom is tilted up and your cervix is right in line with as much semen as possible.

Once you're bored with missionary, try doggy style or rear entry, where your partner attacks from the back. You can be kneeling or lying down or even hanging over the end of a bed if you have a stable and strong foot board. This position also gets sperm closer to their goal.

Lying side-by-side, which is great for orgasm, can also provide good penetration. It's also more relaxing, so don't fall asleep during the process. And speaking of orgasm, it's okay for both of you to have one. Obviously the guy has to, otherwise no sperm would shoot forth in search of an egg. But there actually is research showing that female orgasm, with its muscular contractions, can move sperm up the vaginal canal toward its destination. So tell your guy you want your turn, too.

No matter which position you prefer, some girlfriends and doctors believe you increase the chance of conceiving by lying on your back in bed for thirty minutes following sex, pillow under your butt, legs all the way up. This gives gravity a chance to do its job of dropping the sperm closer to its destination. Julie used to do a modified shoulder stand with her back and legs up the wall. It never worked, but what the heck—try it. Let your partner go get postcoital snacks while you lie there with your hips elevated for a while. At least it's relaxing. For those of you with a uterus that tips backward, you may want to spend your post-sex time in an inverse position, lying on your tummy with a pillow under your pubic bone and your butt up in the air. This position may also help the sperm reach the egg.

Sometimes you even get hurt for the cause. Jessie, a friend who has PCOS, remembers a particularly painful experience in trying to conceive her now one-year-old son.

"We had been doing the 'baby dance' every other night, like good little pregnancy-obsessed couples," says Jess. "One night after sex, I decided to stand on my head against the side of my bed. I wanted to help the little swimmers find the right direction. Instead of flipping up into a headstand the right way, I was being lazy. I had my back on the bed and was easing my head and neck over the side and down to the floor. Well, I slipped or flipped or something and ended up flying off the bed, whacking my leg into the night stand. It's a miracle that I didn't go through the big picture window next to the bed. I finally got into position and held it for twenty-five minutes, but I was in such pain. The next day I noticed a very nasty, eight-inch-long bruise on my leg. It was summer; everyone was wearing shorts, but me. I didn't want to deal with explaining how I got that bruise. It was bad enough telling my doctor what happened when he asked."

Then there's our pal Paige, a West Coast pharmaceutical sales manager, who actually flew to Chicago just to have sex with her husband. "I'm embarrassed to admit I even did that," says the mother of two today. "What was I thinking? I must have just been hormonally addled to spend that much money on that stupid flight."

Her man was there on a business trip. The calendar said *Ovulation! Time for sex! Right now!* Paige was in Sacramento at the time. She hopped the first flight out in the morning, changed planes once before arriving in Chicago, met her husband in his hotel room for a quickie, grabbed a cab back to the airport, and was in Sacramento for a business dinner that night. You can only imagine how stress-free that encounter proved to be. Of course, they didn't get pregnant that cycle, but Paige did get a lot of work done on the plane.

Helping Your Husband Provide a "Sample"

Men love to provide a sample. Orgasm is orgasm. This is orgasm with a cheering section (you) and maybe some assistance from the head cheerleader (also you). Maureen's husband loved providing semen for a procedure because he always asked for—and received—her oral assistance to bring him to climax. Will, like many men, has some fond memories of infertility. He never had it so good.

Some of us add a little zip to the whole procedure in an effort to make our partner feel like more than just a sperm donor. Alma, the West Coast designer trying to get the zing back in her sex life since moving on to IUIs, has even figured out a way to spice up the old deposit.

"I go along with Nate to the clinic when he goes to make his deposit and wear something sexy under my clothes, like thong underwear or stockings and a garter belt," she says. "Anyway, we make a big production of it and in the process we get quite a few laughs. I can honestly say that my husband and I have a stronger marriage and are much closer because of all this. And it takes the edge off what we are doing—the importance of trying to conceive."

Sometimes, even with a little imagination, the whole procedure can fall apart. Our pal Gillian went through infertility twelve years ago. On the day of her insemination, her hubby, Sid, was in a rush to make a plane for another business trip. He literally ran into the clinic bathroom, masturbated in rapid style, and turned to dash out of the room. Unfortunately, he stumbled as he reached for the bathroom doorknob and accidentally spilled the cup. Mortified (and with no time or extra sperm to spare), he scooped the spilled semen up off the floor and back into the cup, along with the dust and dirt on the floor. He never told Gillian what happened until after the insemination worked, and they were into the second trimester. They are convinced this is why the kid never gets sick.

Moving the Goods— or Doing the Semen Shuffle

If your partner doesn't jack off in a small room at the clinic and provide fresh semen on the spot, you will be required to harvest it at home and bring it to the doctor yourself. Once you have procured the semen in that sterile cup the clinic provides, you have limited time in which to get it to the clinic. Here's the trick for successful semen transport—keep the cup warm and drive like crazy.

The following are best places to store semen while en route:

- tucked between your boobs
- snuggled between your legs
- stuffed under your arm
- packed in your pants between your waistband and belly
- perched under your butt like a chicken on an egg

Find the method that works best for you, but be careful not to spill the semen. This is crucial to mention because it happens. One slip-up and the whole cycle is wasted, as Erica found out. She's a forty-one-year-old Boston friend of ours with one year of fertility treatment under her belt.

"It's a forty-five-minute drive from our house to the hospital," says Erica. "Usually, I take Ed's sample to the clinic for our ART procedures by myself, but this last time he wanted to go with me, so we collected the semen at home and jumped in the car. I put the cup in its bag under my arm to keep it warm and away we go. We get there, I give them the bag so they can wash the sperm, and a few minutes later the nurse comes to get me. There's nothing in the cup. Nothing. It's empty."

Erica and Ed looked at each other, which is when Ed noticed his wife's sweater sleeve. "There was a wet stain," says Erica. "The cup had leaked, and my sweater was wet with all my husband's concentrated semen."

Infertility is so unforgiving. They were shuffled into the doctor's spare office to try to collect some more semen for the procedure.

"Poor Ed," says Erica. "He's in there trying to get it up, and he can't. Finally, I had to leave, so he could drum up a little semen. He finally got some more in the cup. It was lucky he decided to come with me that day!"

Why Humor Helps

Of course, there will be embarrassing moments, some private, like Ed's, and some all too public, like our friend Jenna's run-in with the local police.

To set the scene, Jenna was on injectable fertility drug treatment. She and her husband decided to go the movies one night. As fate would have it, the middle of the movie coincided with the time for one of Jenna's shots. No problem. Jenna packed up the medicine and syringes, left them in the car, and went into the theater. When it was time to get her shot, she returned to the car to administer it herself (she's kind of a control freak and wouldn't let her husband give her shots, but that's another story). The plan was for Joe to keep watching the movie and fill her in when she got back in the theater.

So there she is in the car, mixing the powder and the liquid together, filling the syringe. She had just pulled down her pants and was about to stick the needle in when a light shined into her car. It was the police.

"Ma'm," said the officer who thought he had caught himself a drug addict. "Please step out of the car."

"Oh, no," she said, pulling up her pants and getting out of the car. "This isn't what you think at all!"

"Hey, aren't you Joe _____'s wife?" Did we mention Jenna is married to a pretty famous guy in their town?

Finally, the cop got it that Jenna was shooting up fertility drugs, not heroin. After checking her record and finding it squeaky clean, he let her go. When the police officer left she pulled her pants down, quickly gave herself a shot, and ran back into the movie theater. As luck would have it, this was the cycle with which they conceived their darling daughter. Thank God the police officer let Jenna go.

All of us have an Ed or Jenna story—one that makes us cringe, cry, or crow with laughter when we recall it. Something so embarrassing it won't make the baby memory book, but it may make great conversation some day.

Why do we subject ourselves to such indignity? For the sweet smell of a baby's chick-fuzz head, the clasp of their tiny hand around our finger, the toothless yawn. Look, if you don't laugh, you will cry, and laughter beats crying. Laughter is great medicine. Science even says so. You'll survive this. We did.

JULIE

As I relived our infertility experience in writing this book, I kept asking my husband if he wanted to read chapters as they were finished. He kept saying no.

Occasionally, I would share a memory or an anecdote I'd finished working on that day. Sometimes he would shake his head laughing; other times, he'd cringe in embarrassed reminiscence. Still others, he would admit to having totally repressed that particular factoid in our fertility fiasco.

Finally, he said, "Look, don't tell me anymore until it's finished. All I ask is that, when it's through, you'll have left me a few shreds of dignity."

I'm trying, Honey, but as we all know, dignity is the first thing out the window with infertility.

CHAPTER 17

The MAN SHOW

We decided to let the boys tell their tales here.

Robert

At first, I really did not think that much about infertility, even when it didn't come so easily. I figured when it was time, it would just happen, and if not, well, we could always adopt a child or perhaps just travel. Seriously, I found myself not really all that concerned.

But as time went on, I found myself awake at night missing the prospect of not having a blood relative to carry on our family name. I even harbored resentment toward Julie for this, which I never let on to her. More importantly, though, I thought of all the experiences I was going to miss with kids, all those firsts—the first ice cream with my kids, the first movie, the first sunny day by the pool, the first horseback ride, trips to the beach, first day of school, first day of college, marriage, and on and on.

What surprised me the most, however, was the toll this all took on Julie's self-esteem and confidence. I believe she actually thought she was not a real woman because we were having this problem. It was very difficult to watch and very hard to combat.

But from it all here's what I learned—you don't deal with a hormonal wife, you stay the hell out of the way until you are needed, usually for a shot or a specimen. And doctor appointments are not that bad if you don't mind talking about your sex life with strangers. Of course, in this arena, they are only strangers for a very short time! Actually, I thought of it as conception with a tutor or conception by committee.

And I'd tell another guy to memorize these sentences because he's going to be repeating them often if he's smart: Honey, not having children does not make you less of a woman. Yes, dear. Yes, mama. Okay. You bet. I know. You're right. You're great! God still loves you. It will work out. Payable to whom?

Will

In the beginning, when we had trouble getting pregnant, I never thought much about it, attributing it to chance. I'm sure most people do that unless they have some specific information or knowledge of some external fact. In general, I was always philosophical and optimistic. To put it into baseball terms, the "front end" did not create any "pressure," even when "we were in the ninth inning," as amazing as that might seem. The "back end" was the challenging time.

We already had our son, so for me, it was about not being a parent again. When I thought about not having another baby, though, there was a very empty, hollow feeling. Obviously I felt grateful and relieved, however, since we were already parents and would never be childless. However, as much as one might be philosophical—the old "it wasn't meant to be"—I'll tell you, that's pure cover up. It's trying to put the best face on it. Infertility is overwhelmingly disappointing.

You know what surprised me the most? The miscarriages. The disappointment about miscarrying was overwhelming, more than I might have imagined, even after the first one. As much as I was even-tempered and philosophical throughout most of this, it was the complete opposite after the miscarriages. Those were extremely difficult, almost like a death in the family. The sense of loss was very deep. I am literally crying to think of it right now. I think the vulnerability that exists even for a tiny embryo or fetus is something that you feel, especially if you already have a child. The fragility of the whole dynamic is so heightened. I simply don't know what I would do if one of my kids perished somehow. The vulnerability leaves you powerless.

Somewhere during infertility treatment, a woman will wonder how her partner is holding up. In between charting temperatures, coordinating sex with the precision of MacArthur planning battle, and trying to tune out the ticking of our biological clocks, we will look up from an ovulation kit one morning and wonder what the heck the guy in our life is thinking about all this.

What's on His Mind

You may be surprised to discover your man is most likely holding up better than you or better than you give him credit for. Most of us don't expect this. But the truth is, most men are not affected as emotionally or physically by infertility as we women are—unless they are one of the 40 percent who have male infertility. If a guy's plumbing is the problem and he really wants kids, he will usually be as emotionally engaged as a woman. When men are personally poked and prodded by medical professionals, they care. They worry whether or not you still love them. They feel responsible. They feel like us!

But when the semen analysis comes back fine (as it does for 60 percent of the guys), it's a different ball game. He's okay! It's not him! He can relax! There's a sigh of relief, and then he's off to do something else.

Don't get upset by this behavior; it's not personal. That is just how guys operate. Just because he's not worried about himself doesn't mean he's not worried about you, how you feel, or what you're going to ask of him emotionally. He is. But is he in gut-wrenching angst over the possibility of not having kids? Does he feel any less of a man because of infertility treatment? Does he worry you'll leave him for a man with more motile sperm? No. Not really. To survive the nitty-gritty of infertility with your partner, you have to get inside his head. Here, let us help.

Ten Things Not to Expect from Your Partner

1. Total understanding of what is going on.
2. Empathy and compassion about how you are feeling 24/7.
3. Willingness to discuss infertility (particularly yours) ad nauseam.
4. The ability to participate in a conversation on infertility without prompting from you.
5. Unbearable sadness at the possibility of not fathering children.
6. That he and his guy friends will discuss this when you are not around.
7. That he will get tired of having baby-making sex with you.
8. He will think about babies all the time, just like you are.

9. He will happily participate in all infertility doctors' appointments without reminders or prompting.

10. He will tie his manhood to whether or not he sires the next generation.

To be balanced, let's look at the flip side:

Ten Things You Can Expect from Your Partner

1. He is not prepared for the assault infertility treatments have on your body and your sexuality.

2. He will wonder what happened to his wife and want the old hormone-free you back.

3. He will be happy to provide you with all the sperm you may need—and then some—in any position you are willing to try.

4. He will be happy to buy you presents if it will make you smile again.

5. He will be ready for this whole fertility thing to be over way before you are.

6. He will see positive sides of child-free living you can't even imagine.

7. He will not discuss this topic with his buddies.

8. He will do what you tell him to do during this process because he loves you.

9. He will notice how much this whole thing costs sooner rather than later.

10. He is doing this for you.

Do I Really Want to Be a Dad?

Men usually see life much differently from women. While you might not be ready to consider a child-free existence, your man probably figured long ago that no kids means more money, more time, more peace and quiet, and more you for him. From a guy's perspective, what's not to like about that?

Here's what Robert told us: "If they are totally honest, most men really don't want to have kids as soon as their wives want to. I didn't want to have kids as early as Julie did. I didn't want them when Julie was pregnant. I only realized I wanted my kids after we had our first one."

Of course, every person is different. There are men who have dreamed about being a father since they were kids, but our nonscientific research reveals that they are rare. Most men are like Robert; they really don't obsess over having kids. Either they just assume it will happen "some day," or they don't think about it at all. Most men spend the majority of their lives trying not to get some woman pregnant. And as big kids themselves, they understand and embrace the child-free life.

"My husband wasn't always on the same page as I was," says our pal Leslie, who has a precious baby boy after years of infertility treatment. "He was not as anxious to have a child as I was. He wanted one, but he wasn't willing to go as far as I was to get one. He said that he could live life happily without children if need be. In the end, he is happy to be a father and has more respect for what we went through to get our child."

Lesson learned? Lack of interest doesn't mean he doesn't want children. It's just that most men view the world from a different place than women. Men tend to rely on their partners to push the family planning process along. Our friend David, an accountant and therefore a precise, planning-oriented fellow, totally opted out of the family-planning process. He told his wife, Mary, to decide when she thought they should have kids, go off the Pill quietly, and just tell him when the pregnancy test showed two pink lines. They have three little girls conceived that way. He didn't want to know the details, just when the job was done.

The same is true with infertility treatment. Most men won't think to initiate that process, but pushed by their spouse to visit a clinic, they will go along for the ride. Most men step into the doctor's office without really understanding the full effect of what they are getting into. And once there, they spend most of their time nodding, listening while their partner asks questions, and wondering what the heck is going on. They will be surprised to discover fertility procedures are very hit-or-miss. They will be astonished at what's involved. They will blanch at the cost. They won't have much to contribute to the conversation at first—if ever. This is normal.

"Overall, I think men and women think about this kind of stuff differently," says Daniel, who suffers from male-factor infertility. "I can't speak for all men, but I know how I feel sometimes. We are not used to thinking out loud about intimate details unless we are boasting in the locker-room, which are probably lies anyway. My wife and I would often get to the same or slightly different place eventually, but how we got there was totally different. My conditioning, or maybe upbringing, has taught me to pick the shortest line between the points. My wife is more circular in her thinking and stops along the way to evaluate the decisions she is making to get from point A to point B. Neither way is right or wrong—just different.

"Maybe it has to do with the kind of upbringing we have," he adds. "I was never a jock type or a man's man, so I find it a bit easier to emote on these kind of issues, but that is surely not the case with other men that I have met along the way, whether they have male factor or not."

Boys Will Be Boys . . . Even When They Are Men

Now, this is not to say that men are not sympathetic or they don't want to be helpful or supportive. They do. But frankly most men just don't know what to do when their women go nuts while on a wild hormonal ride, plummet into despair over getting their period, or suffer yet another miscarriage. If a procedure doesn't work, men move on. If the doctor tells them there is nothing more than he or she can do, men shrug and go on to the next thing. Many men deal with infertility simply by not dealing with it.

We can't really blame the guys for being wired differently. Most men control their emotions. They tend to be linear thinkers. Your partner may be your best friend and partner in life. In the baby-making process, however, you can count on him to be there reliably with one thing—the sperm. He'll provide plenty of that on command when and where you need it. Of course, you'll probably have to tell him where to be at what time and call repeatedly to make sure he actually gets to the right place with his sample cup. But outside of that, don't expect any more. Then, anything you do get in the way of involvement or compassion is icing on the cake.

Even the most action-oriented guys—the ones running mega-conglomerates, sealing deals in the courtroom, or saving lives in burning buildings—can be reduced to bumbling fools by the infertility process. The simplest situations take on sitcom proportions. Picture burly, muscular "he-men" shaking uncontrollably while trying to stick a hypodermic needle into the skin of an orange in an effort to learn how to give their wife a shot, or a corporate titan jumping out of his car and racing up three flights of stairs to the fertility clinic office while carrying his still-warm semen sample cup in a brown paper bag.

And while we love them until death do us part, men can work our last nerve, which are pretty raw at times during this whole process. Case in point:

JULIE

It's hard for women to wrap their minds around the male psyche, particularly when it comes to infertility. We are consumed by every detail. They aren't.

"What do guys think about when they think about infertility?" I asked Robert. "Nothing," was his first comment, followed by, "Well, they don't really worry about the things you do."

While Robert was waiting for tests on his sperm to come back, did he worry about being infertile? No. He considered how much he disliked condoms.

"I thought about all the condoms I wasted when I didn't need to use one," he said. "I thought that if I was the infertile one, you could go off the Pill, and I would never have to wear a condom again. I was thinking about how great that would be. I never thought about the not-having-kids part. Then, when I wasn't infertile, I was sort of bummed about the thought of having to use a condom again."

Why are men like that?

"I don't know," said my husband, "but we are."

After her husband bungled yet another appointment, showing up late without his sample cup, one girlfriend told the nurse in exasperation, "As soon as I get pregnant, I can get rid of him, right?"

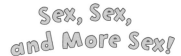

Sex, Sex, and More Sex!

Ah, yes. Infertility sex.

For men, the amount of sex necessary to make a baby is the high point of infertility treatment. It's great that babies are created by the act of intercourse. Otherwise it might be harder to get men's full attention. Fortunately for us, a man's participation in infertility treatment is all about pleasure. They are the sperm providers.

How do you get the sperm? Sex. What do men love almost more than life itself? Sex. Sex by the calendar? Okay! Two, three, four days in a row? Okay! In odd positions that help the sperm reach the egg? Let's go! Ejaculating into a cup? Bring it on!

No matter what he tells you, when it comes to the sexual part, your guy is in heaven. Infertility-induced sex is full of guiltless quickies for the guys. And for the first time, the woman in his life doesn't really mind. Is this great for a guy or what?

Women in the throes of treatment are exhausted and hormonal. We get tired of all that sex much faster than our man. After a certain point in treatment, sex loses its allure for us. We just want to get the semen and be left alone. Men are happy to give us the gold and let us sleep. Actually, it's a pretty good set up for everyone.

Providing plenty of sperm is the one place you can be guaranteed your partner will be very cooperative. In fact, Maureen's husband tried to be even *more* helpful by suggesting they schedule sex more often.

The Sexual Evolution

However, as the months pass, the hormones shift, and there's still no baby on the way, the sex changes. For every woman we talked with, it became a necessary evil. Your partner will worry (if only for a moment) if you still love him or just want his sperm. He may not share that with you, for fear of the answer. But one day he will notice the importance of the sperm at the expense of lovemaking. Be ready.

Men miss the fun and frolic of involved participation. For our guys, there is a link between sex and love. When you don't occasionally act as if you are having fun during sex, it sends the message to your man that you don't love him.

"I think it's pretty common for us to get treated like sperm donors," says Frank, a teacher whose wife has been trying to conceive for a year. "But I don't know that there's much we can do about it. It's ironic, in a way. Men need sex as a relief to the stress, and our wives need to be stress-free in order to participate in sex."

What a vicious circle. And there's more.

Some men, like Frank (and Robert and Will), go to every doctor's appointment with you, handle the financial end of infertility with a smile, and help around the house while you're in hormonal upheaval. Those guys don't mind, as long as they feel appreciated.

"Unlike many husbands, I do most of the cooking, all the laundry, half of the house-cleaning chores, and most of the yard work," says Frank, whose wife is a high-powered, big-city executive. "I don't mind because my wife has a more stressful job than I do and puts in longer hours at it. I've always felt repaid for my efforts in the bedroom, if you know what I mean.

"Now I feel like a slave. All I get from my wife is that I put *too much* emphasis on sex. Well, guess what, that's what's important to me, as I would imagine it is with most men. Without it, I get the feeling I'm just being used. Does this sound weird? It's just so depressing to me."

It's not weird, but it happens to every couple, so let's talk about it.

For the guys: If your wife wants to bypass the sexy part of sex, it has nothing to do with you or her attraction to you. Be patient, please. When a woman is jacked up on hormones and under incredible stress, her lack of desire is mostly chemical- and anxiety-induced and has nothing to do with her devotion to you.

"This was extremely hard for my husband to understand," says our friend Cheryl, who now has two kids (and still no time or energy for sex!). "My whole lack of desire had everything to do with the hormones raging through my body and the anxiety and depression that comes with the whole experience of infertility. Him pushing the issue only added to my frustration. Listen, I missed the desire to *want* to have sex, but honestly there wasn't a whole lot I could do about it. I don't care what the books say, there is no magic switch to 'turn us on.'-"

Katie agrees; "I remember complaining about my husband because I couldn't understand what he was doing and why he wouldn't get involved with our infertility while I was up all hours of the night researching, making the calls, getting the doctor's appointments, finding the perfect specialist, getting finances in order—not to mention my still daily routine of carpooling, T-Ball, cooking, cleaning, taking care of the kids we had, running errands, and so on.

"When it came time for sex, I was put off big time. I was not about to 'give' him anything after all the work I had done, the emotions I have dealt with because of him not being there for me. It was frustrating.

"After talking with my girlfriends and reading some books, I realized I expected my husband to think and feel what I was thinking and feeling, and that wasn't good for him," adds Katie. "He couldn't do it. So we explained to each other what we were feeling in an open forum between us, and amazingly our sex life got better."

Guys, remind yourself that you are dealing with a side effect of a process, not an unloving partner. Also remember she is constantly being poked down in the same area you want to . . . well . . . poke her. Some women get to the point where they just want a break from being poked. You may have to live with a little less than you would like. And think about what's going on around the house. Are you involved, or is your wife doing all the prep work for your future family? Do you stayed glued to the TV while your wife tries to talk about infertility? Katie's husband did because he was insecure about the whole thing, and it ended up irritating Katie to the point that she didn't even want to have that all-important baby-making sex.

For us gals: Like anything in a marriage, this is a two-way street. We need to remember that the desire men have for sex is as strong as the desire we have for a baby. It's actually Mother Nature's way of continuing the species.

Face it, you are probably willing at this point to do just about anything to have a baby. Short of cheating, your partner is most likely willing to do just about anything to get a little lovemaking. So you may have to remind yourself occasionally that he is not an uncaring jerk who only wants one thing, but actually a normal man with normal desires. Smile at him, smooch him, look into his eyes, and tell him you love him. Throw on a sexy nightie. Surprise him. Who knows, you may actually end up having a little fun yourself once you get going. You don't have to do this every time (who has the energy?), but on occasion it will make him happy, and what's better than a happy hubby?

"Men don't have an off switch, and I think the experience of infertility makes them want to prove their masculinity even more," says our insightful pal Cheryl. "I kept telling my husband he needed an anti-Viagra pill. He did not find it very funny. I have to admit that I was not as understanding as I could have been about what he was going through. Honestly, I just didn't understand. I found his sexual desires pretty irritating at the time. The whole issue of sex, or lack thereof, almost put an end to our dream of a bigger family. But it all worked out in the end for us, and I am so thankful my desire to have another baby was as strong as his desire for sex."

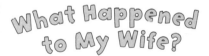

What Happened to My Wife?

Why their partner is acting so weird is probably the number one concern men have during the whole infertility process. We know it's just hormone hell, but the guys don't. When Maureen was on Clomid, there were days when she didn't know who she'd like to strangle first—her doctor or her husband.

"The 'hormonal wife' part is easy to reconcile," says Maureen's husband Will. "Men joke around about 'raging hormones' and the attendant mood swings experienced by women. It's almost like a rite of passage when it happens to you: you know, the flip side of women making fun of men who do stereotypical guy things—like watching sports or living in a dumpy apartment when they're single."

Unlike us, men don't wrap their self-image up in whether or not they can have a baby. But most guys do understand that being a mom is an important part of being a woman, even if you tell him it's not. (And all of us would know you were lying anyway!)

This presents a dilemma to a modern man. Robert was worried about the emotional impact being infertile was having on Julie, but confused because he thought men weren't supposed to consider those elements anymore in defining women.

"I knew she was going to wrap up her whole image of a being a woman in this," he says (and he was right!). "But I've had it drilled into me I shouldn't identify a woman simply by her body. Suddenly, I have a wife who's entire self-image is defined by her plumbing. How do you deal with that in today's politically-correct world? It can be really confusing to a guy."

He's right. What woman in the throes of hormone-induced pathos hasn't suggested her man would be happier with a *fertile* woman? (All of us.) The angst of infertility on you is the hardest part on your partner because he loves you, fertile or infertile, and he wants to make you happy. But you're kind of freaking him out a bit, and he's confused.

Every man we talked with was most unhappy that his partner was unhappy, and he couldn't fix it. The hardest thing to deal with? *Your* disappointment.

Men view their role as being our first line of support. Infertility becomes emotional for men because they can't stand to see their women engulfed in so much hurt. They want to help you cope, but many don't possess the skills.

To understand your partner, you have to get inside his head. This is hard because men tend to keep their emotions under wraps. Particularly when their women are losing theirs.

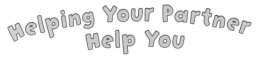

Helping Your Partner Help You

Men are not mind readers. They really want to make you feel better, and they want to get you through this fertility maze, but they need help. You will be happier with your partner's responses to your needs if you tell him what to do. It's like your birthday. After you get four coats in four years, don't you just tell him what you really want? Of course. It's the same thing now. Your man wants help, so help him.

1. Give him directions.

Make it easy. Tell him what you need as explicitly as possible instead of wait-
ing around, hoping he will ask the right question or show up at the right time.
It won't happen, and there's enough frustration in infertility not to add more.
Here are a few examples.

- "I need you to meet me at the doctor's tomorrow at 1:00 P.M., so you can
  learn how to give me a shot."
- "I need to know if you will still love me if we can't have kids."
- "I am unbearably sad and need you to hold me."
- "I need you to read this instruction sheet and follow the directions.
  Here's your sample cup."

Guys do very well with specific missions. Left to their own devices in the
very foreign world of infertility and feelings, they will often revert to what they
do best—sit in a chair and point the remote at the TV in the hope you will not
notice them—unless you need them for sex, that is.

2. Communicate

Men do not want to talk about infertility. It's too uncomfortable for them. We
are discussing intimate details about body parts they consider sex toys. We are
turning their playground into a testing ground. We are talking about adding
kids to the mix. We are talking about feelings. All this is scary to any man. Thus,
you will be the driving force in initiating conversations and pulling information
from your partner.

"I like to talk about my feelings," says Leslie, who had trouble decipher-
ing her husband's feelings throughout the infertility process. "Sometimes Rob
makes the mistake of thinking that I want to be left alone. Often, he wants to
be left alone, and I make the mistake of thinking that he wants to talk about his
feelings. It's very confusing."

It's confusing because our genders are opposites in communicating. We
talk things out. They don't. Men internalize and mull, then act. It's that whole
Mars/Venus thing that author John Gray wrote about in his books.

"I was concerned about my husband's noninvolvement at first," says Stacey.
"It felt to me as though he didn't care and wasn't paying attention to the hurdles
I was encountering with infertility—what doctor to listen to, what protocol was
needed, blah, blah, blah. There's so much information, and it's all so confusing.

I nagged some; I begged some. But then I wised up a little and just waited for a good, quiet moment and asked some simple questions—how did the process make him feel? What was his take on it? That kind of thing."

In a nonthreatening environment, her husband opened up. Stacey learned that her husband felt really powerless and that the whole topic of infertility was really intimidating for him. "When women talk, we want to express our fears and ideas about things that bother us," she adds. "My husband made me realize that men seem to take from that is a request to come up with a solution."

That makes sense. Men have a natural tendency to want to fix things.

3. Question everything.

The biggest surprises for us? Being infertile.

The biggest surprises for Robert and Will? Nothing—because we kept them so well-informed during the whole process. (Well, there were a few surprises, but they were things we didn't anticipate!)

Communication is a woman's job. We want to share feelings and information. We're information junkies. Men want answers, too, but in this realm, they

JULIE

But what happens when your Mr. Fix-It doesn't have a solution? He freaks out and most often retreats into silence.

Men are not referred to as the strong, silent type for nothing. When our doctor told Robert and me that he had done everything possible for us and we might want to consider IVF or surrogacy, we grieved differently. I screamed and ranted with a rage that eventually melted into an unspeakable sorrow. I sobbed for the children we would never have, and the family we would never be. The world felt gray. I felt gray. I talked and churned it around.

Robert said nothing. He never talked about it and went on with his life. He was sad, but more for me and what I was going through. For him, the doctor had closed a door, and Robert, after dusting his hands off, was ready to walk down the hall and try the knobs on the next door. Did we want kids? Okay, what was the next step? Adoption? How do you do that? Who do you call? Child-free living? Whatever. He was ready to move on.

Men are pragmatic. Knock 'em down, and they get up and move to the next thing. You cannot get mad at them for not grieving like you or emoting like you or communicating like you. They're men, for goodness sake.

don't really know the question because they haven't done the in-depth research we have.

Now there are always exceptions to every rule, but generally, men don't ask questions. A guy could have a lump on his testicle the size of an egg and risk his life by waiting to find out if it's cancerous simply because he is too embarrassed to ask. So you will have to anticipate any questions your husband might have and be prepared to ask them for him. Eventually, he may even get into the groove and ask a few of his own.

Because of its anonymity, the Internet offers a great place for men to find answers to their questions.

"As far as expressing our feelings, that has been programmed out of us," says our guy friend Chip. "From a very young age, we are taught to keep that sort of thing to ourselves, and we've become so good at it, we don't even realize that we're doing it."

While women have a need to constantly express themselves, men have an overwhelming need not to show weakness.

"I was the same way earlier in our infertility journey," adds Chip. "Then one day I had a question about something, so I looked it up on the Internet and started reading. I found that our doctor was doing a very poor job of finding a solution to a very obvious problem. Suddenly, it dawned on me I had to keep learning myself because doctors aren't always going to be good problem solvers. That's how I got 'sucked in' to the Internet boards. If it wasn't for the Internet and posting on some of the infertility boards, I wouldn't have found out that a medication I was taking had male sterility as a side effect, and we'd be wondering why we're still not pregnant."

4. Pry open a clam.

If your partner is not communicating at all with you, perhaps he may feel uncomfortable about the way you are approaching the matter.

"Don't bug your husband," says Rex. "Forcing him to communicate his feelings is almost futile. If we men can't fix something, we don't talk about it. That's just us. So pushing a man to talk about his feelings will probably only cause him to communicate less."

For many men, there is some anger and even guilt about this whole process, whether or not they have a male-factor fertility problem. There is also the underlying fear of upsetting you.

"I am sometimes afraid that I will say the wrong thing even if it is what I am feeling," says Randy, another husband with two years of infertility treatments under his belt. "I never intended to make my wife mad, upset, or confused by what I said, but it is just the way I used to approach the situation. After lots of couples' therapy, I have learned to listen and to think before saying the first thing that pops into my head."

The same goes for us girls. If your man clams up like a shellfish when talk turns to fertility factoids, consider when you're bringing up the topic. FYI— infertility is not a turn-on topic before, during, or even after sex.

"While we were in treatment, after a busy day, as soon as I was ready to go to sleep, my wife would bring up a serious topic for conversation," says Daniel, who is the guy with male-factor infertility. "Then if I said something different than what she was thinking, we both got upset. In time we learned to make time to discuss important issues at a time that we were both ready to discuss them."

And definitely not in bed!

If your partner has infertility, he may be even more reluctant to talk. He may feel guilty, like he's letting your down. Take a minute to imagine how you'd feel if you were him. Your man feels the same way—or worse because he is supposed to be Mr. Fix-It, remember?

"Before my wife was diagnosed with having immunological factors and our infertility was solely my problem, no matter what she said, I felt we were not on equal footing," says Daniel. "So I was forever guilty that it was my fault. She was having to do all these things because I could not do what I always thought was just the easiest thing to do—make a baby. After she was diagnosed with an immunological factor, she actually seemed relieved because now were we were equals in infertility again."

What to do? Instead of chatting him up like a girlfriend, try other options. Entice him to write down something on paper. You do the same, then swap letters. Or designate a specific time each week to talk about what's going on. Sit down with a cup of coffee or a glass of wine, ask questions, and listen without offering comment.

5. Nag.

Okay, nag may be too harsh a word, but you get the point. It is your job to remind him as to where he needs to be, why, and when during this whole process. He may be a grown man able to navigate the workday world with ease, but when it

MAUREEN

Generally, I have no problem expressing exactly how I feel. My husband is more reserved. So what happens is that he knows too much about how I feel, and I don't know enough about how he feels.

In dealing with infertility, this was extremely frustrating. I never knew where he stood on certain things, and he was constantly bowled over with where I stood. This theme exists in our wider relationship, but, with something as important as infertility, I could really feel it weighing on me more. It was a lonesome feeling, although I don't believe that was ever his intention.

Thank God Julie came along. She understood, listened, and had a complete grasp of what I was going through. There are certain things you should turn to your partner for, and there are other things that girlfriends are best at.

comes to infertility, he is a babe in the woods. He needs your guidance. He *wants* your guidance. While he probably won't forget that you want him home for sex on Thursday at 2:00 P.M. when you're ovulating, the chance of him remembering a doctor's appointment without your prolific prodding is pretty slim.

Maureen's husband actually missed his appointment for one of her inseminations because he couldn't find a sample cup he had misplaced. He was supposed to drop off the sample two hours before she got to the doctor's office. He assumed he could pick up a sample cup at a pharmacy, so he drove from pharmacy to pharmacy to no avail. Then he went back to his office thinking he'd just meet her later in the day, and they could go together when she went for her appointment. Surely, she'd have a sample cup. When he didn't show up at the clinic, Maureen found him busy and oblivious at work. Since inseminations depend on the male providing the sperm earlier in the day, his snafu caused some major scheduling upheavals. He didn't realize the importance of timing.

First mistake? Maureen figuring she could just hand him the instruction sheet from the clinic without talking him through it. Wrong.

Everyone knows that guys are notorious for not reading instructions. So don't hand your partner a how-to sheet without explanation and expect him to complete the task appropriately. Left on his own, a man is just as likely to show up at the clinic with a sample cup filled up with sperm, and *no* appointment as he is to get it right. Since the life span of sperm outside the body is one to two hours, unexpected semen is not much use if no one at the clinic is ready to receive it.

Bottom line, if you need him to be somewhere or do something, mark it on his calendar, call his secretary, program his Palm Pilot, and/or tie a string around his finger. Provide a map if necessary and any other items he might need—like a sample cup and a brown paper bag. This is not the time to teach him a lesson. You want to be a mother. Here's the perfect place to practice.

6. Remind him that you love him.

Any man doing the fertility fast-dance with his partner loves her. Even if he doesn't talk about his feelings like your best girlfriend, he appreciates what you are doing. Even if he forgets about that ultrasound you really wanted him to be at, you are important to him. More crucial is the fact that even though he tries to hide them, he has feelings and insecurities, too.

Make sure you let him know how significant he is to you and not just to the procreation process. Remember why you hooked up with him in the first place and remind him. You'll be surprised at how much he will appreciate that!

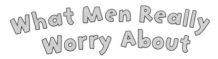

What Men Really Worry About

When men start to stress during this time, they worry about stuff women never consider. At least, stuff *we* never considered.

For example, our friend's husband (who begged to remain anonymous) was stressed because one testicle was smaller than the other one. He was afraid it would prevent him from getting his wife pregnant. Now, different-sized testicles are probably about as common as different-sized breasts (which are pretty common). Though you'll want to confirm it with your doctor, the difference in size should not be cause for concern. The sperm are what's important, and sperm can be made in any size factory. The sperm analysis will then tell you if those fellows are doing their job.

But he didn't want to hear that from us. He went to the doctor (as he should) and heard it from him. By the way, penises come in a variety of sizes as well. Again, size doesn't matter as long as the penis is properly functioning.

Additionally, the stress of infertility and of having to perform on command can cause the one problem men dread the most—impotence, aka the wilted weenie.

"Most men love sex," says Al, a thirty-five-year-old carpenter who suffered impotence when he and his wife were going through infertility treatment.

"When we're eighteen, we're all sexaholics. But infertility treatments can wear you down. Right before our first IVF, I just lost it. I went completely limp. I don't know what was worse—the whole infertility feeling of failure or the impotence feeling of failure."

Even Al knows it could be worse. "Hey, we have some friends, and one minute they're going through IVF, the next thing we knew, they were going through a divorce," he says. "I'd rather stress about impotence than divorce. There's always Viagra."

Ten Questions Guys Ask Themselves Sometime During This Process

1. Will we ever have a child?
2. Is this my fault?
3. What can I do to fix the problem?
4. How will we ever be able to afford this?
5. Why are we going through this?
6. Will I be a good parent?
7. If we can't have our own child, should we adopt?
8. Should we live child-free?
9. How come all these unwed teens can get pregnant, and we can't?
10. How come those people over there don't seem to realize what a blessing their children are?

Been There, Done That

So, what would men who have survived the infertility roller coaster share with guys just hopping on the ride? Here's what we heard.

"You have to be very compassionate, which is hard for us," says Julie's husband, Robert. "But there is an upside. You will get to have lots of guiltless sex while you are trying to conceive."

"Yeah and bring your own magazines!" says Steve, another husband, who also noted he and his marriage survived the whole process with "humor and gin."

Ted, a systems engineer in Florida, definitely thinks infertility affects men differently than it does women. "Be ready for that," he says. "I would feel differently if there was male factor involved in our case. I think I would feel pretty guilty. I definitely don't blame my wife at all. I tell her I love her all the time. I tell her that we're going to get through this together, no matter what the outcome. I tell her that I'll love her the same even if we can't have children.

"I feel incredibly helpless," he says. "I absolutely hate seeing something that hurts my wife so much and get very frustrated because there's nothing I can do to fix it. My instinct is to fix it and make her happy and feel better.

"To tell you the truth, sometimes, we get overwhelmed by it all, and we both cry and hold one another," he adds. "The first time I cried with my wife I was surprised to learn that it helped her see just how much pain I was in, too. I had, for a long time, tried to be the strong husband and be strong for her. But, one thing I've learned is that sometimes you need to break down and show that hurting side of yourself. It's important for the wife to see that she's not alone in her pain."

In addition to sharing her pain, share the stupidity as well. "Keep your sense of humor," says Pete. "Some of the funniest moments during this whole ordeal were telling stories about jerking off in the doctor's office. If you don't laugh, you'll lose it."

In the grand scheme of things, however, it's a learn-as-you-go program. "Much like having children, there is not much one can say," adds Maureen's husband, Will. "Any explanation is largely intellectual and doesn't translate very well. Hence, in my view, the way to convey it is that, like any other 'roller coaster' experience, one needs to truncate the highs and lows and absolutely remain even-keeled and even-tempered. Your wife needs the stability."

"The hell with all that," says Ian, a fifty-year-old newspaper exec. "Make sure there's always a bottle of gin and a shot glass in the house, even if you drink alone."

Well put, boys.

CHAPTER 18

Making Your RELATIONSHIP WORK While Making a Baby

Maureen

Will and I dealt with infertility by trying not to put pressure on ourselves or our relationship. We talked about it. We knew things would be funky for a while and that, eventually, we would be able to get back on track. Accepting that brought us both relief and took the pressure off dealing with our changing relationship.

We looked at it as a new adventure, which doesn't always mean fun! We both tried to infuse some humor and lightness wherever we could. We joked with the doctor and with each other. We found the comedy in the process.

That I suffered from secondary infertility actually helped us. Already having our son made a huge difference in how we dealt with our relationship. We had already given up a great deal of "us" (as it should be) for Quinn. We were already accustomed to lack of spontaneity in our sex life and in our relationship in general. We knew that this too would pass, kind of like our son finally sleeping through the night after four long years. Having survived that, we knew our relationship could survive this as well.

We took seriously the marriage vow that said, "in sickness and in health." I never beat myself up for my infertility. If it had been the other way around, I don't think my husband would have felt guilty, and if Will had considered me damaged goods, I would have thought twice about even trying to procreate with him. It is what it is.

No man should make a woman he loves feel bad. You are guilty of nothing, and if your man is making you feel that way, then perhaps you should reevaluate your relationship and consider taking the infertility journey without him.

Julie

I was married briefly right out of college, a starter marriage that ended in divorce before it really began. I spent a lot of time reflecting on the good, the bad, and the ugly of that marriage in an effort to grow from the mistakes we made.

When I married Robert several years later, I think I was more relationship savvy. I understood the importance of good communication, how to pick your battles, and why it really doesn't matter if a guy leaves the toilet seat up (Robert doesn't, but I couldn't care less if he did.)

I also developed my theory that couples tend to forget the whole boyfriend/girlfriend thing when we get married. I call it the Boyfriend/Girlfriend Clause, and here's how my theory works. We get married and start to think of our spouse as family. Yes, they are part of our new family, but there's a difference. I can be crappy to my brother or my mother, piss them off to no end, and I am still related to them. That person is still my brother, still my mom. We might not speak for ten years, but we are still related.

This is not so with spouses. Think about it. If you're crappy to your husband day in and day out, what are the chances you will still be related? Pretty slim.

Thus, the Boyfriend/Girlfriend Clause: a husband is just a boyfriend who *chooses* to stay (ditto a wife). He wanted to be here with you so much he got married, moved in, or whatever your committed relationship looks like. He chose you to parent with, but he doesn't have to stay. Your brother has to be your brother no matter what. Your mom is stuck, too. Luck of the draw. This is not so for a spouse. A spouse can pick up and move on—get a divorce, leave you.

Speaking for myself, I'm not interested in losing my spouse. I revel in my committed marriage with Robert. So when things get mundane (as they always do in life), I find myself taking my husband for granted (who doesn't?), I get ticked about something small (happens every day), or I really would rather read than have sex (occasionally), I think about my theory. It forces me to remember my boyfriend—this great man I live with, this husband and father, who is really just a boyfriend choosing to stay. When I think about the commitment he has made to me by choosing to stay, well, the small stuff just slips away. I see him for who he is again—Robert, this great guy, this sexy, fabulous boyfriend. Okay, now I remember what caught my attention to begin with, and it catches my attention again.

That's how I keep the love alive in my relationship. I'm married to my boyfriend and, once in a while, I remember to act like his girlfriend.

Ten Ways to Keep Your Marriage Together During Infertility

1. Date your spouse. Go to the movies. Light candles at dinner. Take frequent short vacations.
2. Keep the lines of communication open, no matter what.
3. Have sex when it doesn't fit the fertility calendar!
4. Have sex when you don't really want to, but he does.
5. Force yourself to have a conversation that doesn't revolve around fertility treatments.
6. Listen.
7. Have some fun. Try to laugh as much as you can.
8. Work as a team.
9. Hold hands.
10. Pick your battles.

The Scary Statistics (And How Not to Be One)

Half of all marriages end in divorce, and going through infertility doesn't help matters. We can understand this. The whole concept of lovemaking changes, and anyone who tells you it doesn't is lying. Recreation turns solely to procreation. Sex becomes a line in the Daytimer. Romance disappears amid thermometers, charts, and calendars. Your husband is on call and must be ready to perform on command—anywhere and everywhere. If that doesn't kill your sex life, we don't know what will.

Talk about stress. Talk about feelings of inadequacy, low self-esteem, failure. Infertility supplies all those and more. But there's no need to be a statistic. The trick is to remember why you married in the first place and work to keep the love alive—just as you should do anyhow. You can survive this as well. We did, and so did our friends.

"My biggest discovery was that no matter how bad it gets, you and your marriage can survive," says Louise, an infertility patient who lives in south Texas and recently began adoption proceedings. "Infertility can be awful, but you can't let your failure at conception result in the failure of your marriage or parenting. We celebrated our ten-year anniversary in February, and I can honestly say that we're healing. I'm happier in my marriage than I've been—even with four years of infertility behind us."

Louise is right. Don't ruin your relationship because you can't get pregnant as easily as you would have hoped. To do this, you must first let go of guilt and blame. Like our pal Louise, we both spent plenty of time in the beginning, hashing over with our respective spouses how this could have happened to us. We weren't alone. Other couples have also asked the tough questions—what's wrong with you? What's wrong with me? Would this have happened if you/I had wanted children earlier? Why did you/I put off having kids? Was this caused by something/someone you/I did in college?

This stage, as ugly as it can be, is also normal. Best of all, with a little understanding, patience, tongue-biting, and some deep breaths, this too can pass. And you have to make sure you move out of this stage as quickly as possible. Berating yourself or each other for the situation you are in doesn't make you fertile or happy—and it sure won't get you pregnant any quicker. Frankly, it's pretty hard to have sex with someone you are constantly badgering and blaming. Infertility treatments take enough of the romance out of making babies. Don't let guilt and blame destroy the rest of the fun.

Here's what we learned; you two have work to do, and you need to do it together. You are a team already under the stress of not being able to conceive. Don't add another layer of guilt and blame. That's more stress than you want to shoulder right now. Instead, go ahead and establish a no-fault clause between you and your partner right now. To go forward in a positive way, you have to make an immediate decision that this situation is nobody's fault. Now, that may be an absolute falsehood. Your infertility could be the result of a sexually transmitted disease you or your partner caught years ago before you met each other. You might have blocked Fallopian tubes. Your partner might have a low sperm count. So what? Faulty plumbing doesn't make you a faulty person.

When it comes to facing infertility, you have to forget (or forgive) all that. The sooner you do, the better for your relationship. Forget about the past and focus on your common goal—building your family. To survive and succeed at this insanity that is infertility, you must remain a team. You need each other's love and support to get through the physical and emotional roller coaster you are on. This is a bumpy ride.

If you don't, you might end up with a baby, but lose your marriage—and how fair is that to the child you both desperately want? Forgive, forget, and get going.

Our friend Laura and her husband, Evan, have been through five years of unexplained infertility—multiple inseminations, three IVFs, and thousands and thousands of dollars. They have been married seven years. Their marriage—much of which has been spent trying to conceive—has become stronger during their battle thanks to good communication.

"We were older when we got married," says Laura, who is forty-two, pregnant with IVF twins and ready to deliver any day. "We knew each other and ourselves better; we were more grounded in what was important to us. Evan and I are very good with each other in regard to communication and respect. He doesn't run away when I try to communicate.

"I love him so much, and I believe in my commitment to my marriage," adds the lawyer who plans to become a stay-at-home mom with her twins' arrival. "When we go through something, I am not one to sweep it under the rug. I think if Evan were unable to speak about it, too, we might have had problems. But he has a great gift in listening and that helped us as well."

It was also huge that they didn't play the blame game. Not that they each didn't have plenty of ammo. While they were operating under the "unexplained infertility" moniker, they knew Evan was fertile—he had gotten three women pregnant while in college. All three had had abortions.

"I felt all sorts of things when we first found out there were problems," says Evan, a forty-eight-year-old wine salesman. "I thought, 'Why me? I'm normal—what's wrong with her?' I knew my sperm was good. That my wife was thirty-six when we started to have unprotected sex, and it didn't happen the very first time was sort of strange. Based on what we were told scientifically, there was nothing wrong with either of us. But Laura was in that questionable age, and the doctor told us it was likely that her eggs' outer shell would be more difficult for my sperm to penetrate.

"I started to dwell on the times in my past when I had gotten my then-girlfriends pregnant," adds the expectant father. "I am not proud of these moments in my life. For better or worse, we always opted to terminate the pregnancies. In some cases, this was an extremely difficult decision. These events have always bothered and weighed heavily on me—to this day. I've never revealed this to anyone other than Laura; I'm still on friendly terms with these women, and although we've all gotten over these events, I was always afraid of how that might impact them later in their lives physically and/or emotionally.

"The thought has crossed my mind more than a few times that maybe, on some karmic level, the fact that we could not conceive in my married relationship was because of some karmic revenge," he adds. "I don't generally believe stuff like that, but it crossed my mind occasionally and would sting a bit. How could I blame Laura, when Laura could turn around and point the a finger right back at me?"

The couple used a secret signal throughout the whole infertility process to reconnect when the going got tough. "Before we got married, we came up with this thing," says Laura. "Whenever we go through a tough time, we reach over and take each others' pinky. It's like a sign to each other that we'll get through this, too. Like I said, we are committed to this marriage. If you are, you come out the other side, and you are okay. You don't freak out and leave a situation."

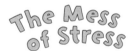

The Mess of Stress

We've already established that stress and guilt can really screw up body and mind. Imagine what that dynamic duo can do to a relationship and your sex life. No need to imagine. All of us have been there. It stands to reason, then, that the stress of infertility will cool any passion faster than water on match.

After years of trying unsuccessfully to conceive, sex starts to be viewed as a cruel joke. The outcome of sex (a baby) doesn't happen for us, while it works for everyone else (at least that's how it feels). When all of us start out trying to conceive, sex is sizzling and so fulfilling. Wow, we're making a baby this time for sure! But month after month of disappointment, of not getting it right, going into years of not getting it right, well, suddenly sex just doesn't hold the same attraction. Sex moves from steamy passion to bada-bing-bada-boom-give-me-that-sperm—and it represents failure.

Our friend Frank and his wife have been fighting infertility for two years. "Whenever I think of sex these days, all I think of is failure. I think of all those

MAUREEN

Sex for us became a chore when we were trying to conceive. We have an incredibly busy life to begin with, so we were doing great just having sex four times a month. I mean, we were just dragging, and really, all I wanted to do was go to bed and sleep. I wanted to say "Will, give me the goods and leave me alone." If we could have put the semen in a turkey baster and done it that way, I'd have been happy. Not only that, but we had Quinn, Mr. Big Ears, in the next room. Age nine, and he's shouting out, "Mom, are you doing the S thing again?" How romantic was that?

After sex, Will would put a pillow under my butt, and I would lay there for as long as possible. Sometimes I'd fall asleep with that pillow still there and wake up with a backache or my leg asleep. I never thought it would come to that . . . so unromantic, so very robotic, so filled with stress. The thought of me with a pillow under my butt, with my son screaming is kind of funny today.

Well, they say the flip side to tragedy is humor. Back then, we just tried to laugh.

years of trying to conceive. I think of how we were wasting our time," says Frank, who is handsome, witty, and bright. "Sometimes now, I have performance anxiety, and I can't even get it up. I just know we have this window, and we have to do it now! And everything just deflates—my ego, my penis, my passion. I feel like such a failure as a man."

Men aren't the only ones who suffer from performance anxiety. Emily, thirty-seven years old, married for five years and trying to conceive for two, finds it hard to get excited for sex as well. "Trust me, it's not easy to try and arouse your man so that he's capable of even having sex when it's fertile time, let alone try and work yourself up into a state of arousal," she says. "Men like to joke that they are sperm donors. Well, we are the egg donors, and believe me, sex when you aren't aroused hurts.

"And of course since the man is dealing with his own head trip, it takes him longer to reach orgasm, which means the woman has to endure pain or discomfort even longer when all she's really wishing is that it would all hurry up and be over now."

It's so horrible to feel this way about making love, and yet, there it is. What should be the most natural act of love evolves into this event both of you actually dread. When lovemaking isn't fun, it doesn't work. We aren't the only chicks who feel this way. In fact, everybody we've talked with feels exactly the same way. Add in the whole high-tech aspect like IVF or artificial insemination . . . well, ejaculating into a cup and have egg and sperm meet in a petri dish is not really hot and passionate. Technology can certainly take the edge off sex. It's safe to say that by the time technology is involved, and you are procreating via committee, most couples have been through the emotional wringer.

That you are exhausted by the prospect of getting it on doesn't mean you love each other any less. And it doesn't mean that sexual desire is gone forever. It just means you're going to have to work (again!) to get it all back in balance. We wouldn't even bother working on keeping it all in balance sex-wise at this point. Infertility sex is what it is. Just remember—this too shall pass.

By the way, some fertility drugs—like Lupron—have been reported by girlfriends to snatch away a woman's sex drive. Lupron can put a woman into a state of temporary menopause—with all the wonderful side effects that implies. Still others pack a few (or a dozen) pounds onto your frame, which may make you self-conscious when you are naked—even though every guy we talked with really loved their fuller-figured partner. The point is, fertility drugs are not necessarily make-me-feel-like-I-want-to-have-sex-with-you-right-now drugs. These drugs are designed to do a job—help get you pregnant. The rest is up to you.

For our friends Cheryl and Seth, sex nosedived when it actually became work. "Prior to actually making love in order to produce a child, our sex life was great," says Cheryl, a thirty-eight-year-old Dallas videographer. "I'll bet if you asked my husband, he'd even tell you I was enthusiastic and energetic. Once we got down to the business of actually having intercourse to conceive, our sex life turned much more regimented—and a lot less joyous. Each month, I felt a little more depressed and desperate as that miracle baby never arrived."

Once the couple started infertility treatments, hope was renewed. "I think we thought, oh boy, everything will be just great now. The doctors will fix this problem!" says Cheryl. "Our sex life saw an uptick, too. After four failed intrauterine inseminations and one IVF, our sex life was back in the tank."

For Cheryl (and others), the biggest obstacles to sex are depression and stress. "When I have hope, my sex drive is back and better than ever," she says. "When I'm depressed, my sex drive is gone. Believe me, I miss it as much as my husband. Without sex, I feel more distant and less connected to Seth. Since my interest is lacking, Seth initiates lovemaking less often. I guess he's probably trying to cope with his own depression and a wife who's shut down. I am painfully aware of this and know this is a big problem. Sex is part of the glue that keeps a marriage together. I don't want to deny my husband, so if there's any glimmer of a spark on my end, I work with it. Sometimes I just initiate sex because I feel sorry for Seth that I'm so uninterested."

Cheryl and Seth are now in the process of adopting a baby girl from China. With the pressure off, they are working to strengthen the sexual side of their relationship.

"Now that I'm on the other side of treatment and we're bringing our daughter home soon, all I want is for everything to be back to normal sex-wise," says Cheryl. "And it's getting there. I guess my biggest message for other women is don't give up hope, there is light at the end of the tunnel. But the tunnel might be kind of long."

It's pretty bad when you can't remember the last time you made love just for the heck of it. Spontaneity? Please. Not when you want to save up the seed for the perfect ovulation moment. But there are ways to jazz up planned intercourse, too. Why can't sex-on-a-schedule be fun some of the time? Rent a sexy, romantic movie. Buy some special fragrance. Light a couple candles. Feed your husband chocolates in bed. Massage him. Let him massage you.

We know what you are thinking. This sounds exhausting to us, too, if you tried to do it every time—but once in a while, why not put a smile on that guy's face. We always found out we were pretty happy afterward ourselves.

If you are suffering secondary infertility and already have children, revving up the romance may be more difficult. Lighting candles and hanging out giving massages will probably be interrupted by, "Mom, can you come and play with me?" or "Daddy, there's a monster under my bed." In those cases, you might need to get Grandma to come spend the occasional night at your house watching Junior while you two sneak away to a hotel for some recreation. Or just buy a lock for your bedroom door. It's cheaper.

If things get really out of sync, take a break—really. Skip a month if you are really getting weary. Yes, you will lose a month—oh well. What's more important—losing a month or losing your mind?

Sometimes you have to put it all into perspective. Pack a picnic. Have sex because you want to, even if you don't want to; once you get started it's usually fun. Or don't have sex. Go to bed, sleep, eat well, and for one thirty-day cycle don't think about babies if you don't want to. It's okay.

The Dating Game

This is the part where we explain in no uncertain terms why you need to get out more with your partner. Focus on fun. Laugh. Be silly. Or be romantic. Or just veg out at the movie theater, eating popcorn and holding hands. It's okay, almost mandatory, to have fun while you are working to build your family. It is totally mandatory to have a conversation that doesn't include the words "baby," "sex," or "infertility."

We bet you were both active people before you found out you were infertile, at least had some common interests you liked to share. There is no need to put your life on hold now, just because you are trying to conceive. Make time to do the things you used to like to do together—before you spent all your time and money trying to make a baby. Go dancing, shopping, or out to eat. Go to a concert or the theater. Throw a party. Pick up a sport or go watch one together. Travel and see things you've always wanted to see—even if it's just in the next town over. Try something new, like dance classes, painting, or sky diving. Just do it together.

If you don't, you will be consumed by infertility insanity. Listen to our pal Thomas, who has been working through infertility unsuccessfully with his wife for two years. "Infertility consumed us for a long time," says the high-tech exec, who lives in Minnesota. "It was all we thought about. Everything my wife ate, drank, and did was in pursuit of getting pregnant.

"Lately we've been getting out of that and trying to find our lives again," he says. "We're at a point right now where we've decided to suspend treatment for a while until my wife gets a job at a company where we know that IVF is covered by the insurance. We've even decided to stop the ovulation predictor test we had been using. We both got so strung out on the calendars and predictor kits and having to have sex that infertility took over our lives."

"It was so bad, we got to a point where we didn't want to go to church when they were baptizing babies because it hurt too much," adds his wife, Lisa, who credits her faith for getting her this far without totally losing it. "We're watching all of our friends effortlessly having babies, and we try to act happy for them, but deep down, it really hurts. We have to find time to find us again—the Tommy and Lisa we used to be. That really fun-loving, cute, happy couple. I know we are still in there somewhere."

If you don't think you have time to find that old you, figure out how to make time. What is more important than you as a couple? Particularly if you want to bring another life force into the picture? You need to date all you can now because once your baby is here, forget it. Even if you can find a babysitter you trust, you won't want to go out for at least a year. You'll be too exhausted to leave and too excited to see just what that cute little human being will do next. We know. It wasn't until their kids were two and five respectively that Julie and Robert even bothered to hire a babysitter for regular date nights. They were (and still are) so enthralled with their kids, they'd rather be home with them then out on the town.

Remember Why You're Together (To Keep from Falling Apart)

You married (or moved in with, or have hung out with) your partner for reasons that had nothing to do with procreation. Maybe you both liked classical music, shared a cultural heritage, were from the same small town, went to college together, or dream the same dreams. You chose to be together as a couple. You had fun together, shared laughs, cried together, and became a family of two. Then, somewhere along the line, you decided it was time to invite some more people to the party . . . your own kids.

"I have no idea how we survived," says our pal Ellen, a schoolteacher with two tykes. "No idea. I guess we just figured it out. My husband could not do the shots for me—he freaks at blood. That kind of hurt me, although I knew I didn't need him passing out on me either. On the other hand, he was very supportive in the ways he could be. He went to seminars with me on adoption and in vitro fertilization, and he tried to understand. He didn't push me when I couldn't handle certain family situations. He put up with the awful beeping basal-body thermometer although he hated it. We did seem to be okay as a couple during infertility even though I felt like a totally different person the whole time, as if all my happiness was just emptied out. Paul couldn't understand that because I was a fairly upbeat person before infertility."

Ellen and Paul became even more of a team. "With our first miscarriage, he was as devastated as I was, and he came home from work to be with me," she says. "After the D&C, we went on a short vacation to get away from the whole thing. He came with me for all my surgical procedures. Really he helped as much as he could. It was a highly stressful time. With the kids and everything, we're stronger for it now."

We're not psychologists; we're just women who survived infertility with our marriages intact. You can, too. Here are a few ideas both men and women can incorporate to help their relationship stay strong while they battle infertility together.

Learn to Listen

Sometimes nobody really wants to hear what you have to say. They would rather you just sit there quietly and listen to them. Not listen and watch TV. Not listen and fold clothes. Just listen, and look into their eyes, and nod appropriately. An occasional "Uh-huh," "Yes," "I understand," or other appropriate comment is also useful. Make time to be a sounding board for each other.

Most of the time, your man won't be the one talking. It will be you. So share with your guy how you need him to take time to just be there with you.

Learn to Talk

Communication is important to any relationship and crucial to yours. Infertility's insanity can cause even the most verbose to clam up. Expressing your hopes, fears, dreams, and desires is good for your health (hey, there are studies that show people who keep their feelings all bottled up don't live as long as those who do express their feelings). Help each other understand the ins and outs of treatment choices and drug impacts. Make decisions as a team—or support the person who does make ultimate treatment decisions or undergoes the corrective surgery.

It is also imperative to make time to talk to each other about more than just infertility and the day's work. What are your dreams? What do you want to be when you grow up? Where would you like to go on vacation? Why do you feel Bruce Springsteen's music still speaks to the world after all these years?

This is all the stuff you talked about when you were dating, right? That's the point. Talk over coffee, in the car, on a walk. Go to the park, sit on the swings, and talk. Meet for drinks after work. Talk in bed.

Hold Hands

This is another old dating technique. Reach out and hold that hand—when you're walking, when you're watching TV, in bed. It's funny how big that small gesture can be. It's reaffirmation of the connection that defines a couple. It's an "I love you" moment.

Be Gifted and Talented

Sometimes you can say more with a little token. Send cards and flowers to let your partner know he or she is on your mind. Cook an exotic dinner. Escape for surprise weekend jaunts. Buy a present just because. Tuck love notes into lunch bags, briefcases, Palm Pilots. Leave dirty messages on each other's cell phones. Why not?

This can even help ease the awful. If you get a call the last IVF didn't produce a pregnancy, consider bringing home the news with some take-out Chinese and chopsticks. After hearing the news via a phone call at work, why not come home with flowers, candy, or a stuffed animal? The bottom line: add an action or item to the process that says to your partner, "I love you no matter what; we are in this together; it is not the end of us."

Battle the Bureaucrats

Volunteer to the be the guy (or gal) who fights the insurance company on what portions of your infertility they are not covering and why. Trade off this position. Support the one making the phone calls (even if you don't agree with their tactic, at least they are in the fight). If one person is doing the drugs, getting the shots, settling in for surgeries, the other can work with those covering the costs. This way, both partners are very aware of what is going on—both physically and financially. Besides, it's all more fun when both parties are involved.

Role Play

You are a team, so act like one. Determine who does what, when, and why. Dividing up the labor worked well for our friend Lee and her husband, Bennett.

"We quickly fell into very clearly defined roles in handling the situation and making decisions," says the thirty-eight-year-old Virginia teacher. "I did all the research, laid out all the options, and reviewed everything with him, and then we'd agree on a course of action. After that, I'd make all the appointments, and he'd be there. I know it's usually the case that one partner is more overtly invested in the process than the other—this didn't bother me though; our professional situations were such that I had more time to devote to it.

"My husband was nothing but supportive," she adds. "He listened, comforted, and had a very pragmatic attitude toward the whole thing, which helped me when I'd get very emotional."

Show up at the Doctor Appointments

This one is really for the guys. Try to come to as many appointments as you can. Obviously, you won't need to be at all of them, but it sure is nice when you are. If you can't make them, help your partner come up with questions to ask. Put a notepad and pen by her purse in the morning. Add an encouraging note. Suggest she call you when she finishes her appointment and fill you in, or meet her for lunch. Be present.

Allow Lash-outs

There will be times when you want to scream, shout, pound the table, and just be pissed off. Or your partner will want to do the same. Have some signal that you are expressing emotion against the infertility gods, so your partner doesn't take it personally. Then, let it out—and let it go.

Remember That Life Is Good

When in the middle of the madness, it is easy to forget infertility is a game we can win. Do not forget that. All of us can be parents if we want. The trick is to remember that until children arrive, you are still a family—a family of two, a couple. You have each other, which is more than some people have.

Our friend Geri and her husband, Ed, now have five-year-old twins, and she looks back at infertility as something that strengthened her marriage.

JULIE

Robert came to many of my fertility doctor appointments. To me, this was such a huge affirmation of his love. I felt very supported in what we were doing—that we were part of a team. He runs his own company, and when you have employees who depend on you, time is money. He never complained, though. To compensate, he would just work later on the days he took time off.

To be fair, Robert didn't make every single appointment I had, but he made all the big ones—the ones where we did surgeries, met with Dr. Cohen, or got results from big tests. On the days I had to swing by the doctor's office to just give blood, he really didn't need to be there, and sometimes he wasn't. If I had a doctor's appointment he couldn't make, he would often meet me after for lunch to talk, or we would meet up at a neighborhood restaurant for dinner and catch-up. Because he was so involved in these appointments, I never felt as if I was doing all the work even though I was the one being worked on.

"Honestly, the entire ordeal brought us closer together and, to my memory, didn't bring any strains on the relationship—other than sex; yes that was affected, but not our connection to one another," says the East Coast academic.

Robert told us that "only a real jerk" would leave a woman just because of her infertility. We like his thought process.

"That's not to say this situation wasn't incredibly stressful. It was. But I guess I learned that in the face of a crisis, I will always want Ed at my side. He is just a rock, and we were absolute partners in facing this.

"I can see how this stress can tear a marriage apart," she adds. "But you can use it as a learning tool, too. You can learn a lot about yourselves as a couple and how you face tough situations together. And, at least in our case, our relationship strengthened and grew even more, as I came to appreciate what a wonderful partner I had."

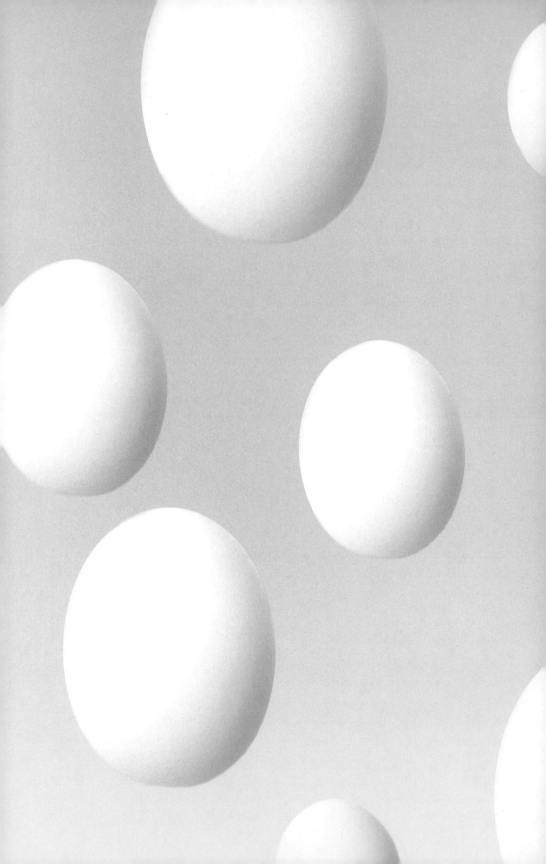

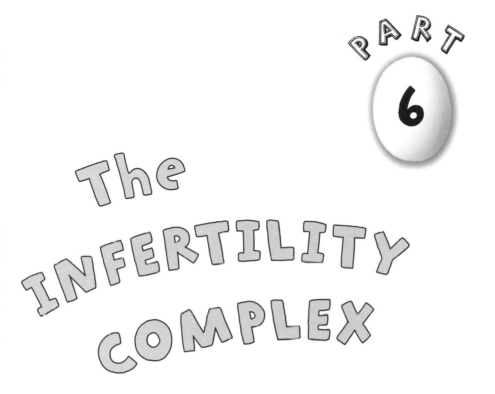

PART 6

The INFERTILITY COMPLEX

Experiencing infertility wipes away preconceived notions faster than a baby goes through diapers. Ideas such as traditional medicine can solve any problem. (It can't.) Or that you will stop thinking about your infertility or worrying about miscarriage once you finally do become pregnant. (You won't.) Or that once you become pregnant and deliver, you have "solved" your infertility once and for all. (Maybe not.) You now have what we call an "infertility complex."

Julie

Here's my take on what happens when you get pregnant after years or months of infertility treatment. You start what should be a blissful experience by worrying through the first three months. Okay. Got past that. Then you worry until the amnio at sixteen or seventeen weeks. Okay. Got through that. Then you worry through the whole second trimester—why do I feel so good? What's wrong? Finally, it's okay, got through that, too. This is how it goes for most of us until we deliver the goods, and the doctor puts that baby in our arms at the end of an exhausting nine months.

For me, I found I finally relaxed a bit at seven months. At seven months, a premature baby can survive in a top notch Dallas hospital. It is obviously not the optimal time to be born, but it is doable. Besides, my brother was born premature at seven months and ten days more than forty years ago in a rural upstate New York hospital. Back then, a neo-natal incubator was probably little better than a flannel-lined shoe box with a lightbulb. Today Richard is a healthy, grown man more than six feet tall. I figured if he could make it premature, so could my child, with all today's modern medical technology.

When I got past the seven-month mark, I felt relief. At my third-trimester, weekly sonogram appointments with Dr. Yarbrough, I started each conversation with "If things look iffy, I'm ready to go in and get the baby." After experiencing infertility and miscarriage, I was ready to do whatever I needed to ensure that baby got out alive.

Luckily for me (and them), Graham waited the full forty weeks for his arrival; Amanda debuted three weeks early. Exhale.

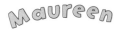

When I had my son, I experienced the magical fantasy pregnancy. I was completely unaware of any of the possibilities of problems. I skated like an Olympic gold medalist—free, easy, and full of delight. I told everyone the day I found out, bought maternity clothes early, filled the closet with baby clothes within the first twelve weeks, painted the nursery in the first trimester, moved couches and furniture into the nursery when I was eight months pregnant, and swam up until the day I gave birth. It was just a dream. I never knew anything else, and I treasure the memories.

After having suffered three miscarriages, I realized how lucky I had been. I knew I would never experience a blissfully ignorant pregnancy again, no matter what. The fear and worry of miscarriage becomes a part of who you are. It's as if you were to get hit by a car and survive. You forever fear crossing the road again, even though you'll probably make it to the other side.

Now I have a problem when someone I know gets pregnant. I hold my breath for them, and they don't even know it. Usually they skate along the way I did in my first pregnancy, while I pray every day they won't crash. Sometimes I express concern, and I get slapped for disrupting their dream. But once you experience a loss, you will never again be able to experience the innocence of pregnancy. It is taken from you much like most of your innocent childhood dreams.

CHAPTER 19

To SOY or Not To SOY?

Julie

In an effort to help my fertility flower, I tried to supplement modern medicine with whatever else I could find. As a result, I ate a tablespoon of molasses daily for its vitamin and mineral boost. I took herbs. I wore healing crystal earrings. I drank raspberry tea to strengthen my uterus. I went back to church. I scrubbed my skin daily with a loofah sponge to exfoliate the body's largest organ, increase circulation, and allow it to breathe in the hope that it would help.

I took a woman's workshop and made a stone and feather doll, drawing a tiny baby on its tummy, then hiding it beneath another flat round stone bound with leather. I was supposed to hide my innermost wish on the doll and then put it away. When my wish came true—as I was assured it would—I was supposed to bury this rock doll in the dirt from which it came, thanking Mother Earth for her blessing. I found the doll in a drawer one day after Graham was born and promptly buried it in the yard.

I say, whatever helps.

Maureen

When I had gallbladder problems, I went to the doctor. I also went to a Chinese herbalist, who gave me a bunch of twigs to boil and then drink. The mixture looked and tasted just like water in which someone dropped a cigarette butt—kind of yellow and bitter. Yuck. My gallbladder problems never went away, even with the cigarette water, and I had to have it removed. I gave it a shot, but perhaps my gallbladder was too far gone for herbs to have an effect.

With my infertility, I never tried alternative treatments. (Wait. I did have a friend of mine who claims to have fertility powers lay her hands over me from time to time. Does that count?)

Ultimately, I realized it all came down to balance between body, mind, and spirit. There are different methods to achieve that, and whatever works for you, go for it. For me, I just needed to slow down and believe.

Ten Reasons to Think Outside the Box

1. Modern medicine may not do it all.
2. There's nothing wrong with making some lifestyle changes.
3. Alternative therapies have helped other couples, or at least they think they have.
4. Miracles do happen.
5. You are what you eat . . . and who really wants to be preservative-and-additive laced?
6. You just never know.
7. What the heck, it probably can't hurt you to try something different—with doctor's approval, of course.
8. Who knows? It could help you!
9. Thinking outside the box opens up more opportunities and possibilities.
10. What do you have to lose?

Alternative Avenues

So what do you do when traditional medicine fails? Rather than give up hope altogether, most of us start looking for something else.

When it comes to alternative therapies, who hasn't tried something? It's like moisturizers. We are convinced that someday someone is going to develop the one that really keeps us young-looking and wrinkle-free. Until then, we'll try them all just so we don't miss out.

That's how our friend Helen approached infertility when technology seemed to be failing her. "I tried just about everything," says the forty-something mother of two, who had unexplained infertility. "I did yoga, which I really believe did a lot of good by relaxing me. I did acupuncture, which definitely helped. I used to go once a week, and it would put me into such a relaxed state—although I can't say whether the relaxation itself was what helped or the actual acupuncture. I also took some of the Chinese herbs the acupuncturist gave me, which looking back, I might not do again—they tasted awful. But at that point, I was at the very end of my rope. I got off caffeine and all artificial sweeteners."

In addition, Helen belonged to a prayer group during most of the three years she suffered infertility. "I think it helped to focus a little on my spirituality rather than only the awful physical stuff I was going through," she says. "I did a lot of praying during that time. Also, I belonged to a RESOLVE support group, and I saw a counselor."

Eventually Helen became pregnant. "I think everything else I was doing in addition to the fertility drugs helped, but since all of these things were overlapping, I can't say really which ones did the trick. Who knows? Maybe it was just the fertility drugs, after all."

We've talked with women who credit herbs, homeopathy, acupuncture, or prayer for their pregnancy. If we learned anything from our experiences with infertility, it is to keep an open mind. Getting your mind, body, and psyche in balance certainly can't hurt anything! Changing your diet, your exercise routine, your stress levels, even your job may be the additional key to your success. Can ancient remedies offer a modern miracle? Why not? We aren't saying you should replace medical intervention. We're just saying you should have an open mind. Science doesn't always hold all the answers for all the people, and lots of women have achieved successful pregnancies by healing themselves spiritually and mentally while pursuing medical treatment.

The lawyers in our families are making us reiterate here that we are not doctors. We aren't suggesting that you do any of these alternative treatments. We are just telling you what others have done. We don't suggest you do anything you haven't run by your doctor first. Okay, now that that's over, let's look at the alternatives.

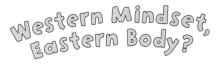

Western Mindset, Eastern Body?

The first thing you must do when moving beyond traditional treatments is to shake off that Western mindset—the realist who wants everything to be concrete, black-or-white, technical, clinical, see-it-to-believe-it. You know, the

American model. Thinking outside the baby-making box means accepting the unseen, finding the gray, believing in magic and higher powers. The goal here is creating a more Eastern mindset body—one driven by a more philosophical mentality and approach. This alternative thought process depends on letting go of the probable and embracing the possible, embracing a more holistic, whole mind/body model. What the heck? If technology, shots, and pill-popping isn't working, why not marry the two?

Harvard has with great results. In 1978, the Mind-Body Institute of Harvard Medical School developed a ten-week group program for women with unexplained infertility. Under the continued direction of fertility expert, researcher, and author, Dr. Alice Domar, the program has taught women how to better cope with stressful issues. They focus on guided imagery, yoga, improved nutrition, exercise, and support group. The shift was away from focusing solely on baby making to living a fulfilled life. It seems to work; they have done many studies that show that the women who complete the program note significantly less anxiety, anger, and depression. Many of them became pregnant within a year of finishing the course. Reduce stress, reduce infertility. Works for us.

Poking and Prodding

Some chicks have gone old school, trying acupuncture, to help their body function more efficiently as a supplement to their Western medicine treatments. Acupuncture is the ancient Chinese treatment of strategically placing tiny needles into the body to stimulate key energy points. These needles, in turn, are supposed to help readjust and regulate the body's balance—spiritually, emotionally, and physically. Acupuncture helps the Qi, or Chi, your body's life energy, flow easily from head to toe. When Qi moves freely, your body is healthy and balance. Clog up the Qi and illness—like infertility—can arise. For a woman facing infertility, an acupuncturist would place the needles in key spots directly affecting reproductive organs.

Studies have shown acupuncture to be beneficial to traditional IVF treatment, increasing the chance of a successful pregnancy. In addition to upping the odds in IVF, some doctors think acupuncture may also work to boost egg production, helping produce one good egg in rates comparable to some fertility drugs. Studies suggest that acupuncture can affect the reproductive hormones and endorphins triggered by the brain, as well as increase blood flow to the ovaries and uterus. Acupuncture, however, cannot fix physical defects like a septum in your uterus or a blocked Fallopian tube.

Our friend Victoria incorporated acupuncture into her fertility regimen. "Well, it hasn't helped in the major way, since I'm not pregnant yet, but it has helped me emotionally I think," says the thirty-four-year-old, who has been trying to get pregnant for six years. "I really like my acupuncturist and the way she approaches things; I have done lots of my own reading and research about alternative therapies, and I'm starting to have less of a frantic approach to the whole infertility thing. I have become more attentive to my diet, to my emotional state, to my body in general. I started with my acupuncturist at the same time as my last IVF attempt and did them concurrently, but I have stayed with her. She reminded me that it takes time for a major change, and I really believe that."

Victoria has also done a series of colonics (irrigating her colon) to detox, juiced daily for a while, and saw a chiropractor three times a week. "I was trying to do it all," she says. "Now I do everything in moderation. I see the chiropractor once in a while for an adjustment. I do see my acupuncturist every week still, and I keep on top of my herbs as well—I actually just switched from capsules to cooked herbs from Chinatown that I drink; that's interesting.

"So, I would like to think that I have gotten to a more peaceful point in my life with it all, definitely less stressful than all the infertility treatments and cocky doctors and being told it's all 'bad luck.' The holistic approach, especially my acupuncturist, has helped me with that. She reminds me to practice positive visualization which I try to do, especially when I first wake up and right before I go to sleep. So we'll see."

To get your Qi flow properly, you may need to go to the acupuncturist once or twice a week, perhaps for several weeks or months. Costs vary depending on the practitioner and where you live, but expect to pay between $50 and $100 for a treatment. Some insurance companies cover the cost of acupuncture, so check out your policy.

Q & A WITH AN ACUPUNCTURIST

Here are some of the things inquiring minds want to know—at least our inquiring minds. We spoke with Victoria's Long Island acupuncturist to clear up a few points. Tish McCrea, M.S. L. Ac., is a licensed acupuncturist, board certified in acupuncture and in Chinese herbology. She has a master's in Oriental Medicine from The

New York College of Health Professions in Syosset, New York, and teaches at the college level.

Q: How can acupuncture help women who are going through infertility?

A: This question is not a simple one; a lot depends on the cause of infertility. Acupuncture can help regulate hormones and the menstrual cycle and even offer help to women who are not ovulating regularly. I am treating a woman now who is in her early thirties and is going through early menopause. Her FSH levels were very high, and through acupuncture and Chinese herbs, she has been able to normalize her hormones. Women should not underestimate the power that stress plays in infertility. Acupuncture can also help with that.

Q: When should a woman seek an acupuncturist and alternative therapies?

A: As soon as possible. They can start acupuncture when they suspect a problem (before IVF, for example), or they can begin acupuncture one to two months before their scheduled IVF—or as far in advance as they want, really. It's best not to wait until the last few weeks before the transfer. Chinese medicine, generally speaking, is a gentle medicine that is trying to correct imbalances. This can't be done quickly. At least, it can't be done quickly in the case of infertility or other chronic conditions. The length and frequency of acupuncture treatment often depends on the cause of infertility and how the patient responds to treatment. I've had a couple of patients who have had trouble holding a pregnancy come a few months before they start trying to get "juiced up" for their pregnancy. A weakness in Qi or blood can often result in a miscarriage.

Q: Why do some medical doctors seem to have a hard time when patients try alternative therapy like acupuncture?

A: Personally, I think it is because they have no understanding of this type of medicine, and therefore they fear it will somehow negatively impact their treatment. It won't. Acupuncture, when done properly of course, can only help a patient.

I think there is so much mystery surrounding Chinese medicine, and patients and doctors think it has no structure to it. Chinese medicine has a very complex and logical philosophy behind it. There are a lot of clinical trials and scientific tests being done on the effects of acupuncture. Unfortunately, because of the nature of the medicine, it is difficult to prove scientifically. Qi is not something that can be measured using a blood test! Nonetheless, the results of these studies are very exciting.

What should a woman keep in mind when working with an acupuncturist on her fertility?

A: Be consistent with your treatments. This type of medicine requires a commitment from the patient. Allow six months, minimally, of consistent treatments before you even think about stopping. A full year of treatment is often needed. Also, keep in mind that it is okay if the places where the needles are inserted are tender or sore during a treatment. This does not mean the acupuncturist is bad; it's a sign that the energy is stagnant and that the needles are doing their job!

The patient should just relax and feel the sensations around the needles and appreciate that they are feeling the Qi moving. Don't resist the needles.

Q: What can a woman do in conjunction with acupuncture to increase her chances of fertility?

A: Chinese herbal medicine is extremely important, in my opinion. I rarely treat an infertility patient without it. Of course, a healthy diet, moderate exercise, plenty of sleep, healthy emotions, and reduction of stress are all important. I try to incorporate Eastern nutrition into my treatments and give diet recommendations to all my patients.

Q: What about women who have unexplained infertility—how can acupuncture help them?

A: These patients often respond to acupuncture the best! Western medicine can't explain their fertility, but a practitioner of Oriental medicine will find the imbalance, and often it is very obvious to us even when doctors are perplexed.

Patients also need to take a good look at their medical history. Sometimes there are past illnesses that may not seem relevant to your infertility but should always be mentioned to your acupuncturist. I had a patient who struggled with unexplained infertility for many years. She has finally had a healthy baby boy, but I remember her telling me that she had a very severe case of bacterial meningitis and almost died! In my opinion, this had a huge impact on her infertility.

Q: How long before someone reaps benefit from acupuncture?

A: Again, it depends on the condition. Generally speaking, chronic conditions take longer to treat, but every patient is different, and I really can't give you an answer to this question. For infertility, I ask my patients to give me six months of treatment (at least) before they try other methods. Really, a year is best. I've seen it work in a month, but sometimes it takes up to two years for a patient to get pregnant. There are a lot of variables.

Q: How can someone find a good acupuncturist?

A: First you want to make sure that the practitioner is licensed (and not just certified) with the L.Ac after his or her name. You also want someone who is board certified and preferable knows Chinese herbology. You can log onto NCCAOM.org to find qualified practitioners. Also, word of mouth is a good start. Don't assume that the practitioner must be Chinese!

Q: What about herbs in conjunction with acupuncture?

A: Each patient needs to choose for themselves, but it makes sense to compliment acupuncture treatments with Chinese herbs. You need someone board certified in Chinese herbology—very important if you want an herbal formula based on the philosophy behind Chinese medicine. There is also a Western approach to herbology, and the herbs or herb combinations can be very different. Then there is Ayervedic medicine . . . again, different philosophy and different herbs.

Q: How much does acupuncture cost, and how long should you expect treatments to last (one month, one year)?

A: I can tell you my fees—the first treatment is $85 and following treatments are $65. Herbs run somewhere between $80 to $150/month. My fees are average for the (Long Island) suburbs. Big-city prices are higher. For infertility, I see patients at least once a week, sometimes twice. It is a financial commitment, too, but a lot less expensive than IVF. How long the treatments last can't be answered. Much depends on the condition of the patient and her lifestyle.

Q: What advice do you have for infertile women seeking alternative treatments?

A: Listen to your gut. If one type of treatment pulls you more than another, go with what resonates with you and what makes sense to you. A woman's intuition is very strong! Be patient and open your mind to unfamiliar things.

Herb Jargon

After your doctor has determined (or not) the causes of your infertility, you can try boosting your body's natural reserves with some herbs. The right herb concoction may enhance your body's hormonal rhythms. Before all these newfangled drugs existed, there were herbs. In fact, many medicines were originally derived from herbs—and trees, bark, flowers, and grasses. There were no science labs and Pergonal back then.

Some herbs are believed to support the reproductive system by restoring hormonal balance and uterine tone. Some herbs are advised to help maintain a pregnancy or limit miscarriage. Often, several herbs may be suggested together to form a tonic of sorts. Herbs can be used and/or ingested in many ways—simmered to make a tea, as extracts added to juice or water, ground into a powder, and put into pill form or as the actual leaves, seeds, or berries.

Julie turned to herbal medicines after her year of fertility treatment found her still baby-free. So have many of our friends. Don't go it alone, however. Some concentrated forms of herbs may be too strong to use for extended periods of time. Talk to herbologists or naturopaths—or the owners of the heath food store in which you are shopping. Don't ingest anything that seems rancid or old. And definitely don't ingest anything until you talk to your doctor first. Herbs can affect the medicines your doctor has prescribed, so it is crucial that he or she be aware of anything else you are ingesting.

Here are a few herbs often recommended to help restore female fertility and tone the reproductive system. Most can be consumed in pill format, though you may want to experiment with teas. Ask your herbologist or naturopath what they suggest.

Dong quai: A root that targets the effects of ovarian and testicular hormones, dong quai is used to treat female issues such as hot flashes, menstrual irregularities, menopause, infertility, and PMS. It is also used to tone a weak uterus.

Licorice: This root helps promote adrenal-gland function and has estrogen-like hormonal effects. This can help women who have low estrogen, elevated testosterone, or polycystic ovary syndrome. Studies have also shown that licorice can improve the regularity of menstruation.

Chaste tree berry: Helps promote ovulation by stimulating the release of LH. This herb also may help return menstrual periods to women who suffer from amenorrhea.

Red raspberry: The bark, leaves, and roots of this plant helps strengthen the uterine wall and relaxes the uterine spasms.

Kelp: The leaves of this plant contain iodine, vitamins A, B, C, and E, and zinc, among other things. The iodine can help improve thyroid function for those with a deficiency.

Ginseng: This root has been used for years to improve fertility by improving adrenal glands, energy, and the immune system and regulating the reproductive hormones, and it boosts overall health. Ginseng can also be used for impotence by stimulating the sex glands.

JULIE

It's hard to forget that Friday afternoon when my husband stood up and introduced Norm to the McKinney Rotary Club as "the man who helped get my wife pregnant." Eighty pairs of eyes shifted from this tall, lanky fellow standing next to Robert to my burgeoning belly. Embarrassed? Yes.

Norm owned an herbal supplement and wellness store downtown. He was my supplier for dong quai, wild yam, black cohosh, licorice, and kelp. He and his wife spent time educating me on the various herbs they recommended and why they might work. Thanks to them, I studied a variety of drug-free remedies that depended on a mix of vitamins, minerals, herbs, and other supplements. Some I still use today for nonfertility related problems. I found the natural approach to be a nice balance to all the high-tech medical intervention.

Did Norm help get me pregnant? Who knows? It didn't hurt.

Black cohosh: Contains estrogen-like compounds and helps enhance your pituitary gland's secretion of LH. As a result, it also helps stimulate your ovaries. Do not take it if you are pregnant!

Blue cohosh: This bitter root can elevate your blood pressure and stimulate your uterus to contract. Considered a uterine tonic, blue cohosh can also relax your uterus and help increase the organ's muscle tone.

Gotu kola: The seeds, nuts, and roots of this plant are used to create a bitter-tasting herb supplement known for its ability to increase sex drive.

Squaw vine: This herb was popular with Native Americans to promote fertility. It helps increase blood circulation to the uterus and improve uterine tone.

Yoga: Stretching Your Imagination

Several of our friends do yoga to help their infertility. Or maybe they do it just to relieve the stress of infertility. Inner peace can't hurt. Neither can stretching, toning, and strengthening the muscles that support all your reproductive organs, realigning your spine, or learning to breathe in a way that brings more oxygen into your system. Most importantly, it helps reduce your stress levels. When we're stressed, we pollute our bodies with chemicals that weaken our immune system. The movements in yoga help flush out the toxins in our bodies. While you are doing yoga, you must focus you mind and body on something other than your fertility.

Here are the benefits of yoga as we see it. If you can better your overall health and relax your mind and muscles by gently stretching your body, then your chances of conceiving probably increase. Some yoga teachers praise yoga for helping regulate menstruation and make ovulation more predictable. Yoga exercises gently work the reproductive organs and pelvis, moving the blood and reoxygenating that part of the body. The breathing techniques yoga teaches bring a more abundant supply of oxygen into the body. The meditation, which is part of the practice, can help you resolve conflicts and angst so present during infertility. Plus, you might just end up with some really well-toned arms when it's all said and done.

None of these things is bad.

We think yoga is wonderful. Julie does it and loves how great it makes her feel afterward. Maureen doesn't, but a lot of her friends do. You can find classes at your local community and health centers; you can rent a tape or read a book to learn the poses. But we can't guarantee that doing downward dog will get you pregnant unless your husband attacks from the back at just the right ovulatory moment. We don't know, it might be fun.

Food for Thought

A diet rich in junk food or packed with preservatives is not good if you're trying to conceive because what you eat is important. Poor nutrition can be a cause of infertility. We think preservatives, additives, and all the other junk in our food can also contribute. Makes sense—if you are deficient in nutrients, your body is out of balance.

When medical science can't find an explanation, look in the pantry. If you see lots of processed, packaged, and canned goods, you're also looking at food soaked in sodium, stuffed with sugar, chock-full of chemicals, and peppered with preservatives. Don't even get us started on the staple of the American diet, fast food—with all its fat, sugar, and sodium. Diet sodas are just flavored liquid chemicals. All of us know that stuff is no good for us. But many of us eat it every day. If you're trying to get pregnant, you shouldn't.

Instead, opt for a diet packed with plenty of organic vegetables, fresh fruits, and whole grains. Eat smaller amounts of animal protein, unless you know where the meat is from. More and more evidence indicates that residues of the hormones (like estrogens) fed to cattle and poultry that end up on our dinner table can interfere with human hormones. All these extra hormones are why we insist that our children drink only organic milk, for example. You should, too.

Occasional junk food is fine—and fun. Just don't make it a habit right now. You'll have plenty of opportunity for the drive-thru once you have kids and no time. There will come a day when you cannot stomach the thought of another french fry. Until then, if you insist on eating crap, at least take a multivitamin.

Vitamins and Minerals

We've heard that the soil in which our food is grown is too stripped of essential nutrients for our food to provide us optimum nourishment. Your body uses some vitamins and minerals specifically for reproduction. It would make sense if your diet is lacking in the proper allotment, your body is lacking, too.

If you can't or don't get all the nutrients you need from your food, you may want to pop a few pills. We mean vitamin pills. Here are few that may help with infertility.

Vitamin B_6: This vitamin may be helpful at relieving PMS and improving a woman's chances for conception. Also called pyridoxine, B_6 is found in dietary supplements and in fruits, vegetables, and cereals. Julie's doctor recommended B_6 to help with the carpal tunnel she developed while pregnant. It worked.

Folic acid: Folic acid is the vitamin recommended to pregnant women to help their developing baby. However, a folate deficiency may also contribute to infertility. Some women report they became pregnant shortly after getting enough folic acid back into their diet.

Zinc: A zinc deficiency messes with fertility by disrupting the normal menstrual cycle. Without enough zinc, your body doesn't produce the right amounts of hormones FSH and LH, which are necessary for reproduction. Semen contains zinc in high concentrations. Adding extra zinc to your partner's diet may improve sperm count. If you don't like popping a pill, snack on zinc-rich pumpkin seeds. These seeds have been long considered a fertility-enhancer. Pumpkin seeds are also rich in Vitamin E.

Vitamin E: This antioxidant vitamin is important for proper reproductive function in both men and women. It improves oxygen utilization, boosts the immune system, and protects hormones from oxidizing. Interesting factoid: Vitamin E's chemical name is tocopherol, which broken down into its roots comes from the Greek words *tokos* (offspring) and *phero* (to bear).

Vitamin B$_{12}$: If you are anemic and suffering from infertility, you may have a Vitamin B$_{12}$ deficiency. Even if you are not anemic, lack of B$_{12}$ may play a contributing role to your infertility, which may be reversed with increased supplements of this vitamin.

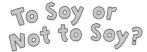

To Soy or Not to Soy?

Let's talk phytoestrogens. Everyone else is. Soy is packed with the mystical, magical phytoestrogens—plant estrogens. Women are consuming vast quantities of soy in this country. Everyone thinks soy is a miracle food. It may be, in moderation. But soy protein is very complex, and so is all the information out there on these legumes.

Soy foods come in a variety of forms, some natural, some heavily processed. In Asia, soy is eaten sparingly—the average consumption is between 9.3 to 36 grams of soy food per day. In America, we tend to like our soy straight-up, and we consume pure soy protein. Let's do some math. A cup of tofu has 252 grams of soy protein. A cup of soy milk has 240 grams. We have friends who regularly consume a couple glasses of soy milk (the chocolate variety is particularly yummy), at least a cup of salted soy nuts, and one or two soy protein bars during the course of *one day*. That's a lot of soy, much more than any Asian woman is consuming.

For us, soy has become a cheap veggie protein to substitute for meat. To make it more of a taste treat, bland-tasting soy is packed with unhealthy sweeteners, salt, artificial flavorings, colors, and monosodium glutamate (MSG). Now, here's what we've learned: too much processed soy in animal feed has resulted in growth and fertility problems in cows, sheep, and guinea pigs. So much so, that farmers limit the amount of soy their animals can eat. Interesting.

On the flip side, a year-long study done at Wake Forest University Baptist Medical Center and Emory University School of Medicine have also shown that plant estrogens, given at twice the amount consumed by Asian women, don't mess up a monkey's fertility. Apparently female monkeys have a similar menstrual cycle to us. However, we have already established that Asian women consume a minimum amount of soy daily—unlike some people we know and love.

We do have some personal knowledge of what soy can do. Julie ate soy nuts and drank soy milk while trying to get pregnant. Once she was pregnant, she didn't consume soy exclusively, but she did eat enough to cause her some concern on how all these phytoestrogens were going to affect her unborn baby boy when she discovered she was carrying a male child. And she quit any and all soy right then.

We also have a good friend Lola, who is a movie producer. When we quizzed her about having kids at thirty-eight, she told us her "body has never been in such great shape," and she didn't "want to ruin it right now by getting pregnant." When Lola turned thirty-nine, she was suddenly in a panic, realizing that forty was around the corner. She and her (much) younger boyfriend tried to get pregnant for six months, with no success. When she finally went to the doctor at our urging (we really do butt into our pals' lives a lot), Lola was told the lining of her uterus was too thick, and it would be hard to conceive. Her estrogen levels were also screwy. The doctor couldn't figure out why. When Maureen asked about her diet, we discovered Lola was a soy junkie with a capital "J." She had consumed vast quantities of soy protein for years. It was her secret to slimness. Her doctor agreed that consuming as much soy as Lola did could indeed alter her body chemistry. By the time she changed her diet and got her levels back to "normal," she was almost forty. She continued to try to conceive, but nothing. In order to qualify for a fertility program, her egg quality was tested, and it was discovered that her egg production had shut down. She was excluded from the program, rendered infertile at the ripe old age of forty. Lola still has her great body and young stud, but no good eggs. For this information, she was not ready.

So, like many thing out there, you are going to find conflicting information. If you have low estrogen, maybe soy will help you. If you are normal or even high in estrogen, you may not want to add anymore estrogens to the mix. Do your research and remember that old adage—all things in moderation.

Back to Work

In addition to bending and stretching for fertility, some women get their spines realigned. Well, why not? Neither of us has ever been to a chiropractor, but we have a few friends who swear by them. Our friend Jess, a mother of IVF twins, is a recently converted chiropractic fan. Jess and her husband, Paul, always wanted more children, but really couldn't justify spending the money on fertility treatments when they were also saving for two sets of braces, college tuitions, and future weddings. Her girls were four years old when Jess decided to visit a chiropractor for her aching back. Five months later, Jess called us to say she was six weeks pregnant!

"I have to attribute it to the chiropractic treatments, but I have no proof," says the thirty-eight-year-old stay-at-home mom. "After I started seeing the chiropractor, my periods stabilized; I felt great. Whatever the cause, I don't care. I'm ecstatic. It's a miracle."

How could this work? Well, according to chiropractors, these treatments work by realigning the spine and physically pulling the body back into proper structural balance. Chiropractors think this may help with reproduction by realigning the reproductive organs and their associated nerves back to their original position, thus helping the egg move down the Fallopian tube more easily. According to chiropractors we quizzed, nerves to the reproductive system run through the spine. Once they're readjusted, fertility may return.

Some studies show that infertile women undergoing chiropractic care—like Jess—have become pregnant. The study we reviewed was a relatively small pool of women in a broad age range, from twenty-two to sixty-five years old. All the women in these studies had misaligned spines or related spinal problems that interfered with the nerves. Many of them got pregnant after undergoing chiropractic treatment. Obviously, the sixty-five-year-old didn't get pregnant, but interestingly to us, after having lost her menstrual periods as a teenager girl following a fall, she began menstruating four weeks after beginning chiropractic adjustments.

Chiropractors are often covered by insurance, and the treatments are less expensive than fertility treatments. However, we'd like to stress again that we would not suggest doing anything without talking with your fertility specialist first. Remember, chiropractors, unlike reproductive endocrinologists, are not fertility specialists.

Power of Prayer

You shouldn't ever think your infertility is some kind of slap by the Supreme Being. God is not out to get us. Sometime stuff just happens . . . to us.

There is no justice in the world—not really. If there were, we'd all get pregnant easily and have all the healthy children our hearts and homes could hold. Additionally, nobody's dog would run loose, and our trash would get picked up on time. Unfortunately, we don't live in that perfect world. We're not going to get all philosophical on you, but life is what it is. The heavens are not singling you out for punishment. This is not some grand scheme to test your spirituality or religion. However, your bout with infertility just might bring you back into the fold. We can promise it will certainly bring you to your knees.

We've already established that you can have a family, just maybe not biologically. Everyone wins at infertility in that regard. The spiritual side of infertility demands that you stop expecting you will get what you want, how and when you want it. Having it your way is only available at certain fast food restaurants. We think faith is more about believing you will get what you need in a way you might never have considered. Faith is believing you will be a parent—somehow.

Julie got pregnant when she quit praying for a baby and began asking God to lead her to her family—to help her find her children, wherever they might

MAUREEN

I believe in God, and I believe in the signs he sends. When we moved to New York and I got my new license plates, I looked down and the plate read AVA 3580. It sounds strange, but at that moment, I just knew I would have a baby girl and her name would be Ava. It spoke to me. . . . yes, God even shows up at the DMV.

And what about the numbers on that plate? Well, I have always had a theory that I was born thirty-five, the woman at the DMV said that was when I last "crossed over," a strange, unscientific theory that people are born the essence of an age. Mine was thirty-five. When I was three, I was thirty-five; when I was eighteen, I was thirty-five: when I was forty, I was thirty-five. I believe my son is at least fifty or sixty. He has always been much older than me. It is a cockamamie theory, but it works for me. In addition, eight and zero are my favorite numbers. I have always adored the roundness of both of them, so the combination of those numbers and the name Ava in front of it just rang out to me. AVA 3580. . . . Ava was calling. I believed this from the bottom of my heart, but it wasn't that easy. I went through all the infertility treatments with failure constantly getting into my car and seeing Ava's name on the plate. When it was time to call it quits, I couldn't figure out where she was, but I had continual faith that she would show up. I had a few conversations with God about it, but deep inside I knew, he had given me a sign and I had to be patient and believe. How strange that it showed up on a license plate. Against all odds I got pregnant, and, when my baby girl arrived, there was no question what her name would be.

be, and to bring them home. Maureen believes God spoke to her when she was issued the license plate AVA 3580—the name she subsequently gave her daughter, Ava. God speaks to us in many ways. We have learned to listen.

It doesn't matter to us if you worship God, Goddess, Buddha, or the moon. Not that it matters, but Julie is Episcopalian, and Maureen is Catholic. Our friends are all over the place religion-wise. But most of them say the same thing—praying, either to God or to a Supreme Being within, can be healing. There are even studies that show the incredible power of prayer on healing, though we couldn't find any reliable ones on the restorative powers of prayer as it refers to healing infertility. We only know the stories our friends have told us and the experiences we have had ourselves.

Being part of a prayer group can help by offering spiritual and emotional support. Praying can put you in touch with your soul and cause you to slow down. Involvement in your church or synagogue can take your mind off your own problems while you focus on the greater good of humankind. It's a chance to figure out what this whole infertility journey is about anyway. What are you learning—about yourself, your partner, your relationship? If you are angry at God, accept it, figure out why, and learn how to get over it. As you come to peace, you will become more peaceful.

We know doctors and nurses who say a little prayer before each IVF, though there is no proof that helps their success rates. "Our doctor's team joined hands and said a prayer before implanting the embryos in me," says our friend Peg, who suffered through six years of secondary infertility before calling it quits. "The IVF didn't take, but I felt better, more secure, with them praying. It was like they knew they weren't God; they were in this with a higher power. They cared."

Quack, Quack, Quack

All practitioners of alternative medicine are not created equal. Some are excellent, knowledgeable professionals, and some are phony-baloney quacks.

The best bet for not getting screwed is doing your homework. Research these options just as you would medical treatment. Look for an acupuncturist, for example, who is trained and licensed. Traditionally, trained acupuncturists must do thousands of hours of training in needle placement—unlike medical doctors who simply dabble in acupuncture. Ditto with a chiropractor or yoga instructor. And if possible, you want people who have experience working with infertile women.

Ask your RE for suggestions. Is there an acupuncturist he or she has worked with in the past? Are there herbs and/or an herbalist he or she would suggest? A chiropractor associated with the hospital or clinic? Quiz your friends—even the infertile ones. It's like finding a good masseuse or nail salon. There are a variety of reasons one would seek alternative treatments, and your pals may know the perfect place.

Make sure your doctors are aware of your alternative treatment plans. They may not agree with what you are doing. If so, ask them why. Certain herbs or procedures might interfere with your medical protocol. Some doctors don't understand the whole "New Age" jargon and may want to be educated on what you are trying to do. Our advice? Do your research, talk to your doctor, weigh the suggestions, and make your decisions.

JULIE

When I was pregnant with Graham, after years of infertility and miscarriages, every church-going friend and family member had my name on a prayer list. My dad had two church groups praying. My grandmother was part of a church group praying. My cousin Carla was praying. Robert and I were praying for a successful pregnancy, for our family.

Did it help? We think it did. We believe in a higher power, and we believe in the power of positive energy. Perhaps our belief strengthened us or relaxed me. Maybe prayer in combination with stellar medical care, good drugs, and a nurturing home environment was the winning combination. Graham arrived here in one piece, so who knows?

P.S.—I was pregnant three more times after Graham. Prayer didn't help with two of them. Or did it? What's that Garth Brooks song—some of God's greatest gifts are unanswered prayers? My second miscarriage made me slow down and be extra careful when I got pregnant with my daughter. My last lost pregnancy made me appreciate even more the gift of the two beautiful children I have.

CHAPTER 20

The BUN'S in the OVEN

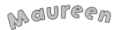

When I think about my pregnancy with Ava, I always go back to her conception.

We had thrown in the towel on ever giving Quinn a sibling. After five months mourning this loss, my husband took me away for a surprise weekend. He wouldn't tell me where we were going—just said to find my passport. This excited me to no end. I had visions of a romantic Caribbean getaway, Paris with the twinkling lights of the Eiffel Tower, or Italy with its rich culture.

So when Will pulled up in front of Air Canada, you can imagine my disappointment. Canada? We're going to Canada? Not just Canada, says my husband, unable to control his great enthusiasm—Ottawa!

Ottawa, I'm thinking. . . . Where is that?

Since I had no choice, off to Ottawa we went.

Ottawa is a short plane ride from New York. What a surprise! It looked more like England than England. We stayed at Chateau Laurier, a castle across from the Parliament, situated on a river that really could have been called Thames. It had accommodated many kings, queens, and movie stars. Our room was large and spectacular with two separate bathrooms—a his and hers (that always works).

Now to note, this weekend was day nine through twelve in my cycle—although I wasn't counting at the time. On a lazy, rainy Monday (day eleven in my cycle), we were awakened from a noon-time nap by clamoring outside. When

I looked outside my window, directly below me was the Queen of England. Yes, Queen Elizabeth. She was in town placing a wreath on the tomb of the unknown soldier, in the rain, under an umbrella, looking up at me in my castle! I waved as if I were a queen, too. Queen for a day. It was magic. The entire weekend was magic. The chemistry was just right. We laughed, we ate, we drank, we kissed, and we made love while the Queen of England was getting drenched in the rain below us. I wasn't thinking about getting pregnant. I was free.

Upon our return I was light in step, like a teenager in love. By Halloween, which was my day twenty-eight, I wasn't feeling well—I was tired with an achy back. I just knew I was going to get my period any moment. When Julie urged me to get a pregnancy test, I was stunned. It had never occurred to me that I could be pregnant . . . never. The thought was absurd. I had accepted it was over for me, that my eggs were officially rotten. When I took the test the next morning on Day twenty-nine, it was more than positive. It wasn't blue, it was purple! Not believing my eyes—or this test—I tested again. Thank God, two come in a pack. Positive! I was pregnant. God bless the Queen of England!

By counting back in my cycle, I figured this baby would most likely be a girl. Not just because of my license plate but also because having sex prior to day fourteen probably meant the sperm had been hanging around for a few days and finally caught up with that one golden egg while I was picking pumpkins at the farmer's market. It *was* Ava . . . AVA3580.

Julie

I remember when I found out I was pregnant with Graham. I had suffered a miscarriage four months prior, and my period was still unpredictable. So it didn't really bother me that my period seemed to be taking a while to arrive this month. But, since I suffered unexplained infertility, I went to my OB/GYN's to check it out. Dr. Yarbrough did a sonogram and said it didn't look like I'd ovulated yet. There was no lining visible in the uterus. He then made an off-the-cuff comment about my left ovary being lower under the uterus. Later in the car, I thought about this comment. Ovary low under the uterus? What's this all about? I didn't know I had this ovarian thing. I chalked it up to yet another thing wrong with my body.

But it kept nagging at me. Low left ovary? Four days later, while getting ready for a big client meeting, I decided to call my RE's office to find out what

Dr. Yarbrough might have been talking about—he should have all the info on this low left ovary. But why didn't anyone tell me about it? The question in my mind should have been, why are you obsessing about a low left ovary that probably doesn't work anyway when you should be pulling your act together for this big client meeting? But there I was, crazed, running around my home office, loading up my materials with one hand and dialing Dr. Cohen's office with the other. (It really had to have been divine intervention.)

His nurse, Lana, came on the phone.

"I need whatever reports you might have on me and my low left ovary," I said. "I haven't had a period in forty days, and I need to figure out what is going on."

"Did you take a pregnancy test?" asked Lana.

"No." Silly Lana! Why would I do that? My last pregnancy was a miracle, remember?

"If I were you, I'd take a pregnancy test. And I'll have Dr. Cohen call you back."

To appease Lana, and because I happened to have one in the cupboard, I took a pregnancy test. After peeing on it and tossing it in the sink, I hopped into the shower. When I got out, I got dressed for my meeting, then remembered the test.

I picked it up and glanced at it. Two pink lines. Two pink lines?! Freaked out, I called Lana back. Much calmer than me, Lana instructed me to contact my OB/GYN.

After hearing my tale, Dr. Yarbrough's nurse told me to come in. Right now.

"I can't, I said, I have a meeting," I said.

"Come after the meeting," she said.

"It's across town. It will be after five when I am done."

"Come after the meeting," she said. "We will wait for you."

I got there at 5:45, waving a pregnancy test stick in a baggie.

"I'm pregnant. What is this all about?" I said, rolling up my sleeve to give blood for a pregnancy test.

"How did we miss this last week?" said Dr. Yarbrough, as the nurse drew out blood.

"Why would we have looked for this last week?" I said. "I'm infertile. Remember?"

My blood test came back positive, as did the next, and the next, and the next—HCG low at first (ninety-eight), but doubling every forty-eight hours. I think I must have been like only a few days pregnant, when I first tested. Maybe I had ovulated late, after my appointment with Dr. Yarbrough? All I know is we discovered this pregnancy early enough that progesterone pills, and suppositories, and HCG shots could help support it until the placenta kicked in.

By the way, I never did find out about this low left ovary. Who cares about it now? But what if I hadn't cared about it then? If I hadn't called Dr. Cohen's office in a huff and spoken with Lana? Would I have lost Graham, too? I don't know.

What I do know is if Graham had been born a girl, his name would have been Lana.

Ten Reasons the First Twelve Weeks are Critical

1. This is the time when, should your doctor advise, you need to support this pregnancy with any drugs, such as progesterone, baby aspirin, or HCG shots.
2. Just because you're pregnant doesn't mean you will stay that way. This is the period in which most miscarriages occur.
3. If you have suffered infertility and are pregnant, you are a high-risk pregnancy—we don't care what your doctor says.
4. If you are over thirty-seven and pregnant, you are a high-risk pregnancy, too. Again, we don't care what your doctor says about this.
5. You may not be aware that you are pregnant.
6. Critical development takes place in the fetus during this period.
7. You need to avoid those with communicable diseases such as fifth disease, the flu, or rubella (if you weren't vaccinated), which can harm a growing fetus.
8. This is the time to avoid hazards, such as changing kitty litter or eating raw beef that can cause problems or birth defects to an unborn child.
9. This is the time to stop smoking, quit drinking, and cut the caffeine.
10. You're finally pregnant, for God's sake.

You Think You're Pregnant

Congratulations! This is the moment you've been waiting for—definitely an "I don't believe it's finally happening!" moment. Because of everything infertile people go through, discovering or simply thinking you might be pregnant causes very mixed emotions. "Normal" couples get all excited and immediately start decorating a nursery. Those of us who have been battered a bit in the baby-making process need to take a slower course of action. Should you get excited, or proceed cautiously? Are you really pregnant, or is this a false positive? Hopes up, or hopes down? Is it really okay to get excited, knowing the flames of fantasy could be doused any minute by a miscarriage? Decisions, decisions.

However, even if you just sorta-kinda-think you might be pregnant, here are a few quick things to consider on your way to the drugstore to buy a pregnancy test (if you don't keep a stock of them in your bathroom cabinet just in case). We call these the I-think-I-may-be-pregnant dos and don'ts.

Do cut back (or stop) caffeine consumption.

Do stop drinking alcohol and diet soda.

Do stop smoking.

Don't change the kitty litter.

Don't eat raw beef and some soft cheeses.

Do stay away from sushi (the hardest for Maureen; no problem for Julie).

Do avoid chemicals and any pesticides.

Don't exercise too much (walking is okay).

Don't take any drugs (even prescription) until you get them okayed by your doc.

Do run and get a pregnancy test.

Do call your doctor. Right now.

How Do I Know I'm Pregnant?

Pregnancy announces itself the same way for every woman whether you get knocked up the old-fashioned way or via high-tech intervention—you miss your period. Or, if you are irregular, you think to yourself, "Boy-oh-boy, this sure seems like a really long time between periods, I better get a pregnancy test."

In addition to missing your period, you may (or may not) also feel some of the following symptoms:

Sensitive breasts	Mood swings
Backache	Exhausted
Nausea	Frequent urination
Spotting instead of a period	Light headedness
Heartburn/indigestion	Constipation
Areolas start to change (get darker, larger, and/or rounder)	

A missed period, coupled with a few of the above symptoms, might be enough to send most women off to buy a pregnancy test. They might be excited. They might be upset (if they weren't planning a pregnancy or if it's not their spouse's baby!). But, because you have battled infertility, you will probably feel a little afraid/excited/confused/concerned about this whole simple process. The angst of simply driving to the drugstore to buy the stupid test was enough to put us over the edge each time. Were we wasting money on this test again? Or are we really pregnant?

Neither of us wanted to deal with the overly friendly sales clerk who always wanted to chat us up while checking us out. "Are you pregnant?" "Your first?" "Ooohhh. Good luck to you!"

How do you share your feelings with some teenager who is just trying to make conversation—"I hope I'm pregnant." "I'm having some challenges getting pregnant, so who knows?" "Yep, good luck to me!"

The confusion and conundrum surrounding a simple pregnancy test seems unfair, doesn't it? After all you've been through, right? Well, hopefully it will make you feel a little better to know all of us felt the same way. Those who haven't faced infertility cannot understand our hesitancy here, but we understand. Boy, do we ever. So go buy the test (or several to have on hand for future avoidance of the agonizing drive and overzealous clerk), then take it.

The Pregnancy Test

At-home pregnancy tests have revolutionized the whole "Am I pregnant or not?" concept. Our mothers had to wait until they were sure their period was late, then make an appointment to see a doctor and have a test, which back in the "good old days" probably had to be sent to the lab (down the hall or across town). Then you waited to find out if the proverbial rabbit died.

Today, home pregnancy tests can be done in the convenience of your own bathroom. You simply pee directly on the testing stick and wait for it to change color. If your urine contains HCG, human chorionic gonadotropin, it will react with the stick and form a colored line in a little window.

All pregnancy tests, whether done in the doctor's office or at home, detect the same thing—the amount of HCG. Once the fertilized egg implants in the wall of the uterus, the placental tissue produces the HCG, which shows up in the blood and urine of pregnant women. A sensitive blood or urine test can detect HCG as soon as eight or nine days after you ovulate. When you are pregnant, the concentration of HCG roughly doubles at least every two days for the first sixty-five days or so. Then it starts to decline.

Why Double Test?

While these home urine tests are pretty accurate, if you don't perform the test just right, you might get an incorrect reading. If you perform the test too early, you might get a false negative. And if they slip out of your fingers and into the toilet while you are peeing on them, forget it. They're ruined.

A false positive test—also known as a chemical pregnancy—is why some women end up at the doctor's office a few days or weeks after doing a home pregnancy test to find out their blood test is negative. That is such a bummer. But home pregnancy tests let you test as soon as you think you might be pregnant, and you actually might have been pregnant when you're first tested. It was just not a pregnancy that was going to last. Who knows why it didn't take—chromosome issues, implantation issues, uterine lining issues, or many other things. Getting pregnant, not having it catch, and losing it around the time of your normal period happens more than we realize. This is the biggest problem with home pregnancy tests, they can get your hopes up when in fact, you really aren't pregnant (or won't stay that way).

This is why doctors do a blood test even when you come in waving a positive pregnancy test. Doctors have to make sure. Blood tests make sure. These doctor-administered blood tests measure the amount of HCG in your body, too, but these tests can detect even very small amounts of HCG in your blood.

Our friend Pam got sucker punched with one those false-positives. Pam, a thirty-eight-year-old schoolteacher who had been suffering from secondary infertility, was seeing an RE and taking fertility drugs. Each month, however, she was so anxious to find out if this was going to be the month that she would test herself early (like the day her period was supposed to start—sometimes even sooner). Once she tested positive only to test negative a few days later at the doctor's office. A day or two following that doctor's visit, her period started. Was she pregnant? Yes, for a few days. But if home pregnancy tests didn't exist, she would never have known. It would have just a been a late period, and she wouldn't have gotten herself so excited only to end up being so upset. Pam did go on to have a healthy baby boy the following year—after she gave up testing herself early every month.

Wow. Now you may be saying to yourself, "Okay, maybe we shouldn't test ourselves early. We'll just wait a few more days and then test." Well, in many cases, you would probably be right. Pam would have saved herself some heartache—and a whole bunch of money on pregnancy tests—if she had waited. But listen to our pal Janet's story.

After trying to conceive for several months with no success, Janet started do a pregnancy test early every month—the twenty-ninth day of her regular thirty-two-day cycle—as opposed to a few days after her period was due.

Here's why: Janet is a veterinarian and understands the medical aspects of biology pretty darn well. She studied her attempts to get pregnant as if she were trying to diagnose one of her own furry, four-legged patients.

After trying to get pregnant for six months with unprotected sex, Janet noticed one month that she didn't feel quite right, kinda different: breasts a little tender and she was a little tired. Her period was due in about three days, so it could be just that . . . premenstrual. But it didn't feel premenstrual. An at-home pregnancy test came up negative. But that didn't satisfy Janet. She then called her doctor and went in for a pregnancy blood test—a test that's much more sensitive to HCG in the body than the home urine test. At first, her doctor balked. He had never tested someone on the twenty-ninth day of a thirty-two-day cycle. But she persisted, and he finally caved. The blood test came back positive. She was pregnant. But three days later, her period began. She wasn't pregnant. Was it a false positive? Turns out it wasn't, because for the next nine months, Janet went in to her doctor's office for a pregnancy blood test at day twenty-nine. For seven months of those nine months, Janet tested positive for pregnancy, only to have her period start sometime the following week.

To her doctor's credit, he referred her to a fertility specialist after just a few months of these false starts. The RE ran a battery of tests, put her on progesterone, monitored her closely, and continued doing the pregnancy blood test every month on day twenty-nine.

Janet eventually became pregnant and was able to support the pregnancy with drugs until her daughter, Ann, was born. Both her OB/GYN and her RE told Janet that had she not noticed something odd about her body (feeling pregnant at day twenty-nine) and insisted on the pregnancy blood test to measure her HCG levels so early in her cycle, they probably would not have caught her fertility issues as soon as they did.

JULIE

The frustrating part about infertility is that there is no one set course that works for every single woman. For most women, I would suggest waiting until your period was several days late to take a pregnancy test. Or double test—early and later—at home before you see your doctor.

Unless you are like me.

I am convinced that I have to catch a pregnancy ASAP if that baby is going to survive. This is based on my own study of my five pregnancies. The ones that have resulted in the two live births were the ones I caught when my HCG was barely in double digits. I was barely pregnant at those moments. I took the test because of a fluke (Graham) or because I was clued in to the fact that I needed to bust my butt to keep my pregnancy viable and sensed I might be pregnant (Amanda). Both times, I was so early that I was able to coddle those pregnancies. I started supporting them immediately with a regimen my doctors designed that worked for me—progesterone suppositories and pills, HCG shots, rest, and baby aspirin. Those pregnancies, caught in their infancy and supported quickly, were the ones that developed into the son and daughter I tuck in at night today. The others, discovered only about two weeks later in their development, never made it.

If I were trying to get pregnant today, I would have a few pregnancy tests in the closet, and I would test as soon as I thought I might possibly be pregnant. I have learned a valuable lesson about me and my body. I have also come a heck of a long way since that pregnancy with Graham!

"I would have gone on for easily a year just thinking my periods were a little late or changing," says Janet. "I was not producing enough HCG to show up on a home pregnancy test, and I was losing those pregnancies very quickly. Really, I could have gone on forever thinking I wasn't conceiving when my problem was actually sustaining the pregnancy."

Ironically, Janet went on to have a second daughter, Jenna, fifteen months later with no problem—in fact, she was thirty days pregnant before she even figured it out. "I was still nursing Ann, so I didn't even think I was ovulating," Janet says laughing. "After all we went through, we never thought I would have such an easy time with a pregnancy as I did with Jenna."

Once again, there is no normal out there for the infertile—not even a "normal" way to do these pregnancy tests! We hate to constantly repeat ourselves, but you have just got to learn to sense changes in your body. Be your own best barometer. If you think you might be pregnant, test yourself. Consider double testing if the results don't seem right. Follow up a positive home pregnancy test (or two) with an immediate visit to the doctor's office to make sure, and support a pregnancy sooner rather than later.

When You First See the Doctor

Once you establish that you are pregnant, be sure you start this journey on the right foot. Not to be a buzz-kill, but the first three months of pregnancy can be tricky—even if you are a "normal" couple who hasn't had any fertility problems. Things can happen. Pregnancies can end. There are ways you can better your chances of supporting your pregnancy to term—and the most important of these is having great communication with your doctor from day one.

Find a competent OB/GYN who has experience with older, higher-risk patients. If you have been seeing an RE, you will probably be referred to one as a matter of course. But the RE may just tell you to go to an OB/GYN, and you might just go back to the guy you've been going to for years and that doctor may just treat you like a normal pregnancy. And you are not a normal pregnancy.

MAUREEN

When I got pregnant with Ava, the first three months were hell. I never thought it would last. I'd been through too many first trimesters that ended in miscarriage. I thought for sure this would end up the same way. With each day that passed I wasn't relieved, I became more concerned that the miscarriage would just happen later in the pregnancy.

Although I was monitored by my reproductive endocrinologist very carefully, I just expected he would look up from a sonogram and tell me the heartbeat had stopped. At twelve weeks, I expected to feel a bit more relieved, but I didn't. I felt worse. Entering into the second trimester made me just think of all the other things that could go wrong due to my age. I was with my RE until I was fifteen weeks along, then I was turned over to a high-risk OB/GYN. That was a hard transition because I had clung to my RE, who monitored me in the first trimester like a hawk.

For the first few weeks, my progesterone was tested every other day, then I had sonograms at least once a week. I was scared to leave that comfort zone, but I had no choice; those were the rules. I moved on to my new doctor—a high-risk specialist who looked like Antonio Banderas. He gave me all the attention I needed, but my heart was in my throat until Ava was in my arms.

Listen, you may feel fine, but if you are older or if you have been going through infertility to get where you are today, you are not a normal pregnancy. You should consider yourself higher risk. You cannot just pop some prenatal vitamins and wait until the end of the first trimester to see a doctor for the first time—like some twenty-two-year-old fertile filly. Your pregnancy might progress in a totally normal, risk-free fashion, but it is our bold suggestion that you consider yourself high-risk and fight to be treated that way.

We may get some flack for this, but we don't care what anyone says. We've both been there, and the following is why we want to label you high-risk:

- If you've had even one miscarriage and they didn't determine why, consider yourself higher risk.
- If you are over thirty-six or thirty-seven and pregnant for the first time, you are a maternal patient with an advanced age. Consider yourself high risk.
- If you suffered unexplained infertility and miraculously get pregnant, you should start off considered high risk.
- If you suffered infertility and had to get pregnant with help, surely we don't have to tell you how precious that cargo is you are carrying. You've probably got the battle scars to prove it without our say-so.
- No matter how great you look, you're at higher risk than that newly pregnant twentysomething chick flipping through *Vanity Fair* next to you in the doctor's office. Act like it. Demand to be treated like it.

Most importantly, reason to consider yourself high-risk and demand the attention from your doctor that this may be your only shot at having a baby. You are pregnant. Right now. Take advantage of this golden opportunity. Act like it may be your only chance. It just may be.

Ten Questions to Ask Your Doctor on Your First "I'm Pregnant!" Visit

1. What signs of possible problems should I be aware of or looking for?
2. What's normal in the way of cramping or even spotting?
3. How can I reach you if I need you—or do I talk with a particular nurse?
4. I've battled infertility—can I get a sonogram at six to eight weeks to observe the uterine lining for my own well-being?
5. How do you check to see if I might have a clotting problem, or should I just start taking a daily baby aspirin as a precaution?

6. How often do I get to see you? Not your nurse—you.

7. How do you normally deal with patients my age?

8. Are there any tests we can do to help prevent miscarriage?

9. What are your delivery procedures?

10. What are your feelings about C-sections, and how often do you perform them?

It's okay to ask your doctor questions. In fact, it's expected, or it should be. You are your own best patient advocate. You are riding around this planet in your body—and now you have a passenger. You have to stick up not just for yourself, but now for your unborn baby. It's your obligation to be as informed as you possibly can to protect this pregnancy and nurture it through nine months. Learn from us and our mistakes.

It really frustrates us when our pals don't take our advice. Not taking our advice doesn't mean anything will go wrong with their pregnancy, but it does mean we have to take extra time out of the day to worry for them—since they don't seem to be doing it for themselves. Here's an example—and yes, we've changed her name to protect our friendship, but she'll recognize herself. Julie's pal Sadie began trying to conceive when she was thirty-nine years old. Even though she has been privy to every fertility fiasco we've jointly been through, she never thought any of it would happen to her. So much so, she doesn't even try to stack the odds in her favor. She makes us nuts.

After going off the Pill and trying to conceive for three months, Sadie got pregnant. She put off going to the doctor for almost ten days until Julie finally convinced her that she needed to confirm the pregnancy (not just tell all her friends, and at thirty-nine, she was considered high risk simply because of her age (her doctor confirmed this).

At her first visit, the OB/GYN drew blood to run a pregnancy test. This was on a Thursday morning. On Friday afternoon, when Sadie hadn't heard back from the doctor, Julie forced her to call to find out the results. The nurse told her she'd have to wait until the following week to get the results. This was no problem for Sadie, but it was a huge flag for us. We worried all weekend. Sadie, on the hand, played tennis with her husband and had a celebratory brunch. Finally, on Monday afternoon, her doctor's office called to tell her that, yes, it looked like she was indeed pregnant, but her progesterone levels were very low—very, very low. So low, her doctor recommended some progesterone suppositories, which Sadie didn't bother to pick up that evening as we begged her to. It was more convenient

JULIE

I keep notes on everything. So it stands to reason I would have in-depth journals on all my pregnancies, recording everything from date and time of an office visit to my blood pressure, weight gain, and baby's size.

I flipped through them while writing this chapter to see how I spent the first three months. In the first twenty-three days after I found out I was pregnant with Graham, I was in my OB/GYN's office eight times, gave blood four times for HCG and progesterone tests, got one shot of HCG, and had three sonograms to check the activity of the ovaries, the uterine lining, and the fetus' development. I then went in every two weeks after that for a sonogram, blood pressure, and weight check. At thirteen and a half weeks, I was moved to the "normal" room (the room with no sonogram). There we heard the fetal heartbeat, but no pictures. It was the first time I had made it to the "normal pregnancy" room. I continued to go see Dr. Yarbrough every two weeks until my amnio at sixteen and a half weeks. Following the amnio, which came back normal, I was bumped to once-a-month doctor visits for the second trimester. At the end of my first trimester, I had seen Dr. Yarbrough fourteen times, and Dr. Jiminez, the amnio specialist, once. Fifteen doctor visits. At the end of my sixth month, I started going every two weeks again, a sonogram at each visit to check the baby and my placenta for possible clots. At thirty-four weeks, I began going to Dr. Yarbrough's every week until Graham was born in week forty.

My pregnancy log for Amanda is about the same for the first trimester, except I got bumped to the "normal" room sooner because hers was my more problem-free pregnancy. And she made her debut three weeks early, cutting off those last few doctor visits. I was a high-risk patient because of my age and my fertility issues. This is how my doctors treat high-risk patients. I wouldn't want it any other way. Would you?

for her to pick them up the following morning on her way to work—even though we urged her to go now. The doctor had also advised Sadie come back into her office in two weeks to have her progesterone tested again and have a sonogram to see what was going on. We suggested she go in sooner. She ignored us. Her doctor, Sadie admonished, was "a really cool woman," and we were being "too intense." Julie was "ruining" this whole experience for her.

We could see her point. But having been there ourselves, we just felt that as a midlife mother-to-possibly-be and a good friend, Sadie should be more aggressive and fight for this pregnancy. We felt her doctor was not being aggressive either, considering Sadie's advanced maternal age. Sadie felt she needed a change of scenery and chose to go to Chicago for a week-long vacation with her husband instead. She was not consistent with her progesterone while in Chicago, forgetting it twice (how do you forget a big suppository?).

You can probably guess how this ended. Sadie came back from Chicago all happy and bubbly, only to go to her doctor's appointment for her progesterone test and sonogram the following week to discover the developing fetus had died. All the progesterone she was taking had prevented her from miscarrying when it happened. She had a D&C the next day; her bubble burst.

Sadie is back to square one, trying to conceive. She lost more than that baby by not taking charge of her fertility; she lost precious time. It hurts us when our friends don't do everything possible to prevent a train wreck.

Wait Three Months to Go "I'm Having a Baby!" Nuts

Having done both the telling everyone "Guess what, we're pregnant!" too-early-scene and the wait-until-we're-really-sure gig, we would advise taking it a little slow here. Julie thinks you should confide in a few close family and friends,

MAUREEN

There's a saying, "You don't know what you've got until it's gone." What I have learned from working with Julie is, "You don't really know what you don't have until you see what you *should* have." Julie has had unbelievable medical care from her doctors. When we share our medical care stories, ultimately my experiences with doctors (with exception of my New York RE and OB/GYN) have been below par.

Here's how it went in California, when I was with a top OB/GYN and trying to figure out why I couldn't seem to keep a pregnancy from miscarrying: Phone calls not returned, questions not answered, being rushed in an appointment because she had to get to another patient, being forgotten, being overlooked, not being heard, being discounted . . . and the list goes on. It is a direct result of all of these things that I believe ultimately led to my losing my babies. Sadly, I thought this was how all offices and doctors worked, until Julie told me differently.

Now I realized that being rushed and discounted by my doctors is not acceptable. I shouldn't have been treated as a "normal" pregnancy as a woman of advanced maternal age with multiple miscarriages under my belt. I should have been treated as if I were high-risk. My care was nothing compared to Julie's.

I spent nine years loyal to my hotshot OB/GYN in California, and she forgot about me. I paid a high price for that.

while Maureen is more inclined to tell no one. Twenty percent of pregnancies end in miscarriage, and most miscarriages happen in the first three months.

When you have been fighting infertility and you get pregnant, you have to think about these things because shit happens. More so, it seems, than for those normal chicks with those normal pregnancies. Hopefully it won't happen to you, but it might, and you should be prepared. You are pregnant with an infertility complex. Sometimes a pregnancy going south can be saved if signs are noticed soon enough and appropriate actions are taken. Those actions could be as simple as lying down or putting your feet up or more complex like taking some drugs to help support the effort or having a stitch to prevent your cervix from dilating too soon.

To keep you on your toes (because every pregnancy is precious), we've compiled a list of signs we experienced while pregnant that were red lights for us that something wasn't quite right. If you experience any of the following—or anything else that seems odd—call your doctor immediately. It's probably nothing, but wouldn't you rather be safe than sorry?

1. Spotting.
2. Loss of any liquid—either clear or bloody—through the vagina.
3. Cramping, no matter how slight.
4. No nausea, no fatigue, no tenderness or swelling of breasts.

Now, to be fair, there are perfectly normal pregnancies where the woman has no nausea or fatigue. Sometimes, slight cramping can simply signal normal uterine stretching. Julie had little breast tenderness with any of her pregnancies. Maureen's breasts, however, are perfect barometers for her. With the pregnancies that "took," her boobs hurt, but prior to her miscarriages, they felt fine. Since she had been pregnant once before, she knew something was wrong.

Why chance it, we say. It is important to know your body and be aware of the intricacies of your system. Don't worry about being a pain in the neck to your doctor. It's not as if you aren't paying for that office visit.

MAUREEN

I got pregnant the second time on June 10. I know because I had unprotected goodbye sex with my husband the night before leaving for New York for the summer with my six-year-old son. Will, who couldn't take two and a half months off from work, was staying in California.

When June 29 came and went (the day my period was due), I ignored it, never considering I could be pregnant. By July 10, I was ten days late and took a pregnancy test. It was positive. I was stunned. I decided not to tell anyone. Instead, I'd wait until I got back to California at the end of August and surprise my husband with the news. Then I'd tell everyone. I called my OB/GYN in California, who told me I didn't need to see them until I was twelve weeks along, which would coincide with my return home. The perfect plan! I calculated the due date to be my mother's birthday. Everyone would be so surprised.

When I returned to California, I tucked the pregnancy test into an envelope with a baby book and handed it to my husband during a romantic dinner. He was delighted. My doctor couldn't see me until the first week of September. No big deal. Once I told Will, I felt free to tell the world—and I did. I didn't really feel pregnant, but just assumed this was an easy pregnancy.

I do remember buttoning my jacket the day of my appointment. It was loose, which seemed odd because I knew I should have been expanding. My breasts weren't tender, either, and I wasn't fatigued. But it never occurred to me that anything could go wrong. I remember driving across the Golden Gate Bridge that day; the sun was sparkling on the water—A perfect day.

At my appointment, I was astonished to find there was no heartbeat. Boom. Just like that, my pregnancy ended. I remember the drive back home across the Golden Gate Bridge. Everything was dark and dead.

In hindsight, I should have been more on top of it. I should have gone directly to a doctor in New York. I shouldn't have just trusted what my doctor's office said and assumed everything was fine.

Don't ever assume . . . ever. It's better to be safe than sorry. Go to your doctor. Tell someone. Even if it spoils your perfect plan. I had a perfect plan. You know what? I stopped making perfect plans in my life after that . . . permanently. That perfect plan, filled with assumption and trust, cost me my baby.

JULIE

I got pregnant the third time at age forty, when our son was barely one year old.

This third pregnancy was fraught with problems from the beginning. I bled and lost small amounts of fluid sporadically almost from day one. But I went in weekly for sonograms and in each sonogram, the baby seemed to be growing. I didn't pay attention to particulars on fluid, or uterine shape, or lining. I asked how it looked. If they said fine, it worked for me.

When we got to week nine, I let out a breath—I was past the time of my first miscarriage. I got more excited each week that passed, even though I was still leaking a little fluid. My doctor directed me to rest, and I tried to as much as you can while tussling with a toddler. I was giddy when I got past the magic twelve-week period. . . . if I can make it past this, I'm sure I won't miscarry. I was beginning to show, and my clothes were getting tight.

We scheduled an amnio for the end of the sixteenth week. The day before the amnio, my husband went to Mumsies, a posh maternity boutique in Dallas, and surprised me with a slew of beautiful new clothes. I remember what I wore to the amnio—maternity jeans and a white knit maternity top. But that office visit went badly. The sonogram showcased things I hadn't paid attention to before—less than half the amount of amniotic fluid necessary surrounding the baby, a misshapen placenta folding over onto itself. The doctor told us our healthy baby wouldn't survive his unhealthy environment.

But wait, I wanted to say, I am past the three-month mark. I am safe. Surely you are wrong. But I just put my new jeans and white top back on and left. I had seen the pictures, too.

The next day I called Mumsies, the store Robert had been to. I told them I needed to return the clothes that I hadn't worn. The salesgirl told me they didn't take returns on maternity clothes. All sales final.

"I lost my baby yesterday," I whispered. "I don't need them anymore, and I didn't wear them. Please take them back. I can't look at them."

Silence. "Let me talk to the manager," she said.

God bless those women. They took back all the clothes—all of them except the jeans and white top. I still have those jeans. The top I wore to shreds practically all through my fourth pregnancy with Amanda Grace. I had no choice, really. I refused to buy any new clothes until I was really sure she was coming.

Wow! I'm Still Pregnant

There will come a point where your doctor will tell you to relax and enjoy your pregnancy. It might be at three months. It might be at six months or somewhere in between. When you know the pregnancy is "sticking," it's time to celebrate your success! Go out and buy all those "I'm Pregnant!" books. Put your feet up. Read them! Take care of yourself. Register for baby shower gifts. Buy some maternity clothes just because you can. Get ready to enjoy pregnancy after infertility.

CHAPTER 21

PREGNANCY After INFERTILITY

Julie

Infertility patients don't get to have a simple, joyful pregnancy. There is an element of worry, fear, and dread that hangs over each trimester like a baggy maternity top. You think every tiny pain signals a miscarriage. You scrutinize every sonogram for something wrong with your uterus, the placenta, or, heaven forbid, your baby.

When I became pregnant with Graham in January 1998 (after being told I would never conceive, then suffering a miscarriage), we held our breath for nine months, too scared to enjoy the new life growing within me. I even waddled into labor and delivery worried—and not just about how I was going to get eight pounds of baby out of my body and into the waiting bassinet. When you have worked so hard to get to a place most women arrive at without much trouble, you can't be smug about any part of it.

From the moment I first held my tiny son against my chest, I have never forgotten that I am one of the lucky ones.

Maureen

When I got pregnant with my daughter at forty-one, I played all these mind games on myself, just trying to keep on an even keel. I told people on a need-to-know basis. Just enough people needed to know, so I could talk with them if I needed to, but not so many that I would go nuts.

My husband, however, immediately went places I didn't want to go—choosing names, talking about future Christmases, and acting like this whole thing was really going to happen. I was hesitant, but he wanted me to be excited. I just wanted to be sure I was really going to have that baby. It really seemed unreal to me. Even after I saw the sonograms, I still felt it wasn't real.

I consider myself to be a fairly normal person with a normal temperament. I can't imagine being a really neurotic woman and surviving those nine months. That would be rough.

Ten Things That Make Your Pregnancy Different from "Normal" Pregnancies

1. When you suffer infertility and get pregnant, you need to consider yourself high-risk.
2. You now realize that normal is a miracle.
3. Once you have suffered infertility, you lose the innocence of pregnancy.
4. You have busted your butt to get pregnant, and you appreciate it more.
5. You will worry for nine months.
6. You will not mind nausea, varicose veins, hemorrhoids, or any other "downside" of pregnancy.
7. You will not complain about being pregnant—at all.
8. You wonder why OB/GYNs don't have in-house counselors for formerly infertile pregnant women to help handle the emotional havoc.
9. You suddenly realize you know way too much about reproduction to survive the next nine months.
10. You will hold back on designing a nursery or buying maternity clothes until the last possible minute just in case.

There is no way to fully describe pregnancy after infertility to anyone who has had a simple (normal?) nine months. It is exhilarating highs (Wow! We did it!) balanced by breath-stealing, fearful lows (no way is this going to make it!).

All babies are miraculous, but infertility babies are true miracles.

The Infertility Complex

Once you get pregnant, you'll forget you were ever infertile. Ha.

If only this were true. Pregnancy after infertility is fraught with worry about the baby's health, your health, and if all the drugs you took trying to conceive

JULIE

After I became pregnant with my son, none of the "I'm Pregnant!" books addressed the fears I had now as a pregnant woman with an infertile past.

For the first three months, I was certain I would lose my baby. I took hormones to support my pregnancy and baby aspirin to prevent clotting, and I visited the doctor every other week for a sonogram to check the baby's progress. Every pain, every muscle spasm found my fingers dialing the doctor's office. Fortunately, Dr. Y. and his staff specialized in cases like mine, so the phone calls never seemed to bother them. At least, they never let on.

When I finally moved into the "normal" category with only monthly doctor visits, I panicked. How would I survive a month without the internal peek at my evolving son the sonogram provided? And by the time I settled into the rhythm, I was back to doctor-ordered weekly office visits to make sure my placenta wasn't breaking down or clotting up.

My husband actually feels sorry for those people who have normal pregnancies. "How do they know what's going on if they don't get to check in on their kid every other week?" he wonders. My husband can't understand how couples with normal pregnancies stand the suspense of not having all these glorious sonograms. I agree. If we are going to go to all the trouble and expense of infertility treatments, I wanted to be able to check in with my unborn babe regularly—clock progress, count fingers and toes, make sure all the organs are working properly. I just wanted to make sure the baby was still there.

This is called having an infertility complex.

will come back to haunt you in some way. Unlike normal pregnant women, you will never forget your infertility. Being pregnant will not be as easy as you would think. You will not mellow out like your coworker who got pregnant by "a lucky mistake!"

We have yet to speak to one infertile woman who, when she finally became pregnant, kicked back and relaxed her guard, not for a moment. We didn't. Not even when our doctor assured each of us we had moved on to the "normal" pregnancy category. Sorry. No such thing for those of us who had to work so hard to do what comes naturally to most people. We focused on the negative possibilities much more. So will you. Welcome to a "normal" pregnancy for formerly infertile women.

Am I Okay?

The sooner you realize and accept that it is normal to worry about *everything* in your pregnancy, the better you will feel.

You will worry at the start of the race, when you move from infertile to fertile, from reproductive endocrinologist to obstetrician. This is scary. We were both frightened by the whole idea of leaving our infertility team and stepping into our OB's office. You will be, too. You will miss your RE and the nurses that have really become your "family" during past treatment. But you will come to love being an OB patient.

To ease the transition, have your RE contact your OB to prep him for your case. Make sure you discuss your high-risk nature with your OB on your very first visit. Demand the attention you need—increased office visits, sonograms, and so on—to ease your anxiety. Continue to take charge of your health throughout this process as well. You're now taking charge for at least two—or more if you are pregnant with multiples.

Even if you are with the greatest OB in the world, you will still drive yourself crazy because you know too much. You will know what it took to get pregnant with this baby. You will know everything that can go wrong. You will obsess over every little thing. Listen, it is better to have all this knowledge than not. On the bright side, you will know the warning signs of possible disaster and be better prepared to stave it off than your uninformed sisters. You will be the one who knows to ask about taking a baby aspirin or progesterone. You will be the one who knows the importance of sitting down and putting your feet up, and you will be the one who actually does it. You will not diet, exercise, smoke, or touch alcohol during your pregnancy. You will be the model patient. You will work this pregnancy as hard as you worked to get pregnant. You may lose the fun and innocence of pregnancy, but that's minor compared to losing your baby.

Is the Baby Okay?

Oh yes, the baby, or as we call it—the Baby.

Now that you realize you will spend the next nine months worrying about your own health and well being, let's turn our attention to the Baby growing in your belly. It's time to start freaking out about his or her health.

Is the Baby okay?

This is a constant question and a constant fear: One you will ask at every appointment. We promise. Again, this is perfectly normal to any infertile-and-

JULIE

Six months after my second-trimester miscarriage, I was (remarkably) pregnant again. Graham was two and more active than ever, but I forced myself to take it very, very easy. I cut back on my assignments, put my feet up as much as possible, delegated responsibility, and prayed to God to let me keep this one.

Again with the progesterone and the hormone shots for the first trimester, and again with the multiple sonograms every week. Everything was looking normal. Everything was looking fine. Everyone was happy—but me. In the back of my mind, I wondered and I worried for nine straight months. Would we make it?

Three weeks before my due date, my water broke. Eight hours later, in the darkness of night, I delivered Amanda Grace. We made it!

The best bet to surviving this new insanity? Listen to your body. You know what it's telling you better than anyone else does. If your body says rest, then lay down and rest. Don't convince yourself (or let others convince you) that you have to first work, weed the garden, clean the house, or anything else. If you're worried, call you doctor—even on a Sunday. Do not hesitate to get things checked out. It's not only okay, but crucial, to feel as if you can ask questions. You need to be informed, proactive, and responsible in your care.

We follow the philosophy of "better to be safe than sorry." Everyone will have an opinion about you and your body. Tell them to keep it to themselves. They are not you, and they are not feeling what you are feeling. If something is alarming to you, act on it and don't feel like you are crazy. There have been too many times when we haven't played it safe, and for that we are eternally sorry. It was a matter of life and death. Don't worry that others may think you're being paranoid or overly anxious by asking questions and raising concerns. Their opinions of you are less important than the life of your baby.

now-pregnant woman. Your friends, however, who had "normal" pregnancies will think you are nuts. They will admonish you to quit worrying. Screw them. They haven't been here before—carrying precious cargo that cost you more pain, suffering, money, and time than they can even imagine—if they are honest with you.

Betsy, the forty-two-year-old paralegal in Boston friend whom we wrote about earlier, got pregnant again at age forty after two miscarriages due to a clotting factor. She worried about miscarriage her entire pregnancy

"I was never able to totally relax," she says. "I spotted for the entire first tri-mester, starting when I was in Greece, with no Western medicine for hundreds of miles. I was a neurotic nut for the entire nine months. It didn't help that a friend lost a baby at thirty-eight weeks (don't ask), and I lived in fear of some-thing similar happening. I was so crazy that for the last two months, I went for weekly fetal monitoring, partly at the suggestion of the hematologist, who was pretty cautious—and partly because I was driving my husband crazy with my concerns."

Betsy is a totally normal pregnant-after-infertility woman.

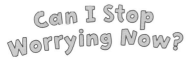

Can I Stop Worrying Now?

So when does the worry go away? When does being a high-risk pregnancy become an everyday mundane thing? It doesn't.

You finally breathe again the minute your baby is out of your uterus and in your arms. The moment you know your baby is healthy and safe is the moment you will finally exhale. It's the moment you will realize you were holding your breath for nine months.

MAUREEN

Here's one that doesn't happen often—one of those surprise things.

Two weeks before I was scheduled for a C-section with Ava, I got a major elec-trical shock. I was thrown across the street when I was closing my metal car door with quarters in my hand as my feet were touching old trolley tracks. It had been a damp day, and an electrical current from work being done up the road came shoot-ing down those tracks in the second that I was closing my car door—Bad timing.

I was stunned, shocked, and driven immediately to the hospital, where they hooked me up to monitors to check my heart and the baby's heart. After surviving the angst of possibly losing this baby for thirty-eight weeks, I couldn't believe this was happening to me now.

Luckily, only my heartbeat was a little erratic and my arm a bit numb. Apparently electricity doesn't travel well through amniotic fluid, and my daughter was all right. On July 1, 2003, Ava was born. She was perfectly beautiful, though her hair tends to stick up a bit . . . static electricity?

JULIE

One of the best things about being a high-risk pregnancy is all the pictures. I had so many sonograms taken weekly, then bimonthly, that my son's baby album actually starts at five and a half weeks after conception. My mother even framed the sonogram shots I sent her, updating every few weeks with the new ones.

These in-utero peeks were my opportunity to be in baby bliss. I got to know my baby in a safe environment—safe because I was with my husband and my fabulous OB, whom I trusted, and right across the block from the top hospital in Dallas should anything happen right then.

The doctor used the sonograms to check the baby's progress—the placental lining, the growth of the baby, whether or not there are any clots forming. I used the sonograms to check out my child—make sure he was still there, alive, well, and that the cord was nowhere near his neck. I did the same thing when I was pregnant with Amanda.

After all the sonograms, I began to recognize habits and sense personalities. Graham would hide his face beneath his forearms in an in-womb version of peek-a-boo. For a year after he was born, my son would snuggle into this same arm-over-the-face position for sleeping. And his feet! They rotated as if he was running in place! After watching him on the sonogram, Dr. Jiminez, who did my amnio, told me to wear my running shoes to the delivery room because it looked like Graham was probably going to hit the ground running. He was right. Graham is action personified—crawling, walking, and running long before the books said he should.

My daughter, however, was so calm in every sonogram—legs crossed oh-so-ladylike, it was hard for us to tell if she was a girl or boy until we had our amnio; hands tucked behind her head; thumb stuck inside her rosebud mouth. After she was born, Amanda remained the same—self-contained, peaceful, and relaxed. She didn't bother walking until she was almost eighteen months old; she was happy to hang out on a blanket, suck her thumb, and watch her brother bounce off the walls.

Ten Fears Pregnant Women with Infertility Complexes Have

1. Fear of losing your baby.
2. Fear of becoming attached to your unborn baby because you are afraid of fear #1.
3. Fear of telling people you are pregnant in case fear #1 comes true.
4. Fear of hearing the worst news possible at each doctor's appointment.

5. Fear the baby will be stillborn.

6. Fear that all your stress about possible harm to the baby is harming the baby.

7. Fear that every time you go to the toilet, you will find blood in your panties.

8. Fear that each pain in your abdominal area is disaster waiting to happen.

9. Fear that everyone else who knows you thinks you're crazy. (Who cares what they think?)

10. Fear that you will not be able to stand the pressure of the next nine months. (You will.)

Surprise!

We don't shy away from the nitty gritty, so here's some news. Sometimes even when you get what you want, there are legitimate concerns. Particularly if you are an older, higher-risk mom-to-be who underwent fertility treatments to get to the maternity ward.

MAUREEN

I was nervous when I went for my amniocentesis at eighteen weeks. When they stuck the needle into my uterus, I watched on the screen as the baby flinched, my uterus contracted, and the needle bent (not supposed to happen!). The doctor was sweating but handled it well. I focused on my baby moving around on the big screen above while he gently maneuvered the needle out of me. Luckily they were able to get just enough fluid for the test.

At that point I had seen my baby so many times in sonograms, I felt as if I knew her. I prayed hard for the two weeks I had to wait to get the results. In that time I worried I would miscarry because of the amnio. I worried about the test results. I worried that my baby had Down syndrome. I worried about congenital defects. I worried about losing this baby later in my pregnancy. I didn't know what we would do if the news was bad. Will and I had never really had that conversation. Bad move! My mind raced, and I suffered in silence.

The phone call finally came, and the news was super . . . no problems. The nurse wanted to know if we wanted to know the sex. Yes, I exclaimed. A girl. She congratulated me and hung up. I was overjoyed and relieved for about one day. Then the fear crept in again. I was watched closely for the rest of the pregnancy. Sonogram, sonogram, sonogram, but I never really felt relief.

For example, if you are pregnant with multiples, particularly fertility-induced, you may end up on bed rest. Actress Julia Roberts spent her last trimester pregnant with twins on bed rest in the hospital and ended up delivering a month early. So did our not-as-famous friend Blair. The East Coast mother of IVF twins had contractions early in her second trimester for a few weeks before she realized what was happening.

"I felt something was not right, but at the same time, friends convinced me I was just skittish and that these were all normal experiences of pregnancy," she says. "They were so wrong. I was hospitalized at twenty weeks with nonstop contractions, put on a terbutaline pump, which kept the contractions at bay at about every six minutes for the next two and a half months. The first month was spent dealing with the potential imminent loss of both babies. The last month was really a matter of pain management. I could get out of bed to go to the bathroom and have a shower every two to three days; otherwise, I needed to lie down in bed, which I did."

So how did Blair survive her two-month hospital ordeal? Thanks to her girlfriends. Blair's pals came to visit often. The obvious care of friends and family and their ability to distract and entertain was invaluable.

"We set up poker night once a week and movie night once a week," she says. "I also hand-pieced my first quilt while on bed rest—I found it a very meditative and creative activity that really got me through some rough hours. Another 'bed rest buddy' from the twins club in my area called me once a week with encouragement, support, and her own war stories. She had been through a similar, perhaps even worse, pregnancy resulting in two healthy kids. She gave me great comfort. The hundreds of people praying for me, thinking about me, sending supportive e-mails, cards, and gifts was truly mind-boggling and made me feel that a larger community of people were joined together in this situation. It gave me great strength."

When you are stuck in bed rest, particularly hospital bed rest, you must realize that you have no control over anything except your mental and emotional states. This is how you will survive—by doing everything in your power to be in the best place mentally that you can be.

"I spoke weekly with a skilled, professional therapist who really helped me deal with a horrible crisis," says Blair. "I also spoke with someone who specialized in meditation and visualization, and she gave me some invaluable tools to deal with the two and a half months of nonstop contractions I was experiencing. I really feel these two people were as responsible for the successful birth of my children as my doctor was.

Normal Really Is a Miracle

Now that you're pregnant and know how much darn work it is to get that bun in the oven, you understand that normal really is a miracle. We should appreciate it more.

Because we know so much(!), we get offended when we see "normal" pregnant women doing all the stuff they are not supposed to do. For example, it makes us livid to see pregnant women do the following:

- Smoking or sucking in second-hand smoke;
- Exercising too much;
- Drinking alcohol;
- Eating crap;
- Not eating so they can stay skinny (this really irks us);
- Complaining about being pregnant (really, really irks us);
- Continuing to be stressed and overworking themselves; and
- Not appreciating the miracle of their pregnancy and not doing everything possible to protect that precious new life growing within them.

We bet you, too, will become a militant mommy-to-be, though you may not stop people on the street and lecture them like we do (bad habit). Welcome to our club. We had a friend who smoked a pack a day during her pregnancy. Maureen actually hounded her to the point of losing the friendship in the hope that she would quit. She didn't quit and had a baby girl born full term, just shy of six pounds. To us, that is an underweight baby, regardless of what the doctors say. To make matters worse in our eyes, she quit nursing after two weeks because it was "just too much work." Sigh. Our friend is still smoking. Her daughter is now three years old and suffers from a very weak immune system. She has been hospitalized twice already—once for pneumonia and once for a stomach virus she couldn't fight. She is constantly sick. This is not a scientific conclusion, but we sure believe smoking and pregnancy don't mix. Ditto second-hand smoke sucked up by a toddler.

Because of our respective businesses, we know of a few celebrity moms we won't name who also smoked during their pregnancies. Their babies weighed in at six or fewer pounds as well. Shame on all these women.

We heard a great story from Julie's current OB/GYN. He told us that years ago he was sitting in the audience when a famous Dallas doctor who lectured and counseled other docs in the Southwest made this analogy:

> If a farmer has a prize heifer and that cow gets pregnant, you don't let that animal run in the pasture with the other cows. You treat that cow special. You put that cow up in the stall with good food, good straw. You make that cow rest. You take extra good care of that cow.

We are paraphrasing the above, but the message is crystal clear. Why should this be any different with women—particularly women who have had a hard time getting or sustaining a pregnancy? So, when you get pregnant, take it easy, rest, put your feet up. Even if you have the most normal of pregnancies, for God's sake, treat yourself as if you were high risk. You are carrying precious cargo.

Why should a prized heifer get better treatment than you give yourself?

Surviving the Suspense

So, knowing you will worry, knowing you will appreciate the nuances of pregnancy more, knowing that you may have to really . . . S . . . L . . . O . . . W . . . down or hit bed rest, how do you enjoying the longest nine months of your life? Sister, with gusto. You deserve to savor every bit of this victory.

Here are the signs of a coveted pregnancy for a pregnant woman who's been through the insanity of infertility.

- You are thrilled with every pound you gain.
- You don't mind throwing up.
- Stretch marks are great signs that the baby is growing inside of you.
- Your hair is turning gray because you can't dye it—and you don't care.
- When you are tired, you actually go lie down.
- Varicose veins? Who cares?
- Your feet swell, and you just buy bigger shoes with a smile.
- Every moment that you feel that baby moving and growing, you are grateful.

What else? Take charge of your pregnancy. Tell your friends and family how you need them to support you during this pregnancy. Communicate your fears and hopes and ask them to respect your feelings. Put off shopping for baby items until the third trimester, if it makes you feel more comfortable.

Cut back on the stress in your life. Don't take on every assignment at the office during the next nine months. Don't volunteer for any civic duty, either. Put your own needs—and those of your unborn child—first.

Cherish the time you have remaining as a twosome with your spouse. Go on that vacation you couldn't take during infertility treatments. Have sex because you want to, it won't hurt the baby! Accept that your pregnancy is real and relish the experience. You deserve it!

In less than a year, you will be parents. We bet you will never take your child for granted. You will rarely, if ever, complain about a 2:00 A.M. feeding. You will enjoy the heck out of your baby and marvel constantly that you really created this precious, perfect human being. You will understand totally that it is a privilege to parent a child. Congratulations! You did it!

MAUREEN

When I was ten days away from my due date, I had a dream that I was giving birth to my daughter in the claw-foot tub we have in our bathroom. The umbilical cord was attached, but she was suffocating and turning blue. I knew I had to cut it, but I couldn't because I was in the tub. I began to bite the cord when I was awakened from this dream quite startled. The next day I was scheduled for a sonogram. After the sono, the doctor told us that my amniotic fluid was low and that it would probably be best if we took the baby sooner than later. We were heading into a holiday weekend, which made me nervous. When I asked the doctor the repercussions of low amniotic fluid, he replied, "compression of the umbilical cord and potential suffocation of the baby."

I was stunned and told him about my dream. He told me we could deliver that day, or we could wait two days later and measure the fluid again. Without really thinking, Will and I decided on waiting. I didn't even have a bag packed.

Driving home, though, that decision didn't feel right. My stomach turned. Halfway home, I turned the car around and drove back to his office. My intuition was screaming. When I returned, my doctor said "I knew you would be back." He called the hospital and scheduled my C-section, and Ava was born two hours later.

My doctor believed in a woman's intuition, and so do I.

The Next Step

Oh, by the way, here are a few tips on giving Junior a sibling. If you want more than one baby—and don't feel greedy if you say "yes"—remember that you are the most fertile in the year following the birth of your child. If you are a midlife mom, if you have had fertility issues, if you think you may want another baby, try to get pregnant in that twelve-month window of opportunity. Just bypass the birth control in any form and have sex as soon as your episiotomy or C-section scar is healed. We've heard those surgeries can take anywhere from two to six months to get better. Okay, we're just kidding; they heal up sooner, but we'll tell you right now, you are not going to want to have sex immediately after the birth of your first child. You will be adjusting to being a family of three (or more, if you have multiples). If you are nursing, you will not want your husband playing with the food supply. But eventually, you will want to have sex again, and if you want to try for more kids, make it protection-free.

And yes, we understand that two kids born close in age may seem overwhelming. If you get pregnant when kid #1 is one year old, it is conceivable you may have two in diapers at the same time. But look on the bright side—you'll have two precious angels in diapers in your house. Wow. How fun!

CHAPTER 22
INFERTILITY
After
PREGNANCY

Maureen

When we lived in San Francisco, having one child wasn't such an issue—it was the norm. When we moved to Long Island, however, I was suddenly meeting women with three, four, even five children. I was stunned.

Quinn's new teachers often commented on his only child status, on how mature and adult-like he was. Everyone from gas station attendants and grocery clerks to new friends would ask if I was going to have another child. Little did they know, I was trying to no avail.

Although it was frustrating going through the treatments, I always wanted to make sure it wasn't taking away from my son. Quinn was actually a real salvation for me and a wonderful comfort when he didn't even know it. Coming home to a child when you are going through infertility really softens the blow of your failures.

Nine-year-old Quinn knew about all my miscarriages. One day, he told me, "Don't worry Mom, I'll give you lots of grandchildren."

Now that we have Ava, he has let go of the burden of providing a lot of grandchildren for us. He realizes what a big responsibility a child is and how much it changes your life. I think he will wait until he is really ready before he provides us with any grandkids!

Julie

I never expected to get pregnant again. Graham was my beautiful, sweet miracle baby, the one who wasn't supposed to happen, the one good egg. I was perfectly, resolutely happy to be a family of three—a family I never thought I'd get to be.

Because I have antiphospholipid antibodies, which increase the possibility of blood clots, I was discouraged from using the Pill. And because I had just come off a few good years of infertility, I never bothered using any other kind of birth control. When Graham was barely past his first birthday, I got pregnant (surprise!) again.

Suddenly, I wanted another baby—desperately, greedily, ecstatically. I finally admitted to myself, my husband, and anyone else who would listen that I wanted more children.

Before this unexpected pregnancy, I had never even allowed myself to think about it. "Don't be selfish; you have a son with ten fingers, ten toes," I would admonish myself. "Who are you to ask for anything more? Some women aren't this lucky. Be happy with what you have." And I was.

But when I took a pregnancy test while out of town for the first time since my son's birth, in Florida for a fortieth birthday trip, and it came back two stripes, I felt a joy I couldn't express. I was so happy I negated the bleeding that was occurring and chose to ignore the concern in Dr. Yarbrough's voice when I phoned him from 1,000 miles away to share the news.

"Bleeding? Get in here as soon as you get back," he said.

Isn't that nice he wants to see me so soon, I thought, forgetting that once high-risk, always high-risk. Once an infertility patient, always an infertility patient.

Ten Tips for Surviving Secondary Infertility

1. Don't feel guilty for wanting another child.
2. If you aren't starting from scratch, pull out your old notes on primary infertility.
3. The child or children you already have will be fine either way.
4. Realize every pregnancy is different to some degree.
5. In your darkest moments, you have a child to hug and kiss.
6. Do everything you can, but realize in the end, what will be will be.
7. Get out of bed every morning.

8. Be patient—it can be an equally complex treatment path the second time around.

9. Don't miss doing things with the child or children you have. It forces you out of yourself.

10. You did it before. You can do it again.

I can't be infertile. I've already got kids. Those with a baby already in the house should never be smug. Just ask us.

There are two types of infertility—primary and secondary. Primary infertility is defined as infertility affecting a couple with no children. Secondary infertility is not being able to conceive or carry a child, even though you already have children.

Oh, No. Not Again.

For some, secondary infertility falls into the "oh, no, not again" category. For others who have had normal pregnancies, secondary infertility is a horrible surprise. But guess what? If having a baby cured this medical condition, there would be no secondary infertility. For some of us, infertility is the gift that keeps on giving. Julie had both primary and secondary infertility. Maureen had secondary infertility. We've seen it all here, too.

Because those suffering secondary infertility already have a child, they are often racked with guilt for being so selfish as to want another. If God had already given us such an amazing child, should we really ask for more? We have found those who suffer from secondary infertility tend to do it very quietly because they understand what a gift they already have. They don't need others reminding them of that fact, either.

Kath and her husband started trying to conceive again when their daughter was six months old. Two and a half years later, Ashlyn is still an only child.

"People tell me to be thankful for what I've got, and I am," says Kath, a thirty-four-year-old, stay-at-home mom in Texas. "Ashlyn is my reason for being, but I know in my heart that my family is not yet complete."

Is that so wrong? Absolutely not. Our friend Caroline was thirty-eight with four children and the desire for a fifth (don't ask us why, but she had always dreamed of five small fry running around her Denver homestead) when secondary infertility hit. Imagine the looks she got sitting in the waiting room of the reproductive endocrinologist or talking to women who were aching for their first when they found out she had four at home already.

"We finally got pregnant with our son just before I turned forty," says Caroline. "People couldn't understand it. A lot of my friends kept telling me to let it go, be happy with the kids we had. We were happy, but it really is none of their business. All they did was make me question myself and feel guilty. Now that Finn is here, my heart and my house is completely full. I'm glad we listened only to ourselves on this one."

Suffering from secondary infertility is tricky. Everyone has their thoughts and opinions about what you are doing. Some, like Maureen's friends, may think you are crazy for wanting another child. Others, like Julie's family, may worry that another pregnancy will be too hard on your high-risk body.

There may be very little sympathy for the struggle to have a second. Most people just think because you have one, you shouldn't feel so bad. The support system you had for your first pregnancy may have disappeared—or at least, shrunk some. The truth is, you will probably wish everyone keep their opinions to themselves. We can promise you will get sick of hearing again and again "Well, at least you have one."

Whether you suffered infertility the first time or sailed through an easy conception, secondary infertility is a shocker for women already raising kids.

JULIE

I hated secondary infertility more than primary infertility. Not just the unfairness of it all, that's a given. But once we realized we could get pregnant again—even though I miscarried—the doctors wanted to run tests to find out the "why" of it all. I didn't want to go through all that testing again. I already knew too much.

The "why" was that my body was not perfect. We had established that, so it felt redundant to have to get the blood work done again. I didn't like having to juggle Graham's schedule with doctor visits. Infertility was more disruptive, if that's even possible, the second time around. I worried about my toddler getting into my syringes or meds.

Eventually, we decided to opt out of any more fertility treatments, enjoy the boy we had, and take our chances if I got pregnant again, which I did eventually. Then, all the knowledge that made secondary infertility such a hateful experience actually helped me—and our baby girl—survive.

The Good News

The silver lining in secondary infertility's dark cloud is that you are not totally hopeless. You got pregnant once! You already proved you can carry a baby and deliver that little bugger. In a way, you're kind of ahead of the game.

If you suffered primary infertility, you will have to go through all the fertility tests again to figure out what's happening this time. Silver lining? You already know the right doctors, and the rigmarole of the testing won't be a surprise.

If secondary infertility is your first trip to the bar, you will need to start at square one, finding a good doctor and getting tested. Be sure to ask if the doctor has experience with secondary infertility. There's a difference. Some doctors really specialize in women who have never, ever been pregnant before. You want a clinic that understands where you are coming from and will help you achieve your goal.

Oh, Yeah, the Kids . . .

Whether secondary infertility is your first experience or a repeat performance, you do have a built in scheduling conflict those with primary infertility don't—your kidlet(s). The balancing act for you will be trying to do everything—doctor visits, shots, med pick-up, sex—while toting along a tot.

Some clinics don't allow patients to bring their kids, which we understand and support. Even if they did, would you really want Junior along for the ride? It's harder to coordinate all the doctor appointments with preschool, carpool, and diaper duty. This is why some people experiencing secondary infertility explore less aggressive treatment methods the second time around.

A little planning, however, makes anything possible. You will need to line up a good sitter or enlist family members to help you juggle your treatment timetable with your child's schedule. You will need to invest in a lock for your door, so your toddler or preschooler doesn't wander in while you are trying to sire their sibling. You will need to buy a spare car seat for your little one that fits in Grammy or Granddad's car to make transportation easier. You will also need to make time to enjoy the child you already have, to keep away the guilt of repeat procreation, and to soothe your soul on this journey.

Why Did This Happen?

It's so easy for couples experiencing secondary infertility to go through the whole questioning phase of infertility again. Could it be something I did?

Probably not. Go back and reread the first few chapters in this book to reaffirm that you are not being punished with secondary infertility.

Secondary infertility is just another one of those "life's unfair" situations. Sometimes you may find coincidences in your past that give you pause. Our friend, Molly, for example, is haunted by a stupid mistake she made in her midthirties.

Molly always wanted a baby, but decided she would wait until she found the right man. When she was thirty-six, he finally showed up. After dating for a year, they got engaged, and within three months, Molly was pregnant. While this should have been a joyous time for our friend, it wasn't. Molly, a native New Yorker with a large Irish Catholic family, couldn't decide if she wanted to keep this baby or not because she wasn't married yet. More important, however, she didn't want to look fat in her wedding dress!

We urged her not to terminate this pregnancy. We told her that she may never get pregnant again. We talked to her about her eggs, and her age, and everything, but she didn't listen. The thought of having a tummy while wearing her wedding dress outweighed having something she had always professed wanting—a child.

When she got to the very end of the legal time limit in which she could still abort the baby, Molly chose to do just that. Now, we want to state emphatically that we are both pro-choice. However, we think Molly's choice was selfish—plain selfish. Her husband-to-be was a wimp, in our opinion, for letting this occur. However, life went on, and Molly looked ravishing and skinny on her wedding day. After she was married for a few months, she announced she was ready for a baby. Sadly, her husband began suffering from unexplained impotence. This went on for over two years. They tried everything, and he just couldn't get an erection—even popping Viagra.

Molly panicked as she turned thirty-eight, then thirty-nine, stunned to be diagnosed with infertility. She neglected to tell her doctor she had had an abortion—she didn't want him to "think badly of her." She wondered to us if having the abortion had hurt her chances of conceiving. Was God getting back at her? We encouraged her to keep trying for the child she wanted.

Finally, using the best technology Manhattan had to offer, Molly got pregnant two months shy of her fortieth birthday. Now that their son is finally here, Molly's husband is ecstatic. His erection has returned! He is a fabulous father.

Molly, however, is not sure about motherhood. She confided in us that "she really doesn't like being a mother—it's too much work."

We guess some things never change—like being selfish.

We give you Molly's story to make two points: first, never take a pregnancy for granted, and second, be careful what you wish for.

If you are over thirty, engaged or seriously dating someone, want to have kids someday, and get pregnant, *have the baby*. Don't worry about how you look in your wedding dress. In fact, don't have a big wedding. Elope. Renew your vows on your anniversary—get a babysitter or bring the baby along, and wear the tightest, slimmest sheath you can find.

Just because you get pregnant once does not mean you can do it again. In fact, statistics show it may actually be tougher to get pregnant the second time around.

Being a mom is a lot of work. Unlike Molly, we just happen to think it is worth it.

Only Children

So infertility strikes again. Some couples quickly come to the conclusion that the one child they have is just fine. They worked hard to bring that baby home, and they want to savor every second of that child's life without the insanity of trying to create a sibling. You know what? That's just fine.

Only children are not an anomaly anymore, though they may seem strange because everywhere you look now, you see midlife moms fresh from the triumphs of IVF pushing double and triple strollers. But during the Depression era of 1920 to 1940, only-child families accounted for 30 percent of the American population. Then came the prolific Baby Boom era, and only-child families slipped to 15 percent of the population. According to the 2003 Current Population Survey, single-child families make up 20 percent of the population, while families with two children are only 18 percent of the population. Only-children families are actually predicted to continue growing as well. Families are getting smaller because people are waiting longer to have children. It's also expensive to raise a child to age eighteen. The U.S. Department of Agriculture pegs the national average cost at about $323,975, with almost $50,000 going for food!

There are other nonfinancial benefits to having a singleton. Your concentration is not split. You can focus on your child without distraction. It's also easier to go places with one child, and there is no energy wasted on trying to teach them to get along with a sibling. There have even been studies to show only children are not really as spoiled as everyone thinks they are. With just one child, when you are done with diapers, you are really done with diapers. Don't underestimate that!

And don't have a child just, so Junior will have "family" when Mom and Dad are long gone. There is no guarantee that siblings will be close. Sometimes they even end up hating each other because of childhood rivalries. Think about your own family tree. Only children never have to deal with that.

Both of us have siblings, so we decided to speak to someone who has seen both sides of the picture—Maureen's son Quinn, now twelve-years-old. He gave us the lowdown on being an only child, as well as how his world changed with the arrival of a sibling.

Quinn's Positives of Being an Only Child

You get more attention.

You get to hang out with your parents and bond more.

Your parents work you hard to succeed.

Your parents have more energy.

When you are sharing with your parents, you always get more.

You have your own space.

Quinn's Negatives of Being an Only Child

You don't always have someone to play with.

Your parents are always watching you.

You can't moan and groan about your parents to someone else who gets it.

The house is quiet.

It can be very boring.

You have to ask your parents to play with you a lot, and they are tired sometimes.

Quinn's Positives on Having a Sibling

They are so cute, especially when they are sleeping.

Their laughter is contagious.

The way they learn to talk and walk is adorable.

They look up to you.

You can play with them and tease them.

They are good to blame things on.

They love you, and you love them.

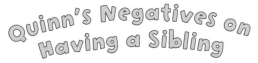

Quinn's Negatives on Having a Sibling

Your parents' attention is not always on you.

Your sibling is much more needy.

Sometimes you can get frustrated with your sibling.

Having a sibling requires patience.

You always have to share with your sibling, and they always get more.

They whine a lot.

MAUREEN

My kids will spend significant time as "only children." Quinn was ten when Ava was born. He will leave for college when Ava starts first grade. She'll then get eleven years as an only child at home.

That Quinn was an only child for so long really shows in his personality. He is more mature, intelligent (we were able to spend lots of time stimulating his mind), able to conduct himself well with adults, and well mannered (we had time to push the manners). Having had an only child for ten years was a delight. I was the baby of five, so it's hard for me to imagine life as an only child. I was always borrowing my sisters' things, and there was always lots of action in the house. I don't function well in peace and quiet. Only children do, and that follows them into adulthood. Quinn has now taken to closing his bedroom door to get away from the commotion of his baby sister. All of those years of peace and quiet have been disrupted.

We were well out of diapers when I got pregnant with Ava. Starting over has its benefits . . . and its downsides. The good parts? I am savoring my daughter because I can and because I am not chasing after a younger Quinn. The bad parts? I am totally exhausted with a baby and a pre-teen, and that affects everyone in my house. But no one ever said it would be easy. At least I know from having had one child that "this too shall pass"—and, unfortunately, just how quickly it does.

Armed with this information and your own gut feeling on what constitutes family for you, you can feel fine about solving your secondary infertility by just saying no more. Make the decision, turn the infertility fund into the college fund, then go guilt-free and take your kid to the park.

What Now?

Once you've determined that you are suffering from secondary infertility and determined you don't want your tyke to be an only child, follow the steps outlined in this book for those going through primary infertility. First and foremost, get a plan for how much you think you can endure financially, emotionally, and physically. This plan may be different because you do already have a child. You may not be willing to spend extravagantly on treatments because you are saving for college as well. You may not want to do all the shots and timetable sex because it interferes with your life now as a family. You may want to jump immediately to the big-gun treatments like IVF because you understand the importance of not wasting time unnecessarily.

You are in a different place from couples without any children. This demands a different plan.

It is still important to look for a program with the highest success rate—in live births, not just pregnancies, per treatment. But this time, ask for information on the clinic's success rates with people your age who experienced secondary infertility. It goes without saying the program should be accredited and meet the standards as defined by the American Society for Reproductive Medicine (ASRM).

Finally, you may decide you want more children, but no more pregnancies. In this case, you may consider adding to your family in another way, such as adoption. The rules of the game here don't change. Secondary infertility doesn't mean you can't increase your family size—it only means you may have to find another way to do it. Bottom line? If you want a bigger family, there is always a way to create it.

There may come a time when the cost—financially, physically, and/or emotionally—overrides baby lust. Are you a "bad" person if you give up trying to have a biological child? Absolutely not! Infertility is a game you can win only if you are willing to look at the next steps necessary to create the family you crave and/or the life you want.

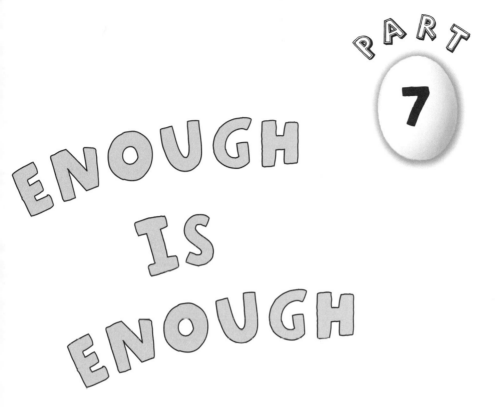

PART 7

ENOUGH IS ENOUGH

When you've done it all, heard it all, and are satisfied you've gotten an honest opinion on your fertility, you may decide it's time to move on to the next step—whether that may be adoption, surrogacy, or child-free living. And you know what? It's totally okay.

Julie

After a year of trying to conceive by committee, we left our fertility specialist. Not because there weren't other things we could try—there were. It's just that Robert and I had put on limit on the pain and suffering up front. We decided from the beginning, if we weren't pregnant after a year of trying everything we could in 365 days, we would move on. We knew our financial and emotional limit and strove to stay within it.

When Dr. Cohen told us that we had unexplained infertility—after a year of poking, prodding, pricking, and pumping me full of hormones—we decided that it was time to move on. No IUIs, IVFs, or AIs for us. Too much money for too little guarantee.

Instead, we began to explore our future, tentatively talking about life with and without children. I don't like the term "childless." Child-free is friendly and more factual. Child-free implies an option. Childless sounds negative and sad.

What we learned from a year of trying to overcome infertility was that we did want to be parents. The year had given us pause for thought. The end result—a child in our family—was more important to us than the process. Just because we couldn't conceive a child didn't mean we couldn't have a child. We began looking into adoption almost immediately.

Maureen

When we reached the end of our fertility journey, we made a decision that we would not adopt. This was personal to us; we felt that it wouldn't be the right thing for our family.

Suffering from secondary infertility is a tricky thing. Although you have one child, it doesn't make it any easier not to be able to have two, yet you feel guilty expressing that pain. You think people will view you as selfish. I suffered silently with this. I never let anyone know just how painful the experience was for me. I felt guilty that I was not able to provide a sibling for my son. I felt guilty that although we were lucky to just have him, I wasn't sure he was so lucky to have just us. Once we were gone, he would be alone, and the thought of that haunted me. I knew he would always have family around him, but not a sibling. I felt tremendous pain about that. My father, an only child, often told me how he always longed for a large family. This is why he wanted five of us.

So in deciding that enough was enough and calling it quits on our infertility journey, we knew that our decision would have lasting effects on our son. My son never longed for a sibling because he didn't know what he would be longing for. When I was pregnant with my daughter, he lay next to me one night and said "Well, Mom, we had a good ten-year run."

I told him a whole new chapter was about to begin in his life, and it has. My husband always wanted four children, and I failed him on that. I didn't want to fail my son in providing him with an experience and love that he would cherish always. Although my children are ten years apart, having the opportunity to watch that bond and love between them is incredible. If all goes well, they will always have each other. Ironically if we hadn't called it quits on our infertility, our daughter wouldn't be here today. I'm forever grateful that we "had enough" when we did.

CHAPTER 23
WHAT ARE My Options NOW?

Julie

There is something liberating about saying "screw you" to fertility treatments. For the first time in a long time, we felt in control of the process again. We were finally free of the infertility frenzy that had controlled our lives—and our wallets—for more than a year. That doesn't mean it was easy to return to normalcy. What is normal, anyway?

When we moved on to the next phase of family building, it was like starting over—again.

I had moved from being a freshman at Infertility College through a pretty intensive education. I felt like I could teach the class on what to expect from faulty fertility, but here I was again back at the beginning. I was a freshman again. Fortunately, there are plenty of adoptive parents ready to share their success stories and help you down that path.

We started with our rector, an adoptive father himself. I can still remember the dinner at a local Mexican restaurant where we shared a bowl of salsa and chips with him and his wife and listened enraptured to their tale of finding their family.

When I discussed the situation with God, I no longer asked him to fix my fertility. Instead, I begged him to lead me to my family. I believed our children were out there somewhere. I just had to find them.

Gathering more information and moving on sooner rather than later was my salvation.

Maureen

Here's how I'm told I can't have more kids—my doctor says he's "throwing in the towel." He's quitting on me! Well, I wonder if he understood how *that* made me feel. After I had given him eight months of my life, it was time for him to move on! Well, thank God he quit on me when he did. He really set me free in doing this and saved me from more useless spending and hardship.

So when do *you* quit? My friend Elena did fifteen IVFs. Fifteen! Her company paid for it, and she finally got twins. Fifteen IVFs was her magic number. Mine was six inseminations. It is different for every woman, but when the clock stops ticking you just know it.

Even though my doctor decided to throw in the towel, I always had the option of finding a new doctor, but somehow I knew he had done everything he could. It was no longer up to science. My infertility was out of my hands. Something much bigger than me was going to make this happen. It was up to God.

When all scientific efforts to get me pregnant failed, I mourned what was lost and began to accept what would be. It took about six months of feeling blue—not depressed, just blue. Then, one morning, I woke up to the feeling of a new beginning. I had finally let go of the past and accepted my future, which I guessed then would not include a second child. I was finally at peace.

Ten Signs It's Time to Stop the Madness

1. Your career is suffering, and that bothers you.
2. You have lost touch with *you* completely.
3. You have run out of money and exhausted all insurance and grants.
4. You want to divorce your husband and have begun taking action.
5. You're a physical wreck, and you're not sure how many more treatments you can stand.
6. You can't get out of bed in the morning, and depression consumes you.
7. You've reached your pre-appointed limit, and you are going to stay within it.
8. You realize you have spent more on trying to conceive than you did on your car, your house, or your college education.
9. You just want to be parents, and you don't care if you get pregnant to do it.
10. You want some control back in your lives.

The End of the Beginning

Just because you can't conceive on cue doesn't mean life is over. While you may have reached the end of the baby-making line, you are just beginning the rest of your life. The end of the beginning really is the beginning of the end. That's a good thing.

Once you are free of the fertility frenzy, you can start taking the baby steps back to a normal life. You can rediscover you. You can reclaim your sanity. You can start building your future—with or without children. It's your choice. The minute you quit fertility treatments, you can begin to look at alternative methods for bringing home baby. Quit this game, and you can still win. You can still create a family. You just have to move on to plan B.

Coming to Terms with Your Infertility

You will know when you have reached the end of the medical line. You will no longer want to fight the fight. One day, you will admit to yourself, maybe quietly at first, that this is it—that you may never get pregnant, ever. You will wonder if you can or want to spend any more of your money on what seems to be an impossible dream. You will want your old self back, even without children. You will be ready to look at the other options before you full in the face—and actually consider them.

It's a tough decision to start infertility treatment. It is even tougher to decide it's time to stop. You should be applauded for the strength you have shown, and the pain you have suffered.

Now it's time to take the next steps. This is the point where hope and dreams smash into the current reality you are living. Where the emotional (what do you mean I can't have a baby? I want a baby!) meets the rational (no matter what we try, I can't seem to have a baby.) for the first time on neutral ground. And they talk.

Hopefully, you and your partner have already discussed the big issues—pregnancy vs. parenting, how far you will go medically, what is your post-infertility plan, how you will achieve this. If not, it's time to address these issues. It's also time to tell all the people who know your conceptual conundrum that you are backing off. If you don't, you will continually hear questions and comments—some meant to be helpful. Once friends know you're on a new track, they might even be able to really help you.

Often, one partner reaches the conclusion that it's time to stop the madness before the other. It's normal, particularly if you didn't discuss it prior to getting involved in treatment. Usually, it's the guy who's ready to move on first. Women tend to tie up a lot of our identity as women in our reproductive capabilities. We are the ones who want to try "just one more time, I know it will work this time, pleeassse." Some of us don't feel like real women if we can't birth a baby. We have to get over that. You are a real woman whether you can procreate or not.

Sometimes, the woman has reached her limit before her partner has given up the dream of seeing his wife's belly bulge with his spawn. We have run across several couples where the woman was tired of being a hormone-injected pincushion and ready to try adoption, but her husband wanted a biological child so badly, he bypassed reason with emotion. He was the one urging one more treatment, when his wife was ready to move one.

In either case, it's time to communicate and come to some type of agreement—not just talk, so you can convince your partner that you're right. You need to discuss your feelings, look at the big picture from each other's viewpoints, understand and accept that you feel differently about this situation, and begin to move on. During your discussions, one of you may be more logical, the other operating on pure emotion. Do not negate your partner's feelings here. There is no right or wrong way to feel. You may not solve the differences in one discussion. You probably won't come to terms until you've had a few discussions. Get a couple of bottles of wine or pick up some good coffee, sit down, and get going.

The Mourning After

Before jumping into the next stage of your family planning, take some time to grieve your loss with your partner. You need the closure. You are grieving the loss of the biological child you may not have. You are grieving the loss of physically being pregnant. You are shaking off the emotional overload of what you have been through to achieve a goal you are now giving up in its present form. Admitting that you may never get pregnant is hard—at least it was for us. By our own inexact calculations, this process will take some time—we each grieved for several months before finally feeling like the old us again. It took our husbands a while, too.

While the pain of abandoning your dreams is pretty raw in the beginning, it fades with time. Really. When you move on to the next step—adoption or third-party reproduction or even child-free living—you will begin to live your life again. The future will look brighter. Almost every woman we spoke with talked about how intense infertility was—how it was all-consuming—until they moved on, either by achieving pregnancy, adopting, or deciding to live without kids. Most say now that they rarely think about it. Some have even repressed the whole infertility experience, much like a woman who has gone through labor and can't remember the pain at all.

Having said that, don't take too much time with your pity party if you are planning on building your family via adoption, surrogacy, donor eggs, or donor sperm. These all take time, so as soon as you feel ready to move on, start putting those wheels in motion.

Now What?

Sometimes, when you've been trying to conceive for a long time, moving on becomes even harder. In addition to wondering if you are quitting too soon, the urgency to conceive may be less than it was at first. Such was the situation with our friend Victoria, who at thirty-four-years-old, already has six years under her belt in the trying-to-conceive category.

"So much time has passed now that I have really lost that sense of urgency," says Victoria. "I have no one to compete with anymore—everyone I know has had their babies and are on numbers two and three, so I am out of the race, and it's kind of nice," says the Long Island shop owner. "There is always that twang of pain when someone else is pregnant, but it's nowhere near as painful as it used to be, and I feel positive that something good will eventually happen for us, whether we get pregnant or decide to adopt. We're not ready to give up yet, but I think we are getting closer to exploring other options."

The other options depend on your fertility issues, your passion for a child who is entirely biologically related to you, and how much money you can or are willing to spend. Adoption is one option. Using an egg donor, a sperm donor, or a surrogate are other options. Foster parenting or living child-free round out the buffet of family-building alternatives.

Adoption Option

Adoption is just that—an option. Whether you choose open, closed, domestic, or international adoption, there is a child waiting for you. While adoption can be more costly and time-consuming than you might have initially expected, it is usually less expensive than years of fertility treatments.

"We pissed away so much money on infertility, I could scream," says Margaret, who estimates her cost of treatment at $30,000. "Finally we adopted, not cheap either, but this has been the best thing. We went through a facilitator, and from beginning to end, we spent about $18,000. Now we have this beautiful baby and could not be any happier."

There are many great books and websites on adoption, as well as support groups and seminars nationwide. Ask your fertility doctor for some suggestions to get you started on your new quest. Ask friends and family members. Often, someone who knows someone just happens to know a young woman looking to place her child in a loving home. That's how our friend Kim found her son.

After years of infertility, a failed attempt with a surrogate, and a botched international adoption, Kim got a call from a friend. The woman worked with an attorney who knew of a nineteen-year-old college student in New Orleans who was pregnant by her boyfriend. The girl had been adopted herself, wasn't ready to be a mom, and wanted to give the baby to a loving home.

Kim and her husband, Ric, put a packet together about themselves, and the woman chose them out of eleven couples. They met the girl, and the three clicked. Three months later, their son was born in Louisiana and brought home to their San Francisco home.

"This child was meant to be my child," says Kim, echoing the sentiment we heard repeatedly from adoptive parents. "It would be hard to love him any more than I do."

Eggs for Sale

Maybe your husband's sperm is great and your uterus user-friendly, but your eggs are old and tired. Your doctor thinks you would have a better shot at IVF or another assisted reproductive technology if you were to use someone else's eggs.

Here are the positives as we see them: the baby would have a biological tie to your partner, and you would get to experience pregnancy and assist in the creation of a baby. How do you feel about that? If the answer is "I can do that!," it's time to buy some donated eggs and move on to the next step. If you can't stand the thought of carrying a child with half the genes of a stranger, you might want to pass on this idea.

So how do you find the perfect donor eggs for your family? The best place to start is with your RE. Some clinics recruit egg donors and handle all aspects of the egg donation process. In some instances, you may have to find your own egg donor with the assistance of an agency that specializes in recruiting donors and matching them to recipients and are responsible for tying up all the legal details. We've also seen ads in college magazines, as well as local newspapers, placed by couples or clinics in search of egg donors. By the way, friends or family members are generally not a good idea as egg donors, for many ethical and practical reasons. You don't really want to be that closely associated to your egg donor for the rest of your life—or have them feel as if they can "hold it over you" when they need a favor. Trust us, this can happen.

Neither of us used an egg donor, but we had lots of questions. Fortunately, we ran into an egg donor who was willing to chat. She's actually a friend of the family, but to protect her identity, we can't tell you which family. Here are some of the questions that piqued our curiosity. We'll call her Alice. When we spoke with her, she was twenty-four years old, a wonderful, witty, loving college student.

Q&A with an Egg Donor

Q: How did you find out about egg donation?

A: My mother told me about it. She saw an advertisement for Dr. X IVF and Egg Donation on the movie screen of our local theater while waiting for a movie to start.

Q: What made you decide to do it?

A: Knowing that I would be helping a couple have a baby. If I were ever in a position like that, I would want someone like me around who would be willing to help me.

Q: What did you have to do to get ready to donate?

A: I had to take a birth control pill every day for about three weeks and then hormone injections in my stomach for about ten days. During the entire process, I wasn't allowed to drink any alcohol.

Q: What did your parents say?

A: They were both 100 percent supportive. My dad was a little worried about the whole thing, but my mom told him all about it. My mom came to every appointment with me—at least the first time I did it.

Q: First time? How many times did you donate your eggs?

A: Three. And Mom was there for all three retrievals.

Q: How does a couple choose you?

A: I believe they tell the nurses at the office what they are looking for, and the nurses then give them a list of women who match the best to their description. I had to fill out a huge packet about myself, my family, and my extended family. The couple pretty much knows everything about me—age, height, eye, and hair color, where I go to school, what I want to do after school, information about everyone in my family, and so on. The only things they don't have are my name and a picture of what I actually look like. The couple isn't allowed to obtain that information.

Q: So what's the whole process? What's involved?

A: We got the information from the ad on the movie screen, then I called them, and they sent me a huge packet of information to fill out. I then had to send that back to them. If everything looks good on paper and I'm what they're looking for, then they call—which they did.

The next step is to set up an appointment to meet with one of the nurses there. The nurse goes over everything you filled out, from beginning to end. After all that, I had to make an appointment with their psychologist. She made me take a few psychological tests to make sure I could handle doing something like this. After you get approved by both the nurse and the psychologist, you then get to meet the doctor. And after all that, I had to wait for a couple choose me, which was extremely quick.

Once I was chosen, I went back to the office to learn how to do the hormone injections. My mother came with me because there was *no way* I was going to be injecting myself in my stomach. So, then I took the birth control pill for three weeks and, after that, waited for them to call to tell me to start my injections. Either a nurse or the doctor called me every day when I was doing the injections to let me know which hormones to mix with which. When doing the injections, I had to go to their office every other day for blood work and a sonogram. Then the last couple of days of the cycle, I started to go every day.

On the retrieval day, there was no eating or drinking anything past midnight. I was given anesthesia, so I was knocked out during the retrieval. It only takes about thirty minutes and then about thirty to forty-five minutes to recuperate. And then you can go home.

Q: How old were you each time?

A: I was twenty-two years old for the first two times I donated and twenty-three for the last one.

Q: How much time did it take?

A: About a month or five weeks each time.

Q: What surprised you about the whole process?

A: I knew everything about the process going into it. But the one thing that really surprised me was how much of a bitch I became when doing the hormone injections. I seriously didn't think I would become as bad as I did. It came to the point where my family members—Mom, Dad, and my two brothers—couldn't wait until it was all over. Little did they know, I was going to be doing it two more times! But they were very good about it.

Q: What would you advise/suggest to women thinking about doing this?

A: It's a wonderful feeling knowing that I was able to make someone's dream of having a baby come true. It makes me feel so great. However, you have to make sure you have the time and strength to do something like this because it does take a lot. You have to make sure you are strong enough to be okay with the fact that part of you is going to be out there somewhere in a person—because some people wouldn't be able to deal with that fact.

Q: Would you do it again? Why/why not?

A: Well, I can't do it again . . . at least not with the doctor I did it with. He only allows a donor to go through with the process three times, and I've done that.

But, if I were able to do it again, I really don't know if I would. And the only reason for that is because I had such a bad experience with the anesthesia the last time I did it. I got very sick, and I didn't like the feeling at all.

Q: How much were you paid?

A: $5,000 for each retrieval. And I didn't pay for the drugs or anything.

Q: Do you think about those eggs out there?

A: Not every day, but yeah, I definitely do from time to time. How can you not? My eggs are out there forming little babies. . . . Of course I'm going to think about that.

Q: Do you know if someone used your eggs and was successful?

A: Well, I know they used them. I actually think there were six couples that used them. The clinic I went to allows two couples to share the eggs they get from each retrieval, and this allows the couple to split the expenses. Therefore, it's not as expensive for them. I just don't know if it was successful. I'm not allowed to know that, which I don't 100 percent agree with because I would like to know if the couple was successful. We both had to go through enough to get to that point.

Donor Sperm

Sometimes your uterus and eggs are just fine, but your partner's sperm is less than desirable. Or he has a genetically transmittable disease. Or he has no sperm at all—despite having tried Epidydimal Sperm Aspiration or Testicular Sperm Aspiration, minimally invasive procedures which take sperm cells directly from the epididymis or testicle, respectively. Your doctor thinks you would have a better shot at artificial insemination or IVF if you were to use someone else's sperm. It's time to consider donated sperm.

This is the male version of the egg donation scenario. Here's how it works with your egg and donor sperm: you would get to be pregnant; the baby would have a biological tie to you; and you would get to have a baby. How do you both feel about that? If your husband says "I can do that!" it's time to buy some donated sperm and move on to the next step. If either of you can't stand the thought of carrying a child with half the genes of a stranger—or if your husband has even minor qualms about you "carrying another man's baby"—you might want to pass on this idea. The male ego is very fragile—particularly when the guy is the reason for the fertility crisis. Be aware of his feelings here and don't push him if he is not comfortable. Find another solution.

Once you decide donor sperm is the way to go, how do you find the perfect match for your family? You go to a sperm bank and make a withdrawal. Actually, you can simply ask your fertility doctor for a recommendation. They know where all the good sperm is anyway. Most sperm banks are associated with universities or medical schools. Any sperm bank you go to must follow safety standards. All sperm is rigorously screened. Donors should be tested two times for all infectious diseases that can be transmitted through semen—like AIDS, hepatitis, and the STDs. It is important to ask what the semen has been screened for as you do not want to acquire any diseases from it during your fertility treatment. Though it is very, very rare, we stumbled across some cases of women being infected with venereal diseases from using donor sperm. So just find a reputable sperm bank and ask a lot of questions.

All donors must have a normal semen analysis, no history of bad genetic diseases, and normal physical traits. Because there are so many donors, you can usually find someone who matches your criteria in hair and skin color, race, body type, and so on. Sperm banks should also provide you with a medical history for your donor and screen out anyone who uses illicit drugs. This industry is pretty tightly regulated, but do your own due diligence in checking out your donor bank's credentials.

MAUREEN

Many moons ago, one of my boyfriends was a medical student. One morning, there was a knock at his door. I crawled out of bed and answered it to find a young man who asked me if I "had the paper bag?"

Paper bag? What paper bag? With that, he appeared a bit uncomfortable. I ran back into the bedroom and woke up my boyfriend, telling him there was a man at the door asking for a paper bag. Frank (not his real name, of course) literally jumped out of bed, ran to the door, and told the guy he would be right back before dashing into the bathroom. Of course, I'm thinking Frank's a drug dealer.

Within five minutes, Frank emerges with the paper bag, hands it to the young man, and shuts the door. This is it, I'm thinking, I'm witnessing a drug deal. Frank never did drugs, but all the good dealers never do, right?

After several minutes of hemming and hawing, Frank finally coughed up the truth. It was a transaction all right, just not drugs. It was a sperm transaction. Frank was a sperm donor—not cocktail conversation in 1984, before the general public had ever heard of sperm donation. Donating a little liquid gold was a quick way for young med students to make a little cash. Frank picked up $50 a pop, and they would come pick it up at your front door to keep you anonymous. I don't know what the going rate is now, but I'm sure there is no home pick-up.

To be honest, as his girlfriend, I was hurt and really miffed by his decision to do this without consulting me. We had been together seven years, and I felt betrayed, as if he was selling the family jewels. It really tweaked me to think he may have had children out there. Eventually, this was one of the contributing factors in our breakup. To me, sharing a lover's sperm was like sharing a lover. I was a lot younger back then, but when I think about it now, I don't feel that differently. I hope those sperm donors out there let their girlfriends know what they are doing up front.

I wonder if he ever thinks about his possible children out there. I sure would.

Once you have the sperm, and depending on your other fertility issues, your doctor will recommend either artificial insemination (AI) or IVF. If you are doing artificial insemination, we suggest you have sex with your partner the day before and the day after the AI. Some doctors we spoke with believe the success rate is actually higher when physical sex is involved around the time of the procedure.

Womb for Rent

Sometimes your eggs are fine, and his sperm is spectacular. It's just your uterus that sucks. To have your own biological child, you will need to hire a surrogate—another woman to go through the pregnancy for you. Today, surrogacy is getting a lot of press, thanks to celebs like TV host Joan Lunden, soap star Deidre Hall, and model Cheryl Tiegs, who are all mothering babies carried for them by another woman. But surrogacy is not always as easy as the celebs make it seem . . . and not an option for everyone. We talked to our less-famous, but more honest, friends to get the real scoop on what's involved when you use a surrogate.

Our friend Megan's story starts with a second marriage. "I had a baby easily in my first marriage," says our Houston, Texas, friend. "When I began trying with my (new) husband several years later, my uterus would not hold the pregnancy. My goal, which I made clear in the beginning, was I would do whatever was necessary until I was forty, then we would put that issue to bed."

Her RE knew Megan's goal. After three IVFs, he said "No more" and put the couple in touch with someone who specializes in surrogates. Megan was thirty-nine at the time.

"I immediately got on the Internet and began researching surrogate agencies," she says.

As Megan discovered, there are actually two types of surrogates—traditional surrogates who contract to be impregnated (using their own eggs) by the infertile couple's sperm and gestational carriers who contract to carry a baby that is created by the infertile couple's egg and sperm or donor egg and husband's sperm. With surrogacy, the father's sperm is almost always used, so the resulting baby is related to at least one member of the couple. If the surrogate is also the biological mother, she signs a form following the baby's birth relinquishing her parental rights. Whether you choose a traditional surrogate or gestational carrier, there is plenty of much legal paperwork that must be completed, and some up front, before the impregnation occurs, while some follows the baby's birth.

Now the big question—why would a woman sign up for nine months of carrying someone else's child? Most surrogates/gestational carriers have their own children and truly want to help other women experience the joy they have found in their families. Others need the money. Still others do it for the white-hot attention they receive for nine months. Megan's gestational carrier, who was thirty-four when she contracted with the couple, had been adopted as a baby and felt this was a way to give back for the loving family she had.

"Having babies was easy for her, and she loved to help other people," says Megan.

No matter why she is doing it, make sure the answer the potential surrogate/gestational carrier gives resonates with you.

To find a surrogate or gestational carrier, you will need to do your homework. Talk to your fertility specialist. Go online. Research agencies. Check their restrictions for surrogates/gestational carriers, which should include age and marital status, as well as psychological testing for everyone involved. Some agencies offer "closed" surrogacies, where there is no contact between the surrogate and the contracting couple. Others are more open, allowing you to build a relationship with the woman carrying your child(ren). Find an agency that feels comfortable to you. Then find a surrogate/gestational carrier who meshes with your mindset

Ten Questions to Ask a Surrogate Agency

1. Where do you find prospective surrogates/gestational carriers?
2. How do you screen them?
3. Do you test them psychologically?
4. How is the surrogate/gestational carrier paid?
5. Does the surrogate/gestational carrier have health insurance?
6. How do you emotionally support your surrogates/gestational carriers?
7. How much contact can we have with our surrogates/gestational carriers?
8. Can we see our surrogate/gestational carrier's medical records?
9. What age range surrogates/gestational carriers do you have?
10. After we contract with the surrogate/gestational carrier, how involved is the agency?

Some couples find their surrogates/gestational carriers without an agency, when friends or family members sign up to take on the task. No matter where you find your surrogate/gestational carrier, you will need a legal contract between all concerned that details all rights and responsibilities. Opt for an attorney who has done surrogate work before.

Ten Questions to Ask a Prospective Surrogate/ Gestational Carrier (And include in your contracts.)

1. How many embryos are you willing to let us implant?
2. How do you feel about having an amnio?
3. How do you feel about selective reduction?
4. How do you feel about C-section? Planned C-section?
5. What are your expectations concerning communication with us during pregnancy?
6. What are you expectations concerning communication with us after the birth?
7. We want to attend the birth. Is that a problem for you?
8. We want to communicate directly with your doctor. Is that a problem for you?
9. What do you expect us to pay for?
10. If there are problems with the fetus, how do you feel about abortion?

If you are a control freak, you may want to be in contact with your surrogate/ gestational carrier more often than someone who isn't concerned over every minute detail. Some women become friends with their surrogates, including them in family gatherings after the baby or babies are born. Others prefer more of a working relationship.

"I didn't care to be close to my surrogate," says Megan. "I will always appreciate what she did for us, but I didn't want the extra burden of friendship. I e-mailed her daily through the process, and my husband called on the phone once a week to touch base."

Our friend Kim, who adopted a little boy from Louisiana, had a different surrogacy experience. Kim, a former Los Angeles wardrobe consultant married to a Silicon Valley honcho, tried for several years to get pregnant. At age thirty-seven, after three failed IVFs, she was diagnosed with a chronic bladder condition in which you have to pee all the time. Her doctor recommended that she not carry a baby and, instead, use a surrogate.

"I found our surrogate through our fertility clinic," says Kim. "They had a binder filled with surrogates with pictures and profiles of them. We chose a thirty-two-year-old married woman with two of her own children. She was an OB/GYN nurse, and we established a great relationship. When we didn't have success at an insemination, I wound up consoling her!" Unfortunately, the inseminations never worked in this instance, and Kim never got her child this way.

Your relationship with your surrogate/gestational carrier will dictate how much you are involved in prenatal care. Suffice it to say, it won't be as much control as you would with your own pregnancy.

"I wasn't as frantic as my husband, who's a doctor and who had never been through a pregnancy before," says Megan, whose daughter was seven during the process. "I relied on the fact that our surrogate had delivered before—both her own children and as a surrogate for another couple. But her diet was horrible. Michael was just appalled at all the hamburgers and french fries she consumed! But we had full access to her doctors. We could call and ask how she was doing. My feeling is, there are certain things you just have to say are out of your control. It was our eggs and our sperm—all our genetics. I figured it would all be okay . . . and it was."

Where your surrogate/gestational carrier delivers drives the whole legal process. Surrogacy is not recognized everywhere, and each state has its own set of rules. If she delivers in some states, the infertile couple has to adopt their child back after delivery—even if they used their own sperm and egg! In other states, the couple's name goes on the birth certificate, but the surrogate's name goes on the hospital records, which makes it tricky to remove the babies before the surrogate leaves the hospital. According to the latest data (which changes constantly), the best laws are in California, where the couple's names go on the birth certificate and things tend to flow smoothly.

Megan and her husband live in Texas. Their surrogate lived on the East Coast. They met with her only a few times during the whole process—once to interview her, one time for the sonogram, and the last time for the scheduled C-section delivery.

"We flew in for the big ultrasound that happens just prior to the amnio," Megan remembers. "It was kind of a tense moment. Our surrogate had agreed in the pre-done paperwork what she was willing to do on our behalf, including amnio. I had firm guidelines—if there were any problems on the ultrasound, we would do the amnio. When we got there, our surrogate was now nervous about amnio, my husband Michael didn't want to risk miscarriage with an amnio, and I was still adamant about doing one. Fortunately, everything looked great, and we didn't need to do it, but that was a stressor."

The couple and the surrogate had determined ahead of time that the babies would be delivered by scheduled C-section because of the distance between them and Michael's work. Megan had also delivered her daughter by C-section and felt it was a good choice.

"As time got closer for delivery, my surrogate's doctor started balking about doing the C-section," says Megan. "He didn't want to schedule it. Finally, we solved that. Another stressor.

"The night before the delivery, we took our surrogate and her husband out to dinner," she adds. "The next morning, we all went to the hospital and all scrubbed up for the delivery. Everyone was there—her husband, the doctor, the nurses, the high-risk specialists, us. Like fifteen people in the room! The hospital had done some surrogate deliveries before, so they were familiar with it all. The babies came out, and, after they had cleaned them off, they handed our daughters to me and Michael. We were also given arm bands that allowed us to go into the nursery because babies' hospital records were put in name of surrogate, even though we are on the birth certificate."

Megan and her husband spent the next few days hanging out with their surrogate and the babies. "When it was time for us to take them home, there was no hesitation on our surrogate's part," says our friend. "Throughout the whole thing, she always reiterated that these were our babies, and she just wanted to do what we wanted. She was just great. When it was time for us to leave with the babies, our surrogate had to ride out the door in the wheelchair carrying our babies and hand them off to us at the curb. Hospital policy."

Megan continued to e-mail her surrogate every few days after she arrived back in Texas with her babies. "Gradually, I began to stretch the e-mails out to every week, our phone conversations to monthly. We had agreed in advance to exchange Christmas cards and, now, three years later, that's where we are at. We are totally open about using a surrogate and plan to tell the girls how they came into the world when they are older. We're fine if they want to meet the surrogate someday."

Surrogacy is not cheap. All told, Megan estimates that she and Michael spent more than $100,000 on the whole process. "I think our surrogate netted about $60,000, including clothes," says Megan. "She did childcare in her home, and when she got pregnant with our twins, she couldn't do that, so we paid her lost income as well. Look, my advice is that you have to have your bankroll determined ahead of time and don't let the nickel and diming that happens get to you. Just write the check and get over it."

Costs are based on what's involved. Megan brought home twins conceived with the first insemination. Kim and her surrogate did a total of five inseminations, and the surrogate only got pregnant once, losing it very early within the first four weeks. Each time, Kim produced eighteen to twenty eggs. Multiple eggs were used each time, with no luck.

"We never tried another surrogate because the doctor told us it was our embryos and not the surrogate's fault they weren't taking," says Kim, whose insurance paid 50 percent of her IVFs, but none of the surrogate expenses which totaled about $15,000 with no pregnancy. "You know, I never got down about that because we had agreed before hand if the surrogate situation didn't work out, we would adopt. That knowledge really helped me. . . . I always felt as if I would have a child someday, so losing along the way wasn't as difficult. Painful, yes, but survivable.

"I'm not the type of woman who had that great attachment to being pregnant and giving birth," she adds. "I just wanted to mother a baby, so using the surrogate never bothered me. I did draw the line at an egg donor, however. For me, that would have been like having a baby that was half my husband's and none of me."

When the last procedure failed, Kim was depressed for a week, then picked herself up and began adoption proceedings. "You know, in hindsight, I think I waited too long to try to have children," she says now. "I was waiting for everything to be perfect before trying. That was stupid."

Ten Tips to Successfully Survive Surrogacy

1. Find a surrogate/gestational carrier who has done it once before. Then you can be assured that she understands what she is getting into.
2. Research, research, research. Control the setting, the doctors, and what is going on with the process as much as you can.
3. Be prepared to be flexible. Things don't always go as planned, and you have to be able to adjust.

4. Hire a lawyer in the surrogate/gestational carrier's state as well as yours and make sure the paperwork is done properly.

5. Choose someone who is married.

6. Choose someone who has her own children.

7. Choose someone who is not doing it just for the money.

8. Outline all expectations upfront and in writing.

9. Communicate your wants, needs, and desires clearly—and in writing.

10. Make sure everyone is clear upfront whose babies these are.

Selfish Surrogacy/Use of Gestational Carriers

Surrogacy in its forms provides an important service to infertile couples. But there's always someone who abuses the system and screws it up for those playing by the rules. Believe it or not, gestational carriers are now being hired by fertile women as well. Not a lot, but enough to make our skin crawl.

We know of another woman, not a friend, but an acquaintance in Los Angeles, who is using a gestational carrier to avoid the pitfalls of pregnancy. We'll call her Perfect Paula. Paula had a problem-free conception and unfortunately spent the last two months on bed rest, but ultimately delivered a beautiful baby girl three years ago. Now that her daughter is older, Paula has decided to hire a gestational carrier to have another baby for her. Her reasons have nothing to do with infertility or carrying the baby. Her doctor has given her a clean bill of health. She's only thirty-one years old. She had a relatively easy pregnancy—except for the bed rest at the end. So what gives?

Paula has a very wealthy husband. She is using a gestational carrier because Paula doesn't feel like "getting fat and ruining her body" again. She doesn't want "the whole mess of being pregnant." Their gestational carrier is currently carrying twins. Once these babies arrive, we are sure Paula will hire a baby nurse to take care of them all night because she needs her beauty bed-rest.

Such selfishness disgusts us and upsets our friends who truly depended on a surrogate or gestational carrier to help build their family. The concept of rich couples hiring surrogates to birth their babies while they party or work through the nine months is frightening, but it is happening. If it continues, we think it will end up tainting the whole system.

But all of us have met those women who want to "have it all" as effortlessly as possible. "After watching us, my sister and her friend brought up the idea of using surrogates to carry babies for them, even though neither of them or their husbands have any fertility issues," says Megan. "We had a shit fit over that—women using a surrogate just because they don't want to get fat or take the time to be pregnant. It's so wrong on so many levels. It's very self-serving, very spoiled brat."

At this point, Megan's husband chimed in. "I have a problem with women who can have their own baby using a gestational carrier," says Michael. "That will drive up the price of surrogacy and make it unaffordable for everyone. There are a limited number of women out there who want to be a surrogate. If our gestational carrier had been busy carrying a baby for some celeb, who just doesn't want to be bothered, she wouldn't have been available for us. That is just wrong."

Just another point to ponder in the insane world of infertility.

Living Child-free

For some couples, not being able to have a biological child puts the kibbosh on having any children. Don't feel sorry for these people. They don't want your pity. They have chosen to have a full life—without kids. They prove it is totally possible!

As one of our friends jokes, you can always tell the child-free couples— they're tanned, in great shape, wearing new clothes, and driving clean cars. Dinner out for them is not the McDonald's drive-thru. They have beautiful, breakable home decor—and it never gets broken. Truth is, without kids, these couples have more money and time to enjoy life. If you choose to join them, jump in with gusto!

There is a difference, too, between being child-free and being childless. Child-free, on the one hand, is a positive word for a choice that denotes a freedom. Childless, on the other hand, has this negative connotation that leaves no room for joy. If no children is your choice, choose child-free.

Our friend Lola, the Hollywood producer who was a soy protein junkie and deemed infertile after much treatment, decided remaining child-free was her destiny. She has made the decision a positive in her life.

"My boyfriend and I both went into the attempt to have a baby as something a couple should do," says Lola. "I think we were interested to see what a baby we'd make would look like, but truthfully, neither of us sincerely wanted to change our lifestyle in the way we would have had to. We are both selfish people who require a lot of solitude and quiet time, which made it easier for us to accept not having a child as best for us. We have friends who have babies now and are unable to continue their work in the same way they used to."

Lola opted out of the infertility game before she had exhausted all the scientific options. "When I was going through the most difficult part of the infertility and feeling punished on some level, I stopped being engaged in my career." Lola said. "Finally, after trying to conceive for several months, my RE did another hormone test that showed my FSH level was too high and had been for too long. My eggs were no good. My only option was to do IVF with donor eggs, which didn't interest me. By that time, I was thirty-nine, almost forty."

After berating herself for a few days about not trying to have kids sooner, Lola came to terms with her future. Her handsome, younger boyfriend, suffered poor sperm motility and so never played the blame game. They are still together.

"I dealt with the loss with meditation and prayer," says Lola "I really took stock of my life and realized that I could be happy without having children. There are a lot of things I enjoy doing [that] I would not be able to enjoy as fully or as frequently being a parent, so I decided to focus on doing those things. I became very clear with how I wanted to spend my life. I would say, the experience, while difficult, has had a very positive affect on me as a person."

Living child-free is a viable alternative for many couples. It's a choice. Like every other aspect of infertility, the possibilities here are also endless.

Families. There is no one definition for families and no single way to build them. Children arrive in a variety of ways—with no intervention, as medical miracles, or through adoption or foster programs. Some parents have only one child, while others have several children. There are families that are made up of both a mom and dad, and families that are made up of a single parent. Some families have no children—made up of couples who are child-free by choice. Each is a family. Each is a success.

In the darkest moments of your infertility, you must always remember that you will emerge a winner in this game. Take charge. Being infertile doesn't mean you can't be a parent. If you want a baby, you will find a way to bring one to your family. Keep thinking of this ordeal as a game—one you will win, just maybe not the way you had always planned. Keep you heart and mind open and the family you so desire will be yours. We promise.

ACKNOWLEDGMENTS

They say it takes a village to raise a child. We think it takes a village to nurture and raise a book. So to our amazing village—thanks for your support, love, and favors. We couldn't have done it without you!

We would both like to extend our deep gratitude to the many people who supported and contributed to this book's birth. To our parents, Rita and Leo Regan and George Vargo and Joan Vogel, for raising us right—and watching the kids so we could write. To Robert and Will, those good eggs we married, who have been there for us—before, during, and after. And to our golden eggs, Quinn, Graham, Ava, and Amanda, who make every day worthwhile.

To our chicks who dished along the way: Dee Dee Liestenfeltz (and baby Pierce), Jill Lynch, Barb Tobias, Christine Onorati, Paula Conway, Cynthia Cooper, Sue Syversen, Erika Rosettie, and Michelle Madonna. Thanks for listening!

To all the women and men who shared their stories with us: Although we changed your names in this book as requested, you know who you are. Your insights and experiences were invaluable. Thank you for your courage and honesty and for dishing with us in an effort to make the insanity of infertility more bearable for others.

This book would never boast its credibility without the help of two physicians. Thank you to Dr. Brian M. Cohen and Dr. W. Michael Yarbrough, who took the time to read each page, comment, correct, and keep us current. You are the kinds of doctors we wish for every woman making this journey. (And thank you so much for helping bring Graham and Amanda into the world.)

We are profoundly grateful to each and every person at ReganBooks. To our publisher, Judith Regan, thank you for your creative genes and genius and for "getting the chicks to the other side of the road." You are beyond brilliant. And by the way, the cover rocks, Auntie J! To our editor, Cassie Jones, whose dedication, tireless effort, and patience with people and words cannot be described. You are a gift. To our art director, Michelle Ishay, thanks for the great eggs. To our publicist, Paul Crichton, thanks for getting it and for working 'round the clock to make sure the Eggs got out. And to Tammi Guthrie, Melissa McCarthy, Vivian Gomez, Kim Hadney, and all the others who supported us every step of the way, thank you.

To everyone in Northport (what a village!), who put my mind at ease by loving and nurturing my children, and to all of you who generously drove Quinn to and from activities so I could write. To Dr. Bronson, what a poet, thanks for being so honest. And to my dear friend Julie Vargo, you're a dream to dish with. **XO Maureen.**

To the village that is Holy Family, and to my support system in McKinney (you know who you are!), thank you for your help and encouragement. And to Maureen Regan, who started off as my agent (the best!), but went on to become not only my coauthor, but also my great friend. What could be better? **XO Julie.**

We most humbly thank all of you from the bottoms of our hearts.
And finally,

To our babies in heaven, may you rest in peace.

The Chicks

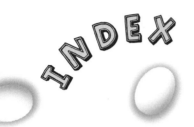